PEDIATRIC INFECTIOUS DISEASE SECRETS

PEDIATRIC INFECTIOUS DISEASE SECRETS

Joel D. Klein, M.D., FAAP

Clinical Associate Professor of Pediatrics
Jefferson Medical College of Thomas Jefferson University
Philadelphia, Pennsylvania
Chief, Pediatric Infectious Diseases
A.I. duPont Hospital for Children
Director, Infectious Disease Laboratory
Christiana Care Health System
Wilmington, Delaware

Theoklis E. Zaoutis, M.D., FAAP

Instructor in Pediatrics
University of Pennsylvania School of Medicine
Attending Physician, Special Immunology
Senior Fellow, Division of Immunologic and Infectious Diseases
Children's Hospital of Philadelphia
Philadelphia, Pennsylvania

HANLEY & BELFUS, INC./Philadelphia

Publisher: HANLEY & BELFUS, INC.
Medical Publishers
210 South 13th Street
Philadelphia, PA 19107
(215) 546-7293; 800-962-1892
FAX (215) 790-9330
Web site: http://www.hanleyandbelfus.com

Note to the reader: Although the techniques, ideas, and information in this book have been carefully reviewed for correctness, the authors, editors, and publisher cannot accept any legal responsibility for any errors or omissions that may be made. Neither the publisher nor the editors make any guarantee, expressed or implied, with respect to the material contained herein.

This book is designed to provide information on the background and modalities used frequently in pediatric infectious diseases and how they are applied by practitioners in the field. It is not intended to be exhaustive, nor should patients use it as a substitute for the advice of their physician. It is strongly recommended that you talk with your own physician about any treatments you use personally and research the area further for safety as it applies to the person you are treating. Before trying/recommending any treatment, the reader should review dosages, accepted indications, and other information pertinent to the safe and effective use of the therapies described.

Library of Congress Control Number 2002109650

PEDIATRIC INFECTIOUS DISEASE SECRETS   ISBN 1-56053-546-6

Last digit is the print number: 9 8 7 6 5 4 3 2 1

CONTENTS

CONTRIBUTORS

Ana M. Alvarez, M.D.
Assistant Professor, Pediatric Infectious Diseases and Immunology, University of Florida Health Science Center; Shands Jacksonville Medical Center; Wolfson Children's Hospital/Baptist Medical Center, Jacksonville, Florida

Edwin L. Anderson, M.D.
Professor of Medicine and Pediatrics, Division of Infectious Diseases, St. Louis University; Cardinal Glennon Children's Hospital, St. Louis, Missouri

Karen R. Beasley, B.S.
University of North Carolina School of Medicine, Chapel Hill, North Carolina

Jeffrey M. Bergelson, M.D.
Assistant Professor, Department of Pediatrics, University of Pennsylvania School of Medicine; Children's Hospital of Philadelphia, Philadelphia, Pennsylvania

Anne Marie C. Brescia, M.D.
Fellow, Pediatric Rheumatology, A.I. duPont Hospital for Children, Wilmington, Delaware

Hal Charles Byck, M.D.
Clinical Instructor, Division of General Pediatrics, Jefferson Medical College of Thomas Jefferson University, Philadelphia, Pennsylvania; A.I. duPont Hospital for Children, Wilmington, Delaware

Kimberly J. Center, M.D.
Clinical Instructor of Pediatrics, Section of Infectious Diseases, MCP Hahnemann University School of Medicine; St. Christopher's Hospital for Children, Philadelphia, Pennsylvania

Aaron S. Chidekel, M.D.
Assistant Professor of Pediatrics, Department of Pediatrics, Jefferson Medical College of Thomas Jefferson University, Philadelphia, Pennsylvania; Attending Pulmonologist, A.I. duPont Hospital for Children, Wilmington, Delaware

Susan E. Coffin, M.D., M.P.H.
Assistant Professor, Division of Immunologic and Infectious Diseases, University of Pennsylvania School of Medicine; Children's Hospital of Philadelphia, Philadelphia, Pennsylvania

Deborah M. Consolini, M.D.
Instructor of Pediatrics, Department of Pediatrics, Jefferson Medical College of Thomas Jefferson University, Philadelphia, Pennsylvania; Staff Pediatrician, General Pediatrics, A.I. duPont Hospital for Children, Wilmington, Delaware

Reza J. Daugherty, M.D.
Fellow, Pediatric Emergency Medicine, University of Pennsylvania School of Medicine; Children's Hospital of Philadelphia, Philadelphia, Pennsylvania

M. Cecilia Di Pentima, M.D., M.P.H., FAAP
A.I. duPont Hospital for Children, Wilmington, Delaware

John Donnelly, M.D.
Chief Medical Resident, Department of Internal Medicine and Department of Pediatrics, Christiana Care Health Services, Newark, Delaware

Stephen C. Eppes, M.D.
Clinical Associate Professor, Department of Pediatrics, Jefferson Medical College of Thomas Jefferson University, Philadelphia, Pennsylvania; A.I. duPont Hospital for Children, Wilmington, Delaware

Henry M. Feder, Jr., M.D.
Professor of Pediatrics and Family Medicine, University of Connecticut Health Center, Farmington, Connecticut

Fred Fow, M.D.
Instructor, Department of Pediatrics, Jefferson Medical College of Thomas Jefferson University, Philadelphia, Pennsylvania; Attending Physician, Division of Emergency Medicine, A.I. duPont Hospital for Children, Wilmington, Delaware

Daniel M. Ingram, M.S.P.H.
University of North Carolina School of Medicine, Chapel Hill, North Carolina

David Lane Ingram, M.D.
Professor, Pediatric Infectious Diseases, Department of Pediatrics, University of North Carolina School of Medicine, Chapel Hill, North Carolina; Acting Staff, UNC Hospitals, Rex Health Care, Chapel Hill, North Carolina; Wake Medical Center, Raleigh, North Carolina

Joel D. Klein, M.D., FAAP
Clinical Associate Professor of Pediatrics, Jefferson Medical College of Thomas Jefferson University, Philadelphia, Pennsylvania; Chief, Pediatric Infectious Diseases, A.I. duPont Hospital for Children, Wilmington, Delaware; Director, Infectious Disease Laboratory, Christiana Care Health Services, Wilmington, Delaware

Shirley P. Klein, M.D.
Clinical Assistant Professor of Pediatrics, Jefferson Medical College of Thomas Jefferson University, Philadelphia, Pennsylvania; Christiana Care Health Services and A.I. duPont Hospital for Children, Wilmington, Delaware

Linda L. Lewis, M.D.
Associate Professor of Pediatrics, Uniformed Services University of the Health Sciences, Bethesda, Maryland; Walter Reed Army Medical Center, Washington, DC

Mark R. Magnusson, M.D., Ph.D.
Clinical Associate Professor, Department of Pediatrics, University of Pennsylvania School of Medicine; Children's Hospital of Philadelphia, Philadelphia, Pennsylvania

James Jeffrey Malatack, M.D.
Professor of Pediatrics, Thomas Jefferson University School of Medicine, Philadelphia, Pennsylvania; Director of Diagnostic Referral Services for Thomas Jefferson University at A.I. duPont Hospital for Children, Wilmington, Delaware, and Thomas Jefferson Hospial, Philadelphia, Pennsylvania

Keith J. Mann, M.D.
Physician, Pediatric Diagnostic Referral Center, Division of General Pediatrics, A.I. duPont Hospital for Children, Wilmington, Delaware

Nizar F. Maraqa, M.D.
Fellow, Pediatric Infectious Diseases and Immunology, University of Florida Health Science Center, Jacksonville, Florida

Edina H. Moylett, M.D.
Assistant Professor of Pediatrics, Section of Allergy and Immunology, Baylor College of Medicine; Texas Children's Hospital, Houston, Texas

Michael J. Muszynski, M.D.
Chief, Division of Infectious Diseases, Nemours Children's Clinic–Orlando; Academic Chairman, Department of Pediatrics, Orlando Regional Healthcare; Pediatric Infectious Diseases, Arnold Palmer Hospital for Children and Women, Orlando, Florida

Sharon A. Nachman, M.D.
Associate Professor, Department of Pediatrics, State University of New York at Stony Brook Health Sciences Center, Stony Brook, New York

Donough J. O'Donovan, M.D.
Assistant Professor of Pediatrics, Section of Neonatology, Baylor College of Medicine; Texas Children's Hospital, Houston, Texas

Elena Elizabeth Perez, M.D., Ph.D.
Fellow, Division of Allergy, Immunology, and Infectious Diseases, Department of Pediatrics, Children's Hospital of Philadelphia, Philadelphia, Pennsylvania

Dwight A. Powell, M.D.
Professor, Department of Pediatrics, The Ohio State University College of Medicine and Public Health; Chief, Section of Infectious Diseases, Children's Hospital, Columbus, Ohio

Amanda Pratt, M.D.
Fellow, Division of Emergency Medicine, A.I. duPont Hospital for Children, Wilmington, Delaware

David P. Regis, M.D., LCDR, MC, USN
Fellow in Pediatric Infectious Diseases, Instructor of Pediatrics, Department of Pediatrics, Uniformed Services University of the Health Sciences, Bethesda, Maryland; Walter Reed Army Medical Center, Washington, DC; National Naval Medical Center, Bethesda, Maryland

Gail L. Rodgers, M.D.
Assistant Professor of Pediatrics, Section of Infectious Diseases, MCP Hahnemann University School of Medicine/St. Christopher's Hospital for Children; Hospital Epidemiologist, Attending Physician, St. Christopher's Hospital for Children, Philadelphia, Pennsylvania

Carlos D. Rosé, M.D.
Associate Professor of Pediatrics, Division of Rheumatology, Thomas Jefferson University, Philadelphia, Pennsylvania; A.I. duPont Hospital for Children, Wilmington, Delaware

Samir S. Shah, M.D.
Fellow, Divisions of General Pediatrics and Immunology and Infectious Diseases, Children's Hospital of Philadelphia, Philadelphia, Pennsylvania

Monica Jain Snowden, M.D.
Resident in Internal Medicine and Pediatrics, Christiana Care Health Services, Newark, Delaware

Kathleen E. Sullivan, M.D., Ph.D.
Associate Professor of Pediatrics, Division of Immunology, University of Pennsylvania School of Medicine; Children's Hospital of Philadelphia, Philadelphia, Pennsylvania

Robert N. Tiballi, D.O.
Director of Pediatric Infectious Diseases, Germbusters, P.C., Hoffman Estates, Illinois; Assistant Clinical Professor of Medicine, University of Illinois College of Medicine, Chicago, Illinois

Charles R. Woods, M.D., M.S.
Associate Professor of Pediatrics, Department of Pediatrics, Wake Forest University School of Medicine; North Carolina Baptist/Brenner Children's Hospital, Winston-Salem, North Carolina

Terry Yamauchi, M.D.
Professor and Vice-Chairman, Department of Pediatrics, University of Arkansas for Medical Sciences; Arkansas Children's Hospital, Little Rock, Arkansas

Lisa B. Zaoutis, M.D.
Clinical Assistant Professor, Department of Pediatrics, University of Pennsylvania School of Medicine; Director of Inpatient Services, Division of General Pediatrics, Children's Hospital of Philadelphia, Philadelphia, Pennsylvania

Theoklis E. Zaoutis, M.D., FAAP
Instructor in Pediatrics, University of Pennsylvania School of Medicine; Attending Physician, Special Immunology; Senior Fellow in the Division of Immunologic and Infectious Diseases, Children's Hospital of Philadelphia, Philadelphia, Pennsylvania

PREFACE

The goal of this book is to address questions commonly asked by physicians about pediatric infectious diseases. The target audience includes general pediatricians, family physicians, nurse practitioners, resident physicians, and medical students. Persons interested in public health as well as other health care professionals also may find this book useful and informative.

The emphasis is on common infections, but information is included about "hot topics" and emerging issues in infectious diseases, such as bioterrorism, Lyme disease and other tick-borne infections, West Nile virus, "mad-cow disease," and cat-scratch disease. In addition, the text discusses new diagnostic approaches to infectious diseases in children and new drugs for the treatment of influenza.

The text is not intended to be a comprehensive review of the specialty. It includes questions and answers in an informal manner and may come in handy as a board review. Contributors are experts in pediatrics and infectious diseases who often are asked similar questions in their practice.

We hope that you find our book entertaining as well as useful. We certainly did!

Joel D. Klein, M.D., FAAP
Theoklis E. Zaoutis, M.D., FAAP

ACKNOWLEDGMENTS

We gratefully acknowledge the help of our mentors, who taught us the joy of teaching.

We are indebted to the contributing authors, who took time from their busy schedules to participate in this project. As editors, we have made some changes in the chapters in an attempt to be consistent with the spirit of the book and appreciate the authors' understanding.

Special thanks go to Lisa B. Zaoutis, M.D., and Shirley P. Klein, M.D., esteemed authors and spouses.

Finally, we thank Hanley & Belfus for giving us the opportunity to write this book and the support needed to succeed.

Joel D. Klein and Theoklis E. Zaoutis

Individually I would like to thank Joel D. Klein and Stephen C. Eppes for being my mentors and friends since medical school. They inspired me to pursue the rewarding field of pediatric infectious diseases. They taught me how to take care of patients and the importance of teaching. A special thanks to Joel for allowing me to write this book with him.

Theoklis E. Zaoutis

I. Primer on Pathogens and Antimicrobial Therapy

1. BACTERIA

Reza J. Daugherty, M.D., and Stephen C. Eppes, M.D.

1. **Match the organism with its most important virulence factor.**

   a. *Streptococcus pyogenes*   1. Endotoxin
   b. *Pseudomonas aeruginosa*   2. Cytotoxin
   c. *Streptococcus pneumoniae*   3. Exotoxin
   d. *Escherichia coli* 0157 H7   4. Shiga-like toxin
   e. *Clostridium difficile*   5. Capsule
   Answers: a, 3; b, 1; c, 5; d, 4; e, 2.

2. **Many aspects of the immune system are involved with the host response to bacterial infections. This process has obvious relevance to congenital and acquired immunodeficiency. Match the immunologic abnormality with the most likely pathogens (one best answer for each; all responses to be used).**

   a. Deficiency of complement 1 (C1))   1. Catalase-positive organisms
   b. Deficiency of C5–C9   2. Bacteria and certain fungi
   c. Neutropenia   3. Various encapsulated organisms
   d. Deficient oxidative burst (PMN)   4. *Neisseria* species
   e. Asplenia   5. *Streptococcus pneumoniae*
   Answers: a, 5; b, 4; c, 2; d, 1; e, 3.

3. **Gamma globulin deficiencies (e.g. ,IgA and IgG deficiencies) cause susceptibility to a variety of pathogens. Which group of bacteria are most likely to be problematic?**

   a. *Streptococcus pneumoniae, Haemophilus influenzae, Moraxella catarrhalis*
   b. Staphylococci
   c. Enterobacteraciae
   d. Intracellular bacteria
   e. HACEK group (*Haemophilus, Actinobacillus, Cardiobacterium, Eikenella, Kingella* spp.)
   Answer: (a). These organisms may cause mucosal disease (e.g., otitis, sinusitis), lower respiratory tract infection, and, in the case of pneumococci, severe and invasive disease in patients with antibody-deficient states. Staphylococcal infections and Enterobacteraciae are likely to be problematic in patients with neutrophil abnormalities, quantitative or qualitative. Intracellular bacteria may evade phagocytic cells and certain antibiotics. The HACEK organisms are fastidious bacteria associated with infective endocarditis.

4. **The presence of certain organisms in clinical specimens should call to mind particular disease processes. Match the culture result with the disease for which it is a "red flag" or sentinel organism.**

   a. *Burkholderia cepacia* in sputum   1. Colon cancer
   b. *Salmonella* sp. in bone   2. Cystic fibrosis
   c. *Serratia marcescens* in tissue   3. AIDS
   d. *Clostridium septicum* in blood   4. Chronic granulomatous disease
   e. *Rhodococcus equi* in blood   5. Sickle cell disease
   Answers: a, 2; b, 5; c, 4; d, 1; e, 3.

5. Match the organism with its description (characteristics that a microbiology technologist may mention).

a. *Staphylococcus aureus*
b. *Streptococcus pyogenes*
c. *Enterococcus faecalis*
d. *Escherichia coli*
e. *Proteus mirabilis*
f. *Klebsiella pneumoniae*
g. *Haemophilus influenzae*
h. *Fusobacterium necroforum*

1. Growth on chocolate, not blood agar
2. Swarming
3. Weak catalase-positive, nonhemolytic
4. Golden colonies, beta-hemolytic
5. White-to-gray colonies, beta-hemolytic
6. Green sheen
7. Anerobic growth only
8. Mucoid colonies, short gram-negative rods

Answers: a, 4; b, 5;. c, 3; d, 6; e, 2; f, 8; g, 1; h, 7.

6. What did Hans Christian Gram do in 1884?

Hans Christian Gram was a microbiologist from Denmark who developed the Gram stain. By applying an iodine solution to cells previously stained with crystal violet and treating them with mixtures of alcohol and acetone, he was able to differentiate bacteria based on their permeability. Gram-positive organisms retain the iodine-dye complex, causing them to appear purple, whereas in gram-negative organisms the dye is washed away. A counter stain (safranin) is then added to make the gram-negative bacteria appear red.

7. How can you tell whether a specimen has been properly stained?

Any surrounding cells or tissue should be stained red (i.e., gram-negative). If other nonbacterial cells appear purple, particularly the nuclei of nearby neutrophils, the specimen has not been appropriately decolorized and the Gram stain may be inaccurate.

8. Certain bacteria are not well seen with Gram stain. How are the mycobacteria and spirochetes visualized microscopically?

Because of the lipids contained in their cell walls, **mycobacteria** must be visualized using a special technique known as the acid-fast stain. They are exposed to highly concentrated dyes for a prolonged period and treated with heat. They are unique in that they are resistant to decolorization with acids and ethanol after they have taken up the dye; hence the term acid-fast. **Spirochetes** must be visualized using a technique known as darkfield microscopy. The microscope focuses light in such a way that only reflected light (i.e., that which strikes the organism) reaches the observer's eye. As a result, a vivid aura of light surrounds the bacteria against a black backdrop.

9. The laboratory technologist may report that a culture is growing a gram-positive "this" or a gram-negative "that." What are the major shapes that bacteria can assume?

Bacteria come in a multitude of shapes and sizes. In addition to staining, differentiating them starts with defining their shape. If they are round, they are referred to as **cocci** (e.g., staphylococci and streptococci). If they are rod-shaped, they are called **bacilli**; some are short, plump rods (e.g., *Klebsiella* sp.), whereas others are long and thin (e.g., *Pseudomonas* sp.). If they are somewhere between a rod and a coccus, they are sometimes called **coccobacilli** (e.g., *Haemophilus* sp.). A bacillus with very narrow ends is described as **fusiform**. Finally, spiral-shaped bacteria are commonly known as the **spirochetes**.

10. True or false: All bacteria possess a cell wall.

False. The cell wall is common to almost all bacterial species except *Mycoplasma* spp. In fact, the presence of a cell wall is one of the distinguishing features of prokaryotic cells. It gives bacteria their individual shapes and helps protect them from chemical and mechanical insults. Because *Mycoplasma* spp. do not have a cell wall, they do not stain with Gram stain. *Chlamydia* and *Rickettsia* spp. also do not possess cell walls.

11. How do some antibiotics use the bacteria's own house-keeping mechanisms against them?

In contrast to mammalian cells, bacteria are packed with enzymes that can break down peptidoglycan, the main constituent of bacterial cell walls. Bacteria must be able to expand their murein sac in order to grow. This process entails hydrolyzing some bonds so that new chains can be inserted. Some antibiotics work by interfering with this usually delicately balanced mechanism and allowing potentially toxic enzymes to run rampant.

12. The microbiology lab reports that the patient has a positive spinal fluid culture. Gram-positive cocci grew within 24 hours. The technologist may be able to give you some information over the phone that helps you determine what the organism is likely to be and how urgent the situation is. Most of the following questions are reasonable. Which one would make the technician laugh?
1. Does the Gram stain show pairs, chains, or clusters?
2. Is it a lactose fermenter?
3. Is it catalase-positive?
4. Can you do a rapid coagulase test?
5. Does the organism show alpha, beta, or gamma hemolysis?

Answer: (2). Lactose fermentation is used to differentiate certain gram-negative bacilli. The other answers would help you narrow down what the gram-positive coccus is likely to be.

13. The lab reports that the blood culture in a burn patient is growing an oxidase-positive, gram-negative rod. The technologist's voice has a trace of alarm, because she can tell from the organism's morphology, odor, and rapid biochemical test that it may be a serious pathogen. You recall that the patient had been placed on antibiotics immediately after the culture was drawn and you hope that it was which of the following:
1. Ceftazidime and gentamicin
2. Ampicillin/sulbactam
3. Trimethoprim/sulfamethoxazole
4. Ceftriaxone
5. Ampicillin, gentamicin, and metronidazole

Answer: (1). *Pseudomonas aeruginosa* is fairly easy to recognize in the lab. Although other gram-negative organisms may be oxidase-positive, most would not be confused with *Pseudomonas* species. The antibiotic regimen most commonly used is an antipseudomonal beta-lactam and an aminoglycoside (although alternatives are available).

14. A 2-year-old child is discovered by computed tomography to have a periappendiceal abscess. The bacteriology of the abscess is likely to include multiple fecal organisms. Which of the following regimens would have the best activity against the likely pathogens?
1. Ampicillin and gentamicin
2. Ampicillin and metronidazole
3. Clindamycin and gentamicin
4. Ampicillin/sulbactam and gentamicin
5. Ceftazidime and gentamicin

Answer: (4). Ampicillin combined with the beta-lactamase inhibitor sulbactam provides excellent activity against anaerobes (including *Bacteroides fragilis*) and many aerobic gram-negative bacilli. In combination with gentamicin, ampicillin is generally active against enterococci, although resistance may occur. The other regimens have some activity against the array of pathogens, but none provides equally comprehensive coverage.

15. What mechanism is responsible for beta-lactam resistance in *Streptococcus pneumoniae*?
1. Decreased cell wall permeability
2. Decreased binding of beta-lactam antibiotics by the cell wall
3. Beta-lactamase production

4. Inoculum effect
5. Overuse of quinolone antibiotics
Answer: (2). The penicillin-binding proteins of the bacterial cell wall have been genetically altered so that beta-lactam antibiotics (e.g., penicillins, cephalosporins) do not bind well and cannot exert their effect on the growth of the cell wall. Twenty to 50% of *S. pneumoniae* in the U.S., depending on geographic location, have reduced susceptibility to beta-lactams.

16. Describe the mechanisms involved with macrolide resistance in *S. pneumoniae*.
The macrolide antibiotics, including erythromycin, clarithromycin, and azithromycin, have also become less active against *S. pneumoniae*. There are two main mechanisms. In the U.S., three-fourths of the resistance is mediated by the macrolide efflux pump, encoded by a *mef* gene. This generally low level of resistance may be overcome by higher doses of the drug. One-fourth of the resistance is associated with an *erm* (erythromycin ribosomal methylase) gene, which causes the ribosomal binding site for macrolide antibiotics not to allow binding. This is high-level resistance, with cross-resistance to clindamycin; thus, macrolides should not be used for these organisms.

17. The following bacteria are human pathogens but frequently are associated with an animal source. Match the organism and the animal source. (Use each answer only once.)
a. *Coxiella burnetii*   1. Mice
b. *Pasteurella multocida*   2. Rats
c. *Streptobacillus moniliformes* 3. Shell fish
d. *Salmonella* species   4. Cattle
e. *Francisella tularensis*   5. Sheep
f. *Bacillus anthracis*   6. Reptiles
g. *Borrelia burgdorferi*   7. Rabbits
h. *Vibrio parahaemolyticus*   8. Cats
Answers: a, 5; b, 8; c, 2; d, 6; e, 7; f, 4; g, 1; h, 3.

18. Match the organism with its likely source (the answers to these questions in the patient's social history may offer a clue to the etiologic agent).
a. *Aeromonas hydrophila*   1. Chitterlings
b. *Mycobacterium marinum*   2. Lake water
c. *Vibrio fluvialis*   3. Sea water
d. *Listeria monocytogenes*   4. Soft cheese
e. *Yersinia enterocolitica*   5. Fish tank
Answers: a, 2; b, 5; c, 3; d, 4; e, 1.

BIBLIOGRAPHY

1. Holt JG, Krieg NR, Sneath PHA, et al: Bergey's Manual of Determinative Bacteriology, 9th ed. Philadelphia, Lippincott Williams & Wilkins, 2000.
2. Mandell GL, Bennett JE, Dolin R (eds): Principles and Practice of Infectious Diseases, 5th ed. New York, Churchill Livingstone, 2000.

2. VIRUSES

Stephen C. Eppes, M.D.

1. **"It's just a virus," said the pediatrician to the mother of the febrile child. Although many childhood viral illnesses are usually benign, others have caused worldwide, often fatal human disease. Name five viruses which fit in the latter category.**

    Measles, influenza, smallpox, rotavirus, and human immunodeficiency virus (HIV).

2. **Classic virologic methods involve cultivating viruses in cell culture, in which viral cytopathic effect (CPE) can be observed, often over a period of days to weeks. Many rapid viral diagnostic techniques now are available to clinicians. Name five viruses for which such technology exists and the method commonly used.**

Respiratory syncytial virus (RSV)	Enzyme immunoassay (EIA)
Influenza viruses	EIA
Herpes simplex viruses (HSV) 1 and 2	Direct fluorescent assay (DFA)
Varicella zoster virus (VZV)	DFA
Rotavirus	EIA

3. **Which of the following statements about accurate diagnosis of viral disease is *not* true?**

    a. Precise diagnosis allows accurate reporting to public health authorities.

    b. Rapid diagnostic tests can assist hospital infection control coordinators to isolate and cohort patients with specific viral diseases.

    c. Families often appreciate knowing the exact diagnosis rather than "viral syndrome."

    d. Viral cultures are generally of no value, because the results often return after the patient's illness has resolved.

    e. Knowledge of which viruses are in the community at a given time can assist clinicians in presumptive clinical diagnosis of these infections.

    Answer: (d).

4. **Match the virus to its *predominant* route of transmission (numbered choices can be used more than once):**

a. HIV	1. Exposure to blood
b. Yellow fever virus	2. Direct contact with infected secretions
c. Rotavirus	3. Sexual transmission
d. Influenza viruses	4. Fecal-oral transmission
e. RSV	5. Mosquitoes
f. Hepatitis A virus	6. Respiratory droplets
g. Hepatitis C virus	
h. Ebola virus	
i. HSV-1	
j. HSV-2	

    Answers: a, 3; b, 5; c, 4; d, 6; e, 2; f, 4; g, 1; h, 2; i, 2; j, 3.

5. **All of the following viruses are both sexually and perinatally transmitted except (a) hepatitis B, (b) HSV-2, (c) HSV-1, (d) HIV, (e) human papilloma virus (HPV), or (f) lymphogranuloma venereum.**

    (f). Lymphogranuloma venereum is caused by a bacterium, *Chlamydia trachomatis*.

6. Match the virus to the clinical finding that is commonly associated with fetal infection.

a. Rubella virus   1. Hydrops fetalis
b. Parvovirus B19   2. Slowly progressive liver disease
c. Hepatitis C   3. Heart defect
d. Cytomegalovirus (CMV)   4. Intracranial calcification
Answers: a, 3; b, 1; c, 2; d, 4.

7. Hepatitis is associated with the named hepatitis viruses (e.g., hepatitis A, B, C). Name five other viral infections that can involve the liver as part of a systemic illness.

Epstein-Barr virus (EBV), CMV, parvovirus B-19, HIV, and neonatal HSV are examples commonly seen in the United States. In tropical and developing countries, virulent infections such as ebola, dengue, and yellow fever can cause severe hepatitis.

8. All of the following viruses can cause encephalitis except (a) HSV, (b) EBV, (c) human herpes virus type 6 (HHV-6), (d) influenza viruses, (e) parainfluenza viruses, or (f) mumps virus.

Answer: (e). Parainfluenza viruses cause infection limited to the respiratory tract. HSV type 1 causes central nervous system (CNS) infection manifested by fever, altered sensorium, seizures, cerebrospinal fluid (CSF) pleocytosis (sometimes hemorrhagic), and temporal lobe changes on imaging studies (in neonatal disease, other areas of the CNS may be involved). EBV causes a spectrum of neurologic disease; the encephalitis is usually not severe and often has a good prognosis. HHV-6 is the most common identifiable cause of febrile seizures and is associated with encephalitis in a minority of infants. Influenza, particularly influenza A, sometimes can cause severe encephalitis. As many as 5 in 1000 cases of mumps are associated with encephalitis.

9. Name three viruses associated with malignant neoplasms. Specify the neoplasm.

EBV   Lymphomas, nasopharyngeal carcinoma
HPV   Cervical carcinoma
HHV-8   Kaposi's sarcoma

10. Many antiviral therapies have been developed over the past two decades. Match the infection with an effective treatment. (There may be more than one correct choice for each infection; numbered choices may be used more than once.)

a. HSV   1. Interferon
b. RSV   2. Lamivudine
c. CMV   3. Acyclovir
d. Influenza   4. Gancyclovir
e. Hepatitis B   5. Ribavirin
f. HIV   6. Oseltamivir
g. VZV   7. Nelfinavir
h. Lassa fever   8. Saline nose drops
Answers: a, 3, 4; b, 5; c, 4; d, 5, 6; e, 1, 2; f, 2, 7; g, 3; h, 5.

11. The immunologic response to viral infections is often complicated and can involve various arms of the immune system. Which of the following is typically *not* important in handling viral infections: (a) neutrophils, (b) T lymphocytes, (c) B lymphocytes, (d) antibodies, or (e) cytokines?

(a). Neutrophils are phagocytic cells primarily involved with handling bacterial and fungal infections. In people with isolated neutropenia, viral infections tend not to be a major problem.

12. Postexposure prophylaxis is sometimes used to prevent certain dangerous viral infections, especially in high-risk patients. Prophylaxis often uses gamma globulin injections that contain high titers of antibody to the particular virus. Hyperimmune globulin

products are also available for preventing or managing viral infections in high-risk patients. **Name four hyperimmune globulin products and explain how each is typically used.**

1. Rabies immune globulin: used in conjunction with rabies vaccine after potential rabies exposure.

2. Varicella-zoster immune globulin: used to prevent varicella after exposure of high-risk (e.g., immunocompromised) patients.

3. RSV immune globulin: the plasma-derived product is less commonly used than the newer monoclonal antibody; both protect high-risk infants and children (e.g., premature infants, children with chronic lung disease) against severe RSV infection

4. CMV immune globulin: used for prevention and management of CMV disease in bone marrow and solid organ transplant recipients.

13. Some viral infections are contained within mucosa-lined organs, such as the upper respiratory tract or intestines. Others go through a viremic phase, with dissemination to multiple tissues and organs. Name five viruses that cause bloodstream infection and dissemination.

Measles, varicella, EBV, CMV, and HIV.

14. Various immunologic mechanisms are involved in the host response to viral infections. Which of the following organisms requires an appropriate antibody response to prevent chronic infection: (a) herpes viruses, (b) enteroviruses, (c) hemorrhagic fever viruses, (d) influenza viruses, or (e) parainfluenza viruses?

Answer: (b). Enteroviruses (echovirus and coxsackie viruses, in particular) can result in serious infections in persons with agammaglobulinemia and hypogammaglobulinemia. In fact, chronic enteroviral meningoencephalatis may develop in such patients. Abundant experimental evidence also demonstrates the importance of specific antibody in the host response to enteroviral infections. Of the choices listed, the only other viruses that cause chronic infection are the herpes viruses, all of which cause latent chronic infection.

15. The immune response to infection is often responsible, at least in part, for the clinical manifestations. Name a virus whose disease manifestations occur well after peak levels of viral replication and are the result of immunologic mechanisms.

Parvovirus B19 replicates mainly in erythrocyte precursors. The rash, which is recognizable as erythema infectiosum (fifth disease), and the arthritis, which is usually seen in older girls and women, are postinfectious phenomena.

16. Name the herpes viruses.

Herpes simplex 1 and 2, varicella-zoster virus, Epstein-Barr virus, cytomegalovirus, human herpes virus (HHV)-6, HHV-7, and HHV-8.

17. Which of the following is not readily cultured in the clinical virology laboratory: (a) influenza viruses, (b) CMV, (c) EBV, (d) RSV, or (e) coxsackie B viruses?

Answer: (c). EBV can be identified by various means (classically, the ability to immortalize cells; more recently, the use of DNA technologies), but it is not culturable in the usual sense.

18. All of the following, if positive in a serum specimen, are considered diagnostic of active or recent infection in unimmunized people *except* (a) hepatitis B surface antigen, (b) IgG antibody to rabies virus, (c) IgM antibody to EBV, (d) IgG antibody to hepatitis A virus, (e) HIV DNA, or (f) HIV IgG antibody in an 18-month-old child.

Answer: (d). IgG antibody to HAV is seen in a significant percentage of the population (varying by country of origin) and is most commonly associated with remote infection. IgG antibody is diagnostic in the case of rabies, because it is a disease with almost no seroprevalence in a population. The presence of IgM usually signifies that an infection is active or recent, although there are occasional exceptions. The presence of antigen is likewise associated with the presence of disease, in most cases. Viral nucleic acids in a specimen generally are associated with active or recent infection, but in latent infections such as EBV or CMV, low viral nucleic acid loads are often seen in healthy people with remote infections. Remember that IgG is transplacentally passed, and its presence in a child under 18 months of age may be of maternal origin and cannot be used to diagnose infection.

19. Match the virus with the illness with which it is most closely connected.

a. Influenza virus	1. Cough, coryza, conjunctivitis
b. Parainfluenza virus	2. Pharyngoconjunctival fever
c. Respiratory syncytial virus	3. Febrile respiratory infection
d. Adenovirus	4. Croup
e. Rhinovirus	5. Herpangina
f. Coxsackie virus	6. Gingivostomatitis
g. Herpes simplex virus	7. Bronchiolitis
h. Measles virus	8. Common cold

Answers: a, 3; b, 4; c, 7; d, 2; e, 8; f, 5; g, 6; h, 1.

20. What is the Monospot test? How is it useful in the diagnosis of EBV infection?
    The Monospot test is a rapid test for heterophile antibodies, which are antibodies not directed against specific antigens but are an excellent marker for acute EBV infection. It is based on the observation that serum from patients with infectious mononucleosis will agglutinate red blood cells from other mammalian species (e.g., horse and sheep). Current tests use latex particles, which agglutinate in the presence of heterophile antibodies. When performed properly, the Monospot test is highly specific for acute or recent EBV infection, but the sensitivity of the test varies with the age of the patient and duration of infection. Young children may never have a measurable heterophile response, whereas adolescents become positive in > 90% of cases, usually after the first week of symptoms.

21. Corticosteroids are sometimes given to college students who have infectious mononucleosis, and their use is associated with more rapid clinical improvement, but the practice is controversial. Name five situations in which steroid medications are likely to be of benefit in EBV infection.
    1. Airway compromise due to tonsillar hypertrophy and/or cervical lymphadenopathy
    2. Hemolytic anemia associated with acute EBV infection
    3. Idiopathic thrombocytopenic purpura associated with acute EBV infection
    4. EBV encephalitis
    5. Virus-associated hemophagocytic lymphohistiocytosis (LHR)

22. Match the virus with the virologist.

a. Rabies	1. Gallo
b. Influenza	2. Henle
c. EBV	3. Pasteur
d. Measles	4. Whitley
e. HIV	5. Enders
f. HSV	6. Smith

Answers: a, 3; b., 6; c, 2; d, 5; e, 1; f, 4.

23. Effective antiviral therapy is available for each of the following except (a) RSV, (b) Lassa fever, (c) CMV, (d) yellow fever, (e) rabies, or (f) hepatitis C?
    Answer: (d) and (e). Rabies and yellow fever are not treatable conditions. Thus effective postexposure prophylaxis and other methods of prevention are especially important.

24. Explain the derivation of the names for the common enteroviruses.
    Coxsackie comes from the town in New York where some of the early work on the virus was done. Echo stands for **e**nteric **c**ytopathogenic **h**uman **o**rphan.

25. A 17-year-old girl from New York state presents in August with a 5-day history of fever, lethargy, and anorexia. Physical findings include mild cervical adenopathy and tenderness in both upper quadrants of the abdomen. She is sexually active. She recently visited family in Puerto Rico. There is a pet cat in the home. Laboratory studies show the following results: hemoglobin, 12.6 gm/dl; white blood cell count, 4200/mm³; platelet count, 130,000; alanine aminotransferase, 150; bilirubin, 1.5; and sedimentation rate, 65. Which of the following tests would have the lowest yield: (a) Monospot test, (b) CMV IgG antibody, (c) antinuclear antibody, (d) hepatitis A IgM antibody, (e) HIV IgG antibody, (f) hepatitis B surface antigen, (g) *Toxoplasma gondii* IgM antibody, (h) ehrlichiosis serology, or (i) Dengue serology?

Answer: (b). Because IgG antibody to CMV is found in at least half of adult women in the U.S., its value in diagnosing acute infection is minimal. The patient may have a mononucleosis syndrome; the differential diagnosis includes EBV, CMV, HIV, and toxoplasmosis. Hepatitis viral infection, Dengue viral infection, ehrlichiosis and systemic lupus erythematosus are also possibilities.

BIBLIOGRAPHY

1. Mandell GL, Bennett JE, Dolin R (eds): Principles and Practice of Infectious Diseases, 5th ed. New York, Churchill Livingstone, 2000.
2. Pickering LK (ed): 2000 Red Book: Report of the Committee on Infectious Diseases, 25th ed. Elk Grove Village, IL, American Academy of Pediatrics, 2000.
3. Remington JS, Klein JO (eds): Infectious Diseases of the Fetus and Newborn Infant, 4th ed. Philadelphia, W.B. Saunders, 1995.

3. FUNGAL INFECTIONS

M. *Cecilia Di Pentima*, M.D., M.P.H., FAAP

1. Mycoses, the term broadly used to include infections caused by fungi, was coined by which of the following scientists?

1. Agostino Bassi in 1835
2. Robert Remak in 1835
3. David Grub in 1941
4. R. Virdow in 1856
5. Hans Christian Gram in the late 1800s

Answer: (4). Bassi and Remak were the first authors of publications associating fungi with animal and human disease. Grub first isolated a fungus from a patient with ringworm and reproduced the disease by inoculating the fungus into normal skin.

2. Define the two main groups of fungi.

Yeasts, which are unicellular fungi that reproduce by budding or fission, and molds, which are multicellular fungi that grow by filamentous threads.

3. Do fungi have chlorophyll?

No.

4. True or false: Fungi can reproduce sexually or asexually.

True.

5. What is a conidium?

A conidium (plural = conidia) is an asexual spore produced by fungi at the tip or side of a hypha.

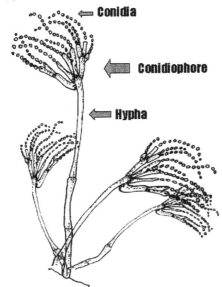

Fruiting heads of *Penicillium* species are composed of conidiophores, forming a brush that contains small spherical or oval conidia.

6. What is a hypha?

The tubular filament representing the vegetative unit that characterizes molds (see figure in question 5).

7. What is a pseudohypha?

A thread of cells (simulating link sausages) resulting from budding.

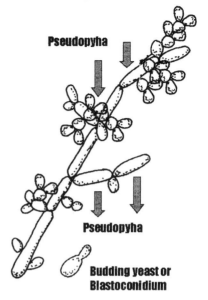

Pseudopyha

Pseudopyha

Budding yeast or Blastoconidium

Candida spp. with pseudohypha and budding yeast or blastoconidium.

8. What is a conidiophore?

A conidiophore is a hyphal structure that contains conidia (see figure in question 5).

9. What is a blastoconidium?

Blastoconidium (pleural = blastoconidia) refers to the asexual formation of conidia by blastic conidiogenesis, also known as budding forms (see figure in question 7).

10. Define dimorphism.

Dimorphism is the ability of certain fungi to display two morphologic types, one in the environment and one as an invasive pathogen. In the laboratory, dimorphic fungi grow as a mold at 25°C (room temperature) and as a yeast at 37°C.

11. What are the clinical implications of dimorphism?

Dimorphism is essential in the pathogenesis of some fungal infections. For example, Chlamydia albicans can switch from unicellular yeast to a filamentous form, a skill that increases its virulence. The pathogenic mechanisms are not clearly understood. One possibility is that the yeast form is used for proliferation, whereas the filamentous form allows the pathogen to evade the immune system.

12. Of the following, which is a yeast and which is a mold?

a. *Malassezia* spp.   d. *Zygomyces* spp.
b. *Aspergillus* spp.   e. *Penicillium* spp.
c. *Histoplasma* spp.
Answers: a, yeast; b, c, d, and e, molds.

13. Match the species with the correct genus or family.

a. *Lusitaniae, glabrata, krussei, tropicalis*   1. *Zygomyces*
b. *Fumigatus, flavus, niger, terrus*   2. *Candida*
c. *Rhizomucor pusillus* and *R. arrhizus*   3. *Histoplasma*
d. *Capsulatum, dubois*   4. *Aspergillus*
Answers: a, 2; b, 4; c, 1; d, 3.

14. Classify the following mycoses based on their location as superficial cutaneous, subcutaneous, or deep mycoses.

    1. *Fusarium* spp.   4. Chromoblastomycosis
    2. *Mycetoma* spp.   5. *Trichophyton* spp.
    3. *Microsporum* spp.

Answers: 1, deep; 2, superficial cutaneous and subcutaneous; 3 and 5, superficial cutaneous; 4, subcutaneous.

15. Glucan and chittin are the main constituents of

    1. A traditional Indian dish   4. Fungal enzymes
    2. Fungal ribosomes   5. None of the above
    3. Fungal cell wall

Answer: (3).

16. Which fungal infection is also known as farmer's lung?

Aspergillus fumigatus.

17. Blastomycosis is also known as (a) New Orleans disease, (b) New Yorker's disease, (c) Chicago disease, (d) Long Island disease, or (e) none of the above.

Answer: (c).

18. What is piedra?

    1. Spanish word for rock   4. (1) + (2)
    2. Fungal infection of the skin   5. (1) + (3)
    3. Fungal infection of the hair

Answer: (5).

19. Match the regions shown in the map with the endemic fungal infection.

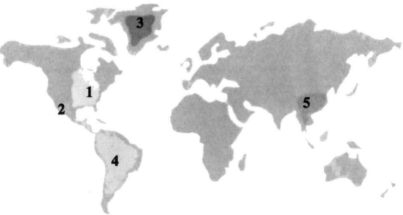

    a. *Histoplasma capsulatum*   d. *Coccidioides immitis*
    b. Paracoccidiodomycosis   e. None of the above
    c. *Penicillium marneffei*

Answers: a, 1; b, 4; c, 5; d, 2; e, 3.

20. Which of the following is used as fungal media?

    1. Sabouraud dextrose agar   4. Inhibitory mold agar
    2. Sterile bread   5. All of the above
    3. Brain-heart infusion agar

Answer: (5).

21. Most routine fungal cultures require incubation at 30°C for 3–4 weeks before they are discarded. However, you tell the laboratory to hold respiratory and/or tissue specimens for 12 weeks when you suspect that your patient is infected with which of the following?

a. *Trichophyton* spp.   d. *Mucor* spp.

b. *Blastomyces dermatitidis*   e. *Histoplasma capsulatum*

c. *Candida parapsilosis*

Answer: (e).

22. Which of the following accomplishments is attributed to the Scottish physician, Sir Alexander Fleming,?

a. Extraction of a chemical from *Saccharomyces cerevisiae*

b. Use of intravenous penicillin in soldiers wounded in World War II

c. Creation of the first pharmaceutical company

d. Observation that growth of *Staphylococcus aureus* was inhibited by *Penicillium* spp.

e. Development of nystatin, the first antifungal agent

Answer: (d).

23. A positive germ tube test indicates the presence of which of the following:

a. *Candida albicans* infection   d. Any fungal infection

b. *Candida* spp. infection   e. None of the above

c. Mold in his nose

Answer: (a). However, it is important to remember that approximately 5% of *C. albicans* are germ tube-negative.

24. Match the fungus with its microscopic appearance

a. *Aspergillus* spp.   d. *Cryptococcus neoformans*

b. *Paracoccidioides brasiliensis*   e. *Candida* spp.

c. *Blastomyces dermatitidis*   f. *Histoplasma capsulatum*

1. Oval or slightly elongated yeast cells (3–5 μm) with a single narrow-based bud, seen within macrophages or extracellularly

2. Small and dichotomously branching hyphae at 45° angle with cross-septa

3. Large yeast forms (8–20 μm) with thick, double contoured wall and single broad-based bud

4. Round-to-oval encapsulated budding yeast cells with narrow base

5. Mother yeast cell with narrow-based budding yeast in "pilot wheel" or "Mickey Mouse" configuration of approximately 2–30 μm

6. Hyphae and pseudohyphae with budding yeast forms (see figure in question 7)

Answers: a, 2; b, 5; c, 3; d, 4; e, 6; f, 1.

25. Diagnosis by antigen detection is available for which of the following fungi?

1. *Cryptococcus neoformans*   4. *Histoplasma capsulatum*

2. *Coccidioides immitis*   5. All of the above

3. *Candida albicans*

Answer: (5).

BIBLIOGRAPHY

1. Feigin RD, Cherry JD: Fungal diseases. In Feigin RD, Cherry JD (eds): Textbook of Pediatric Infectious Diseases, vol II, 4th ed. Philadelphia, W. B. Saunders, 1998.

2. Hoog GS, Guarro J, Gene J, Figueras MJ (eds): Atlas of Clinical Fungi. Central Bureau voor Schimmelcultures, Universitat Rovira i Virgili, 2000.

3. Kwon-Chung KJ, Bennet JE (eds): Medical Mycology. Philadelphia, Lea & Febiger, 1992.

4. PARASITIC INFECTIONS

M. Cecilia Di Pentima, M.D., M.P.H.

1. How are parasites classified?

Parasites can be divided into two large groups based on the complexity of their morphology: protozoa and helminths.

The word **protozoa** derives from the combination of two Greek words, *protos* (first or primary) and *zoon* (animal), meaning the simplest of all parasites. Protozoa are unicellular organisms and, unlike most helminths, can replicate inside the host, which explains their ability to survive and the severity of human infection after a single exposure.

The word **helminth** derives from the Greek word *helmins* (worms). Helminths include the more complex, multicellular parasites. Almost all helminths lack the ability to multiply inside their host.

2. What is the difference between incidental and intermediate host? What are the clinical implications?

Parasitism is usually the result of a long evolutionary interaction between parasites and different host species. **Incidental hosts** are those that are accidentally infested by a parasite that normally infects other species. Accidental or incidental parasites usually do not survive in the wrong host, and because the host is not well adapted to the new intruder, consequences of this interaction may be harmful for both. A clear example of this dreadful mistake is toxocariasis or visceral larva migrans. Human infection is a suicidal road for the unaware larvae of *Toxocara canis* with potential serious complications for the unguarded human host. Because the larva cannot mature, it migrates for months, until the host inflammatory response overcomes the lost pilgrim and it dies.

Intermediate hosts are required to complete parasite development. Survival of the species is key to maintain the survival of the parasite. Examples of intermediate hosts are different species of snails. *Schistosoma* spp. evolve into infective forms that penetrate human skin when we swim or bathe in fresh water contaminated with both *Schistosoma* spp. and their favorite snails. No snails, no schistosomiasis! Sounds simple, but without the snails, schistosomas would need to find another suitable host to complete their development. As a matter of conveyance, intermediate hosts are usually not harmed by the parasites.

3. Name the two major pathogenic groups of protozoan parasites.

Sophisticated names for two important groups of parasites: apicomplexans and kinetoplastids. Both names are derived from distinct parasitic organelles seen only under electron microscopy.

The **apicomplexans** have evolved to live only intracellularly; examples include *Plasmodium* spp., *Toxoplasma gondii*, and *Cryptosporidium parvum*. The apical complex is a combination of distinct organelles that play an important role in the process of host cell invasion.

The **kinetoplastids** include a large group of parasites that can live either extra- or intracellularly and can infest everything from humans to plants. The most important species that infect humans are *Trypanosoma* and *Leishmania* spp. The kinetoplast is a DNA-containing organelle whose function is not clearly understood (see figure on following page).

4. What are the most clinically important protozoa? Which organ systems do they commonly affect?

See table on following page.

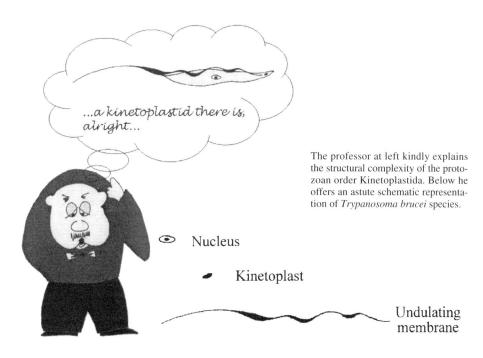

...a kinetoplastid there is, alright...

The professor at left kindly explains the structural complexity of the protozoan order Kinetoplastida. Below he offers an astute schematic representation of *Trypanosoma brucei* species.

Nucleus

Kinetoplast

Undulating membrane

Clinically Significant Protozoan Parasites

	FLAGELLATES	SPOROZOA	COCCIDIA	AMOEBA	CILIATES
Gastrointestinal	*Giardia lamblia*		*Cryptosporidium parvum* *Isospora belli* *Cyclospora cayetansis* *Microsporidium* spp.	*Entamoeba histolytica* *Blastocystis hominis*	*Balantidium coli*
Pulmonary		*Pneumocystis carinii*			
Central nervous system	*Trypanosoma* spp.	*Plasmodium* spp.	*Toxomplasma gondii* *Microsporidium* spp.	*Naegleria fowleri* *Acanthamoeba* spp. *Balamuthia mandrilaris* *Entamoeba histolytica*	
Blood/systemic	*Trypanosoma* spp. *Leishmania* spp.	*Plasmodium* spp. *Babesia* spp.		*Balamuthia mandrilaris*	
Skin	*Leishmania* spp. *Trypanosoma* spp.				
Genital	*Trichomonas* spp.				

5. Describe the risk factors associated with congenital toxoplasmosis.

Primary maternal infection is the most important risk factor. If previous infection has occurred, maternal antibodies are protective for the fetus. Because primary infection always precedes fetal infection, the risk is higher in countries with low endemicity. The risk of acquiring primary infection during pregnancy is higher when rates of seroconversion are low during childhood.

Primary *Toxoplasma gondii* infection is acquired by ingestion of infective oocysts, which are mainly shed in cat excrement. Risk factors for primary maternal infection correlate with exposure to oocysts by handling kitty litter, gardening, and playing with children in sandboxes. Another risk factor is ingestion of infected meat that has not been properly cooked. In the United States, it is estimated that 10–80% of beef, 20% of pork, and 30% of lamb at grocery stores is infected

6. Name three intestinal parasites that can be diagnosed by antigen detection in stool samples.

Rapid antigen detection tests are available for *Giardia lamblia, Cryptosporidium parvum,* and *Entamoeba histolytica.*

7. What are the current therapeutic options for *G. lamblia*?

Metronidazole is effective in 85–95 % of cases and remains the drug of choice. Furazoline, although less effective, is the only drug available as a pediatric suspension. Paromomycin, because it is not absorbed, also can be used safely during pregnancy. Albendazole, as a single daily dose administered for 5 days, is as effective as metronidazole. About 10–20% of cases fail to respond to therapy. Reinfection is the most common contributor, but poor compliance, infection with a resistant strain, or an underlying immunodeficiency may explain failure to respond.

8. Treatment of invasive *E. histolytica* infections, such as colitis or liver abscess, requires combination therapy. Which is the drug of choice for invasive amebiasis? Why is a second drug always recommended?

Invasive amebiasis should be treated with metronidazole, a highly effective amebicidal agent that reaches adequate concentrations in most tissues. Eradication of intestinal colonization cannot be achieved with metronidazole, because luminal concentrations are almost undetectable. Treatment of invasive infections should be followed by a second agent. Paromomycin, iodoquinol, and diloxanide furoate are poorly absorbed, reaching high luminal concentrations and reducing the risk of relapse from residual intestinal infection.

9. *Entamoeba dispar* is not a human pathogenic parasite. In an ova and parasites (O&P) examination, *E. dispar* and *E. histolytica* are morphologically indistinguishable. How do you determine whether your patient needs treatment?

When ingested erythrocytes are present in the cytoplasm of the microorganism. there is no doubt that the parasite is *E. histolytica*. This finding is also consistent with invasive colitis, and patients should be treated accordingly. In the absence of erythrophagocytosis, specimens should be submitted for further enzyme immunoassay analysis to differentiate the two species.

10. Name the three major clinical syndromes associated with *Leishmania* spp. Which are seen in Latin America?

Leishmania spp. can cause cutaneous, mucocutaneous, and visceral leishmaniasis. All three clinical entities can be seen in the Americas, but the involved species differ in each continent. In endemic countries, children are often affected with visceral leishmaniasis, the most severe form of the disease.

11. What is the Romaña sign?

Unilateral, painless palpebral edema (sometimes associated with conjunctivitis) seen at the portal of entry of *Trypanosoma cruzi*, the etiologic agent of American trypanosomiasis or Chagas disease.

12. What are the major groups of helminths?

Helminths are subdivided in three main categories: (1) nematodes or roundworms, (2) cestodes or tapeworms, and (3) trematodes or flukes.

Clinically Significant Helminths

	INTESTINE	TISSUE	BLOOD AND TISSUES
Nematodes	*Ascaris lumbricoides*	*Toxocara canis* or *catti*	Filarial worms
	Enterobius vermicularis	*Ancylostoma brasiliense*	*Wuchereria bancrofti*
	Ancylostoma duodenale	and *caninus*	*Brugia malayi*
	Necator americanus	*Angiostrongylus cantonensis*	*Brugia timori*
	Strongyloides stercolaris	and *costaricensis*	*Loa-loa*
	Trichuris trichiura	*Gnasthostoma spinigerum*	*Onchocerca volvulus*
	Capillaria phillipensis	*Anisakis* spp.	*Mansonella ozzardi*
			Mansonella streptocerca
			Mansonella perstans
			Dirofilaria immitis
Cestodes	*Hymenolepsis nana* and *diminuta*	*Taenia solium*	
	Taenia solium and *saginata*	*Echinococcus granulosus* and *multilocularis*	
	Diphylobotrium latum	*Spirometra mansonoides* and *mansoni*	
	Diphilobotrium caninun		
Trematodes	*Fasciolopsis buski*	Liver	*Shistosoma mansoni*
		Fasciola hepatica	*Shistosoma haematobium*
		Clonorkis sinensis	*Shistosoma japonicum*
		Opisthorcis viverrini	
		Lungs	
		Paragonimus westermani	

13. Which intestinal parasites are known as "the unholy trinity"?

"The unholy trinity" includes the three major soil-transmitted intestinal nematodes that frequently can be found infecting the same child. Also known as geohelminths, they include:

1. *Trichuris trichiura* (whipworm)
2. *Ascaris lumbricoides*
3. Two species of hookworms, *Ancylostoma duodenale* and *Necator americanus*.

14. True or false: Cutaneous larva migrans (CLM) and visceral larva migrans (VLM) refer to the same parasite with different organ involvement.

False. CLM is caused by invasion of the skin by larval nematodes. The most frequently encountered parasite is *Ancylostoma braziliensis*, a cat and dog hookworm. *Toxocara canis* is the single etiologic agent of VLM in the Western Hemisphere. Rare cases of VLM can be attributed to *Capillaria hepatica* in Southeast Asia.

15. Can neurocysticercosis be acquired by eating infected undercooked pork?

No. Neurocysticercosis is acquired by ingestion of food or water contaminated with eggs of *Taenia solium*. After ingestion of eggs, larvae hatch in the intestine, invade the mucosa, and through the mesenteric vessels spread to different organs. In this case, humans accidentally replace pigs as intermediate hosts. Ingestion of undercooked meat containing cysticerci (larvae) allows only the adult worm to develop, which remains quietly attached to the small intestine (see figure on following page).

	SOURCE	HUMAN HOST	LIFE CYCLE		END RESULT
A	Ingestion of undercooked meat containing cysticerci	**DEFINITIVE** CYSTICERCOSIS	Cysticercus develops into adult tapeworm	Gravid proglottids hatch and pass with the feces	**Eggs** are ingested by pigs
B	Ingestion of food or water with human feces contaminated with eggs	**INTERMEDIATE** CYSTICERCOSIS	Eggs hatch, and oncospheres emerge	Oncospheres spread by the mesenteric vessels	**Cysticercus** develop in target organs

Life cycle of *Taenia solium*. (From DiPentima MC, White C: Neurocysticercosis. Semin Pediatr Infect Dis 11:262, 2000, with permission.)

16. Is *Strongyloides stercolaris* endemic in the United States?

Yes. Strongyloidiasis is endemic in the southeastern United States.

17. Hyperinfection syndrome is a chronic, disseminated, life-threatening *S. stercolaris* infection affecting immunocompromised patients What is the most common infectious complication in such patients?

Gram-negative septicemia, most frequently due to *Escherichia coli* and other enterobacteriaceae. Secondary bacterial dissemination occurs in approximately one-half of patients. Although the mechanisms involved are not completely clear, the accepted explanation is active transmission of enteric bacteria across intestinal mucosa by invasion of filariform larvae.

18. How is *Enterobius vermicularis* infection acquired?

Ingestion of pinworm eggs is the most common route of acquisition. However, because eggs are only 57×28 μm, they can be easily spread into the air, where they are only a breath away from the human oropharynx. Swallowing pharyngeal secretions or phlegm containing the eggs completes the short road trip for the lightweight pinworm. The egg hatches in the small intestine and becomes an adult worm as it goes through the lower ileum and ascending colon and copulates near the cecum. The adult worm releases thousands of eggs in the anorectal area and dies soon thereafter. The entire journey takes approximately 6 weeks.

19. Crawling creatures under the skin: name three parasites that can cause a migratory rash.

Any of the parasites that cause cutaneous larva migrans can produce a migratory rash. The classic creeping eruption that presents as a serpiginous rash is more frequently seen with *Ancylostoma brasiliense*. This parasite can move 1–2 cm per day. *Ancylostoma caninum* and *A. duodenale* are also common, but they usually clear spontaneously within 1–3 weeks.

Gnathostomiasis, caused by *Gnathostoma spinigerum*, is characterized by intermittent episodes of migratory skin swelling, pruritus, and burning sensation.

Loa-loa can crawl beneath the skin, producing similar manifestations as cutaneous larva migrans or a transient, localized area of subcutaneous, nonpitting edema known as calabar swelling.

In chronic infections, the larvae of *Strongyloides stercolaris* can invade the skin, leading to a migratory, serpiginous, and urticarial rash known as larva currens.

20. Fulminant parasitic central nervous system (CNS) infections in immunocompetent hosts are rare. Which parasites are almost invariably associated with a fatal outcome when they invade the CNS?

Although rare, amebae can invade the brain, causing a fulminant infection in both immunocompetent and immunocompromised patients. *Entamoeba histolytica*, the most frequent amebic pathogen in humans, more commonly causes invasive infection of the colon and liver; brain abscess or cerebral amebiasis is rare. However, the mortality rate for reported cases is 100%. The most important among the many species of free-living amoeba are *Naeglaria fowleri*, *Acanthamoeba* spp., and *Balamuthia* spp. *N. fowleri* is associated with a devastating and almost always fatal CNS infection known as primary amebic meningoencephalitis (PAM). *Acanthamoeba* and *Balamuthia* spp. more often cause a progressive, subacute, or chronic infection known as granulomatous amebic encephalitis (GAE).

21. What is hydatid cyst disease?

Hydatidosis or hyatid cyst disease is a zoonosis caused by *Echinococcus granulosus*, a canine cestode or tapeworm that incidentally infects humans.

22. Which parasites cause hypereosinophilia?

Some parasites cause hypereosinophilia because eosinophils play an important role in resistance to their tissue-migratory larvae. The severity of eosinophilia has a direct correlation with the degree of tissue invasion by the intruder. Eosinophilia is seldom seen with protozoan parasites that are mainly intracellular. Helminth parasites with life cycles that involve tissue invasion (e.g., toxocariasis, filariasis, strongyloidiasis, trichinosis, schistosomiasis) are among the most frequent causes of parasite-related eosinophilia. Eosinophilia may be transient, depending on the extension of the migratory phase.

23. Explain the origin of the word *malaria*.

During the eighteenth century the word *malaria* was coined to replace the old term *ague*. Malaria derives from the Italian phrase *mal aria* (bad or poisonous air).

24. Which parasite is responsible for the disease known in Texas as "red water fever"?

Texas fever or red water fever is a zoonosis caused by *Babesia* spp and characterized by febrile hemoglobinuria; it affects mainly cattle.

25. Which is the longest parasite known to infect humans? How long does it get? How many years does it live?

Taenia spp. can measure up to 20 meters and can live up to 25 years inside the same human host (as seen on Ripley's *Believe It or Not*).

26. Why does treatment of *Enterobius vermicularis* require two doses of antihelminths given 1 week apart?

Antihelminth agents effective against *E. vermicularis* are active only against adult worms— not the eggs. A second dose given 2–3 weeks after the first dose destroys any adult worms that have hatched from eggs during this period.

27. Match the parasite and the route of acquisition.

a. *Paragonimus westermani*	1. Walking bare foot on a Caribbean beach
b. *Strongyloides stercolaris*	2. Eating sushi at a cheap restaurant in Japan
c. Free-living amoeba	3. Swimming in Lake Malawi, Africa
d. *Shistosoma* spp.	4. Swimming in a southern pond on a summer day
e. *Toxocara* spp.	5. Playing in a sandbox in Central Park
f. *Angiostrongyliasis cantonensis*	6. Eating sushi in Acapulco, Mexico
g. *Ancylostoma brasiliense*	7. Eating watercress salad on a sheep farm in France
h. *Gnathostoma spinigerum*	8. Eating raw salad or sushi in Jamaica
i. Hookworms	
j. *Fasciola hepatica*	

Answers: a, 2; b, 1; c, 4; d, 3; e, 5; f, 8; g, 1; h, 6; i, 1; j, 7.

Eating raw fish is risky! *P. westermani*, a lung fluke, is acquired by eating uncooked infected fish. Although the parasite has a worldwide distribution, the three endemic foci of human disease are Asia, Africa, and South America. It is most prevalent in Japan, Korea, China, and Taiwan.

Gnasthotomiasisis also acquired by eating uncooked fish, mainly in Asia; most cases are reported from Japan and Thailand. However, outbreaks of *G. spinigerum* have been increasingly reported among travelers to Central and South American, particularly Mexico and Peru.

Larva stages of hookworms (*Necator Americanus* and *Ancylostoma duodenale*), *A. braziliense*, and *S. stercolaris* that contaminate soil and/or water can penetrate intact skin. These parasites have a worldwide distribution, but they are more prevalent in developing countries where hygienic conditions are inadequate. Walking barefoot in contaminated soil in the Caribbean islands or throughout Central and South America represents a risk for acquiring infection.

Free-living amebae, including *N. fowleri* and *Acanthamoeba* spp. can be acquired by swimming in contaminated, warm, fresh, or brackish water and even in swimming pools with inadequate chlorination. These infections are more common during the warm months.

Schistosomiasis is acquired by swimming or walking barefoot in contaminated water. Lake Malawi is highly contaminated with the infective larva or cercariae of *S. hematobium*, which can easily penetrate intact skin. Several other species of bird schistosomes distributed throughout the

United States, Canada, and Mexico also may infect humans, causing limited disease (usually only cercarial dermatitis)

Toxocara canis or *catti* is the second most common helminth infection in North American children, who became infected by ingestion of eggs, mainly from exposure to contaminated soil in public parks. Puppies and kittens can shed up to 200,000 eggs per day by the time they are 1 month of age.

Children and adults can became infected with *A. cantonensis* by eating food that contains the third-stage larvae—especially raw vegetables contaminated with snails, slugs, or mollusk secretions; infected hosts such as crabs or freshwater shrimp; or improperly cooked snails or slugs. Angystrongyloidiasis is common in Southeast Asia and the Pacific Islands. A recent outbreak was reported among United States medical students returning from a trip to Jamaica.

F. hepatica is acquired by ingestion of uncooked contaminated plants, particularly watercress, in sheep-raising areas where fascioliasis is endemic. *F. hepatica* is widely distributed throughout tropical and temperate areas.

28. Match the parasite with the correct vector.

a. *Babesia microti*	1. *Anopheles* spp. mosquitoes
b. *Plasmodium* spp.	2. *Ioxides* spp. ticks
c. *Onchocerca volvulus*	3. *Simulium* spp. or black flies
d. *Leishmania brasiliensis*	4. *Chrysops* spp. or tabanid or red flies
e. *Trypanosoma cruzi*	5. Sandflies
f. *Trypanosoma brucei* spp.	6. *Triatoma* spp. or kissing bugs
g. *Wuchereria bancrofti*	7. *Glossina* spp. or tsetse flies
h. *Loa-loa*	8. *Anopheles, aedes,* or *culex* spp. mosquitoes

Answers: a, 2; b, 1; c, 3; d, 5; e, 6; f, 7; g, 8; h, 4.

B. microti, the primary agent of babesiosis in the United States, is acquired by *Ioxides* tick bites. Malaria, the most important human parasitic infection, is caused by four species of *Plasmodium: vivax, ovale, falciparum,* and *malarie*. The route of transmission is the bite of an infected female anopheles mosquito, the definitive host of the genus.

Onchocercaiasis, also known as river blindness, is acquired after been bitten by a black fly (*Simulium* spp.) infected with *O. volvulus.*

Sandflies are responsible for the transmission of the protozoan parasites of the genus *Leishmania.* In the Americas, parasites responsible for leishmaniasis are transmitted by sandflies of the genus *Lutzomyia,* whereas in Europe transmission is by the genus *Phlebotumus.*

American trypanosomiasis or Chagas disease is transmitted to humans by *Triatomes* spp. infected with *T. cruzi.*

T. brucei rhodesiense and *gambiense,* the etiologic agents of sleeping sickness or human African trypanosomiasis, are transmitted to humans by the genus *Glossina,* which includes more than 22 species of tsetse fly.

W. bancrofti, which causes one of the oldest filariases and is responsible for the disease known as elephantiasis because of the severity of lymphatic obstruction (particularly of the lower extremities), is transmitted to humans by the bite of *anopheles, aedes,* or *culex* mosquitoes.

Loaiasis is acquired when an infected tabanid or red fly takes a blood meal, injecting the filariform larvae.

29. Which of the following parasites frequently identified in stool samples from children are not considered pathogens?

a. *Endolimax nana*
b. *Endolimax grandpa*
c. *Chilomastix mesnili*
d. *Entamoeba coli*
e. *Entamoeba hartmanni*

Answer: all of the above except b.

30. What about *Dientamoeba fragilis*, which is also commonly identified in stool samples from children?

If *D. fragilis* is identified in the stool, treatment with iodoquinol, paromomycin, or metronidazole is recommended if symptoms warrant.

Pearl: Look for pinworms in these patients. The life cycles of both parasites may be related.

BIBLIOGRAPHY

1. Feigin RD, Cherry JD (eds): Textbook of Pediatric Infectious Diseases, 4th ed. Philadelphia, W. B. Saunders, 1998.
2. Strickland TG (ed): Hunter's Tropical Medicine and Emerging Infectious Diseases, 8th ed. Philadelphia, W. B. Saunders, 2000.
3. Schmidt GD, Roberts LS (eds): Foundations of Parasitology, 5th ed. Boston, William C. Brown Publishers, 1996.
4. Cook GC (ed): Parasitic diseases in Clinical Practice. London, Springer-Verlag, 1990.

5. ANTIMICROBIAL AGENTS

Reza J. Daugherty, M.D., and Stephen C. Eppes, M.D.

1. What does it mean if an antibiotic is described as bactericidal vs. bacteriostatic?

Certain antibiotics are capable of killing susceptible organisms without intervention from the host's immunity. Examples of common bactericidal antibiotics include the penicillins and amino-glycosides. These antibiotics are particularly useful in patients with infections who have de-pressed cellular or humeral immunity, such as neutropenia or HIV. Bacteriostatic drugs, such as the sulfa drugs and tetracyclines, act by hindering vital metabolic functions of the organism, thereby preventing further growth or replication. Hence, it is ultimately the responsibility of the host immune system to destroy the microorganism.

2. Describe how antibiotic susceptibility can be determined.

The two main methods are disk diffusion and use of serial broth dilution. In the broth dilu-tion procedure, a fixed amount of bacteria is added to decreasing concentrations of antibiotic and incubated. The smallest concentration of antibiotic required to prevent growth, identified by lack of turbidity in the tube, is defined as the minimal inhibitory capacity (MIC).

3. Who is Kirby Bauer?

Kirby-Bauer actually refers to a disk diffusion technique for determining susceptibility. An agar plate is inoculated with the bacteria, and multiple paper disks impregnated with antibiotics are applied to the plate. While bacteria grow confluently on the rest of the plate, a zone of inhibition appears around the disk. Standardized criteria for common bacteria and antibiotics allow correla-tion of the diameter of inhibition around the disk to define susceptibly. It is less labor intensive and less costly than the dilutional technique but still gives a relatively accurate semiquantitative result.

4. What do the terms *sensitive* and *resistant* commonly mean when used to describe a par-ticular bacterial organism?

The diameters of inhibition around the disks in the Kirby-Bauer method are converted to these terms based on standards established by the National Committee for Clinical Laboratory Standards. Bacteria described as **sensitive** are inhibited by the antibiotic at doses that are rou-tinely used in clinical practice (i.e., usual dosing achieves blood levels that exceed the MIC). If bacteria are **resistant**, the antibiotic (at usual dosing) does not significantly exceed the MIC.

5. True or false: If sensitivities show that a bacteria is resistant to a given antibiotic, that antibiotic cannot be used.

False. In some cases increasing the dose of the antibiotic, and hence raising serum levels to exceed the MIC, can overcome relative resistance. Obviously this approach must be done with caution and is useful only with antimicrobials that have a wide therapeutic index (e.g., peni-cillins). In addition, some antibiotics achieve massive levels in the urine even when dosed nor-mally. An organism that appears resistant in vitro may in fact be adequately treated when it is present in the urine because of this fact.

6. True or false: The Eagle effect occurs when bacteria are transmitted to humans by large predatory birds.

False. In 1952 Dr. H. Eagle observed that in some severe cases of *Streptococcus pyogenes* infection, penicillin was ineffective. Theoretically, if infection is heavy, production of penicillin-binding proteins may be downregulated because the bacteria have entered the stationary phase of the growth cycle. In such cases, antibiotics that work by protein synthesis inhibition, such as clin-damycin, may be more efficacious. Clindamycin is routinely added to penicillin in severe invasive streptococcal infections for this reason. In addition, group A streptococcal toxins, the main virulence factors for the organism, are proteins whose synthesis may be reduced by clindamycin.

7. What are the *Streptomyces*? Why may they be one of the most helpful microorganisms to humans?

Streptomyces is a genus of gram-positive bacteria commonly found in soil and fresh water. Different isolates have been used to produce the tetracyclines, erythromycin, chloramphenicol, and, of course, streptomycin.

8. What are the beta-lactam antibiotics? What do they share in common?

The two main classes of antibiotics in the beta-lactam group are the penicillins and cephalosporins. They all share a similar ring structure (called the beta-lactam ring) and differ mainly in their side chains. The side chains distinguish the different compounds and determine their pharmacodynamics, spectrum of activity, and mechanism of bacterial resistance. They all share a common mechanism of bactericidal action, mainly disruption of bacterial cell wall synthesis. The monobactams (e.g., aztreonam) and the carbapenems (e.g., meropenem) are related compounds with less cross-reactivity to penicillins in terms of allergic reactions.

9. Name four general methods by which bacteria may be resistant to an antibiotic.

1. Decreased uptake of the antibiotic because of either alteration in the bacterial structure or active transport of the substance out of the cell (e.g., the macrolide efflux pump, by which *Streptococcus pneumoniae* develops resistance to macrolide antibiotics).

2. Alteration or removal of bacterial target proteins, thereby decreasing antimicrobial affinity (e.g., genetically mediated alterations in the penicillin binding proteins [PBPs] leading to resistance to beta-lactam antibiotics).

3. Novel metabolic pathways to circumvent inhibited enzymes (e.g., the folate pathway for trimethoprim-sulfamethoxazole).

4. Production of a substance that binds to the antibiotic and either prevents target binding or outright inactivates the agent (e.g., beta-lactamases, which destroy the beta-lactam ring).

10. Define the terms *additive*, *synergistic*, and *antagonistic* as they refer to antimicrobials.

These terms reflect the relative interactions of antibiotics with one another when used in combination. **Additive** describes a situation in which the cumulative effect of the drugs is equal to the sum of the individual antibiotic activities (1 + 1 = 2) (e.g, nafcillin and rifampin used against some strains of staphylococci). **Synergistic** expresses the finding that some antibiotics when used in concert have an effect that is greater than the sum of their individual effects (1 + 1 > 2) (e.g., ceftazidime and gentamicin against some strains of *Pseudomonas aeruginosa*). Finally, antibiotics that have an **antagonistic** effect on one another other have less efficacy than the sum of their individual effects (1 + 1 < 2) (e.g., penicillin and tetracycline are no longer recommended for treatment of bacterial meningitis).

11. True or false: Penicillin-binding proteins (PBPs) bind to all beta-lactams, not just to penicillin.

True. PBP is a bit of a misnomer in that the proteins may bind to many different beta-lactams. Bear in mind that PBPs are not simply one protein. They are a diverse mix of many proteins that, in general, share a common function of bacterial cell wall maintenance, although some have no identifiable function at all. The beta-lactams act by binding to PBPs and interfering with their activity, effectively punching holes in the cell wall. This effect allows water to pass into the bacteria unhindered and to kill the microorganism by cell lysis.

12. What is the incidence of allergic cross-reactivity between penicillin and cephalosporins?

Approximately 10–15% of patients who are allergic to a cephalosporin are also allergic to penicillin. A recent study, however, suggests that the different side chains may play an important role in determining allergenicity. Thirty-eight percent of patients who were allergic to amoxicillin were also allergic to cefadroxil, but none were allergic to cefamandole. Amoxicillin shares a common side chain with cefadroxil but not with cefamandole.

13. What are the four main classifications of the penicillins?

The penicillins can be subdivided based on their spectrum of activity. It should be noted that many bacteria have developed mechanisms of resistance to antibiotics despite the antimicrobial's inherent activity against them (e.g., methicillin and methicillin-resistant *Staphylococcus aureus*).

CLASSIFICATION	COMMON EXAMPLES	ANTIBACTERIAL ACTIVITY
Narrow spectrum	Penicillin G (parenteral) Penicillin V (oral)	Many gram-positive cocci, a few gram-negative cocci, and *Treponema pallidum*
Penicillinase-resistant (aka antistaphylococcal)	Methicillin (parenteral) Nafcillin (parenteral) Oxacillin (parenteral) Dicloxacillin (oral)	Same as narrow-spectrum penicillins but possess inherent resistance to penicillinase produced by *S. aureus*
Aminopenicillins	Ampicillin (parenteral, oral) Amoxicillin (oral)	Same as narrow-spectrum penicillins but with some added gram-negative coverage
Extended spectrum	Piperacillin (parenteral)	Same as narrow-spectrum penicillins with increased gram-negative coverage and some inherent anti-pseudomonal action

14. Describe the spectrum of activity for each of the generations of cephalosporin.

The cephalosporins are categorized based on their spectrum of antibacterial activity. Within each generation, however, there maybe a wide range of activity against certain organisms. The following table is a general outline of their spectra of activity that makes them easier to learn. As they increase in generation, they gain activity against gram-negative organisms at the cost of some gram-positive coverage.

GENERATION	COMMON EXAMPLES	ANTIBACTERIAL ACTIVITY
First	Cefazolin (parenteral) Cephalexin (oral) Cefadroxil (oral)	Excellent activity against gram-positive cocci and good activity against *Escherichia coli, Proteus mirabilis,* and *Klebsiella pneumoniae*
Second	Cefuroxime (parenteral) Cefoxitin (parenteral) Cefuroxime axetil (oral) Cefprozil (oral) Cefaclor (oral) Loracarbef (oral)	Members in the same group have particularly wide variability in action. In general, they maintain good activity against gram-positive cocci and have improved activity against *Haemophilus influenzae, Moraxella catarrhalis, Streptococcus pneumoniae, Neisseria meningitidis* and *gonorrhoeae,* and *Bacteroides fragilis* (cefoxitin only)
Third	Cefotaxime (parenteral) Ceftriaxone (parenteral) Ceftazidime (parenteral) Cefpodoxime (oral) Cefixime (oral)	Maintain some activity against gram-positive cocci, but some have particularly strong activity against species of Enterobacteriaceae and, in the case of ceftazidime, *Pseudomonas aeruginosa*
Fourth	Cefepime (parenteral)	Restores excellent gram-positive coverage, has broad activity against the Enterobacteriaceae and is very active against *P. aeruginosa*

15. What mechanism of penicillin resistance is used by *S. pneumoniae*?

S. pneumoniae possess six penicillin-binding proteins, named 1A, 1B, 2A, 2B, 2X, and 3. The resistant organism has acquired one or more mutated genes from other bacteria that cause alterations in the conformation of the proteins. These changes decrease penicillin's affinity for them and hence its activity. The more proteins that are altered, the more resistant the organism. This resistance sometimes may be overcome by increasing the dose of antibiotic. Resistance in this case has nothing to do with production of a beta-lactamase. Hence, addition of a beta-lactamase inhibitor has no benefit (a common mistake in practice).

16. Match the antibiotic with the organism from which it was first derived from. Some answers are used more than once.

a. Penicillin
b. Cephalosporins
c. Erythromycin
d. Tetracycline
e. Aztreonam
f. Gentamicin
g. Polymyxin

1. *Streptomyces*
2. *Cephalosporium* mold
3. *Bacillus* species
4. *Chromobacterium violacium*
5. *Penicillium* mold

Answers: a, 5; b, 2; c, 1; d, 1; e, 4; f, 1; g, 3.

17. True or false: The suicide inhibitors are a small group of militant freedom fighters that engage in guerilla warfare and kamikaze tactics.

Sort of true. In fact, they are beta lactams that have no intrinsic antibacterial activity but inhibit the activity of many types of beta lactamase. They do so by binding irreversibly to the beta-lactamase and inactivating its activity. They are destroyed in the process; hence the name suicide inhibitors. They are commonly combined with a penicillin to extend its spectrum of activity. Currently, four combination antibiotics that possess beta-lactamase inhibitors are in common use: amoxicillin/clavulanate (Augmentin), ampicillin/sulbactam (Unasyn), ticarcillin/clavulanate (Timentin), and piperacillin/tazobactam (Zosyn).

18. Match the antibiotic class to its mechanism of action.

1. Macrolides
2. Trimethoprim
3. Tetracyclines
4. Metronidazole
5. Aminoglycosides
6. Rifampin
7. Quinolones
8. Sulfonamides
9. Beta lactams

a. Inhibit DNA gyrase
b. Bind 30S ribosomal subunit and inhibit protein synthesis
c. Inhibit cell wall synthesis
d. Inhibit DNA-dependent RNA polymerase
e. Bind 30S and 50S ribosomal subunits and inhibit protein synthesis
f. Bind 50S ribosomal subunit and inhibit protein synthesis
g. Para-aminobenzoic acid (PABA) analog
h. Block anaerobic metabolic pathways
i. Inhibit dihydrofolate reductase

Answers: 1, f; 2, i; 3, b; 4, h; 5, e; 6, d; 7, a; 8, g; 9, c.

19. Match the following antibiotics with a common or significant adverse effect.

1. Gentamicin
2. Tetracycline
3. Rifampin
4. Penicillin
5. Erythromycin
6. Ceftriaxone
7. Metronidazole
8. Imipenem
9. Chloramphenicol
10. Sulfamethoxazole
11. Vancomycin

a. Most common allergic reaction
b. Orange-colored urine
c. Pseudotumor cerebri
d. Inhibits liver metabolism of some drugs, raising their levels
e. Biliary sludging
f. Disulfiram-like reactions with alcohol
g. Gray baby syndrome
h. Red man syndrome
i. Lowers seizure threshold
j. Ototoxicity and nephrotoxicity
k. Hemolytic anemia in patients with G6PD deficiency

Answers: 1, j; 2, c; 3, b; 4, a; 5, d; 6, e; 7, f; 8, i; 9, g; 10, k; 11, h.

20. What four properties constitute the pharmacokinetic profile of a drug? Give an example of how each can influence the selection of antibiotics to treat a given infection.

1. **Absorption** is the fraction of an administered dose that is delivered to a given site. With parenteral therapy, absorption is generally high. For oral drugs, absorption is often incomplete, and high systemic levels may be difficult to achieve. Certain drugs have relatively poor absorption (low bioavailability) and are generally not recommended; for example, ampicillin is not well absorbed, but the chemically altered amoxicillin is well absorbed.

2. **Distribution** refers to the exchange of drug between various body compartments and tissues. Usually it means distribution from plasma to a certain anatomic site or tissue, such as the central nervous system, middle ear, or prostate. Drugs that do not cross the blood-brain barrier very well, such as aminoglycosides, may be less effective in treating bacterial meningitis.

3. **Metabolism** occurs for certain drugs, whereas others are eliminated largely unchanged. Metabolism of drugs often occurs in the liver via the cytochrome p450 system. Drug interactions may occur as a result; for example, erythromycin can elevate theophylline levels, and rifampin can interact with a number of drugs.

4. **Excretion** of drug and drug metabolites eliminates them from the body, commonly through the urine or bile. High concentrations of active drug may be obtained in these fluids. However, if bile or urine flow is obstructed, toxic accumulation of drugs may result. A familiar example is the toxic level of aminoglycosides in the setting of renal insufficiency.

21. Why and when should antibiotic levels be checked?

When used properly, serum antibiotic concentrations can optimize treatment regimens and decrease dose-dependent side effects. Ensuring adequate peaks maximizes efficacy, and ensuring appropriate troughs minimizes dose-dependent adverse events. As a general rule, the dosing interval is changed to affect the trough (remember timing and trough). For example, if the trough is too high, you increase the dosing interval. In general, drug dosing is altered to affect the peak (there is no trick; just remember timing and trough). For example, if the peak is too low. you increase the dose. Interval and dose have a complex interaction with drug levels based on pharmacodynamics, and both affect peaks and troughs to some degree. For aminoglycosides, both peak and trough should be monitored, especially with prolonged drug administration. For vancomycin, peak levels do not routinely need to be monitored in patients with normal renal function, but trough concentrations should be measured to help avoid toxicity.

22. Antibiotic usage can be categorized as empirical, specific, and prophylactic. Define these terms.

Empirical antibiotic therapy refers to starting an appropriate antibiotic based on clinical findings (in some cases with laboratory and imaging data) without precise knowledge of the offending organism(s). In significant infections, empirical antibiotics usually are given after appropriate cultures have been obtained. Empirical therapy should be done with knowledge of the following: likely pathogens and their susceptibility patterns, pharmacokinetics of the drug, clinical guidelines or results of clinical trials, safety and tolerability, and cost.

Specific antibiotic therapy is provided when culture and susceptibility information can guide the choice of agents.

Prophylactic antibiotics are given to avert the possibility of a significant infection (e.g., surgical wounds, animal bites, and recurrent urinary tract infections).

23. Match the in-patient situation to the appropriate empirical antibiotic.

a. Neonatal sepsis	1. Vancomycin and ceftriaxone
b. Ruptured appendix	2. Oxacillin
c. Osteomyelitis	3. Ampicillin and cefotaxime
d. Community-acquired pneumonia	4. Ceftazidime
e. Bacterial meningitis	5. Ampicillin, gentamicin, metronidazole
f. Fever and neutropenia	6. Second- or third-generation cephalosporin

Answers: a, 3; b, 5; c, 2; d, 6; e, 1; f, 4.

24. Match the ambulatory infection to the empirical antibiotic therapy (one best answer for each).

a. Cellulitis
b. Acute otitis media
c. Otitis media with effusion
d. Community-acquired pneumonia
e. Urinary tract infection
f. Shigellosis

1. Trimethoprim-sulfamethoxazole
2. Azithromycin
3. Amoxicillin
4. Cephalexin
5. No therapy
6. Cefixime

Answers: a, 4; b, 3; c, 5; d, 2; e, 6; f, 1.

25. Antibiotic resistance has become a huge problem in both the ambulatory and hospital settings. Which of the following can clinicians do to help manage the problem?

1. Avoid treating viral infections with antibiotics
2. Select the correct drug, dose, and duration
3. Avoid prolonged prophylaxis
4. Use preventive measures, including immunization
5. Develop effective infection control procedures
6. All of the above

Answer: (6). And don't you forget it!

BIBLIOGRAPHY

1. Antimicrobics and Chemotherapy of Bacterial and Viral Infections. In Ryan (ed): Sherris Medical Microbiology, 3rd ed. Norwalk, CT, Appleton & Lange, 1994.
2. Cephalosporins. In Mandell, Bennett, Dolin(ed)s: Mandell Principles and Practice of Infectious Diseases, 5th ed. New York, Churchill Livingstone, 2000.
3. Gubbay AJ, Isaacs D: Pyomyositis in children. Pediatr Infect Dis J 19:1009–1012, 2000.
4. Miranda A, Blanca M, Vega JM, et al: Cross-reactivity between a penicillin and a cephalosporin with the same side chain. J Allergy Clin Immunol 98:671–677, 1996.
5. Penicillins. In Mandell, Bennett, Dolin (eds): Mandell Principles and Practice of Infectious Diseases, 5th ed. New York, Churchill Livingstone, 2000.
6. Romano A, Mayorga C, Torres MJ, et al: Immediate allergic reactions to cephalosporins: Cross-reactivity and selective responses. J Allergy Clin Immunol 106:1177–1183, 2000.
7. *Streptococcus pneumoniae.* In Mandell, Bennett, Dolin (eds): Mandell Principles and Practice of Infectious Diseases, 5th ed. New York, Churchill Livingstone, 2000.
8. Zimbelman J, Palmer A, Todd J: Improved outcome of clindamycin compared with beta-lactam antibiotic treatment for invasive Streptococcus pyogenes infection. Pediatr Infect Dis J 18:1096–1100, 1999.

II. Upper Respiratory Tract Infections

6. SINUSITIS

Samir S. Shah, M.D.

1. Describe sinus anatomy.

There are four pairs of paranasal sinuses (air-filled cavities within the skull): maxillary, ethmoid, sphenoid, and frontal. Each sinus is lined with respiratory mucosa that is contiguous with that of the nasal cavity and communicates with the nasal cavity through various ostia.

A

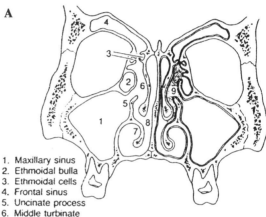

1. Maxillary sinus
2. Ethmoidal bulla
3. Ethmoidal cells
4. Frontal sinus
5. Uncinate process
6. Middle turbinate
7. Inferior turbinate
8. Nasal septum
9. Osteomeatal complex

Coronal (*A*) and sagittal (*B*) sections of the nose and paranasal sinuses. (From Wald ER: Sinusitis in children. N Engl J Med 326:319–323, 1992, with permission.)

B

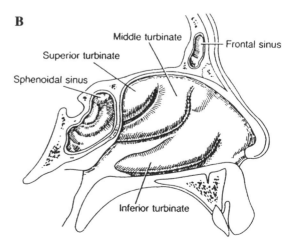

Middle turbinate
Frontal sinus
Superior turbinate
Sphenoidal sinus
Inferior turbinate

2. At what age do the sinuses develop?

The maxillary and ethmoid sinuses, which develop between the third and fourth months of gestation, are present at birth. The sphenoid sinuses develop by 5 years of age. The frontal sinuses are last to develop. They appear at 5–8 years of age but are not fully developed until adolescence.

3. Define sinusitis. How is bacterial sinusitis classified?

The term *sinusitis* describes inflammation of the paranasal sinus cavities. Sinusitis can be allergic, viral, fungal, or bacterial in etiology. Bacterial sinusitis is classified as follows:

- Acute bacterial sinusitis: duration < 30 days.
- Subacute bacterial sinusitis: duration of 30–90 days, after which symptoms resolve completely.
- Recurrent acute bacterial sinusitis: episodes of bacterial sinusitis, each lasting < 30 days and separated by intervals of at least 10 days during which the patient is asymptomatic.
- Chronic sinusitis: duration > 90 days. Patients have persistent residual respiratory symptoms such as cough, rhinorrhea, or nasal obstruction.

4. Explain the pathogenesis of sinusitis.

Normal sinus function is related to three factors: (1) patency of the sinus ostia, which are narrow, tubular structures; (2) function of epithelial cilia; and (3) quality of secretions, which are required for the normal function of cilia. The paranasal sinuses are sterile, but their contiguous areas (nasopharynx and nose) contain microbial flora. Normal ciliary movement and mucus flow keep the sinuses clear of pathogens. Insults that alter ciliary function or mucus viscosity cause the sinus ostia to become obstructed with mucus. The resultant negative intranasal pressure allows large numbers of pathogens to accumulate in the sinuses, which can lead to infection. Remember the mucociliary escalator. It is not the stairway to heaven.

5. What conditions predispose children to sinusitis?

CATEGORY	CONDITIONS
Inflammatory	Viral upper respiratory infections Irritants (tobacco smoke) Allergic/nonallergic rhinitis Gastroesophageal reflux
Local/anatomic	Nasal septal deviation (congenital or traumatic) Swimming/diving Adenoid hypertrophy Nasal foreign body Nasal polyp/tumor Nasogastric catheter/nasotracheal intubation Craniofacial abnormality
Systemic diseases	Cystic fibrosis Ciliary dyskinesia (immotile cilia) Primary immune deficiency Acquired immune deficiency

6. How common is sinusitis in children?

The true incidence of sinusitis in childhood is unknown, but 0.5–5% of upper respiratory tract infections are complicated by acute sinusitis.

7. Which sinuses are infected most often?

The ethmoid and maxillary sinuses are the most frequently infected, probably because the narrow-caliber draining ostia are prone to obstruction after moderate inflammation from viral respiratory infection and allergy. Isolated frontal or sphenoid sinusitis is rare in children. Their infection is usually part of pansinusitis.

8. Name the most common bacterial pathogens responsible for acute sinusitis in children.

The principal bacterial pathogens are *Streptococcus pneumoniae*, *Haemophilus influenzae* (nontypable), and *Moraxella catarrhalis*. *S. pneumoniae* is recovered from approximately 30% of children with acute bacterial sinusitis. *H. influenzae* and *M. catarrhalis* are recovered from about 40% (20% each). In the remaining 30% of children, aspirates of the maxillary sinus are sterile. *Staphylococcus aureus* and respiratory anaerobes are not usually recovered from children with acute bacterial sinusitis.

9. Name the most common bacterial pathogens responsible for chronic sinusitis in children.

S. aureus and anaerobic organisms are recovered more frequently in chronic sinusitis. Common anaerobes include *Bacteroides* species and peptostreptococci. Other isolated organisms include viridans group streptococci, *H. influenzae*, *M. catarrhalis*, and *S. pneumoniae*. Sixty-percent of *S. pneumoniae* isolates from children with chronic sinusitis are penicillin-nonsusceptible.

10. What are the signs and symptoms of sinusitis?

Acute bacterial sinusitis has two common clinical presentations:

1. Persistent respiratory symptoms (> 10 days), including either nasal discharge of any quality (thick or thin; clear, mucoid, or purulent) and a daytime cough, which is occasionally worse at night. Malodorous breath is often present. Young children may have painless morning eye swelling but rarely complain of facial pain and headache.

2. Severe symptoms, including high fever (temperature > 39.0°C) and purulent nasal discharge for at least 3 days.

Patients with **subacute or chronic sinusitis** present with a history of protracted respiratory symptoms (lasting 30–90 or > 90 days without improvement). Nasal congestion, rhinorrhea, and cough (day and night) are common. Headache and fever are uncommon. Malodorous breath is occasionally present. It is important to distinguish between protracted and recurrent symptoms (there will be a test on this point).

Older children may complain of hyposmia (a diminished sense of smell), facial pain or pressure (often exacerbated by bending forward), fatigue, otalgia, and frequent throat clearing.

11. Describe how sinus transillumination is performed to diagnose sinusitis.

Sinus transillumination should be performed in a completely darkened room. Place a high-intensity light beam either in the mouth or against the cheek (for the maxillary sinuses) or under the medial aspect of the supraorbital ridge (for the frontal sinuses) and assess the transmission of light through the sinus cavity. If transillumination is normal, sinusitis is unlikely; if the transmission of light is absent, the maxillary or frontal sinus is likely to be filled with fluid. Good luck in trying to perform this procedure on toddler-age patients.

12. How reliable is sinus transillumination for the diagnosis of maxillary or frontal sinusitis?

The sensitivity of transillumination for the diagnosis of sinusitis in children ranges from approximately 50% to 75%. Transillumination is most useful when there is asymmetry between the sinuses and when a sinus is either completely opaque or completely normal. It is less useful when the finding is dull transillumination. In the absence of a suggestive history, the isolated finding of abnormal sinus transillumination is not sufficient to diagnose sinusitis.

13. What is the stethoscope-tuning fork (ST) test (Ahmadizadeh test)? When is it considered positive?

The ST test, used to diagnose sinusitis, is based on the physical property of sound, which is heard louder when transmitted through solid materials. Place a vibrating tuning fork (256 or 512 Hz) in the middle of the patient's forehead and listen to the tone over each maxillary sinus with a stethoscope. The louder vibration occurs over the side filled with fluid or pus. The test is considered positive when asymmetric sound transmission is present. If you knew the answer to this question, please close the book and contact the editors about a job.

14. What is the best way to diagnose sinusitis?

Bacteria are recovered from an aspirate of the maxillary sinus in approximately 60% of children with symptoms of sinusitis (persistent or severe, see above) and 75% of children with symptoms of sinusitis plus an abnormal sinus radiograph. Therefore, the diagnosis of sinusitis should be based on clinical criteria. Imaging studies should be reserved for evaluation of complicated, recurrent, or chronic sinus infection.

15. List the imaging modalities used to evaluate the paranasal sinuses.
• Plain skull radiograph (anteroposterior, lateral, and occipitomental views)
• Computed tomography (CT)
• Magnetic resonance imaging (MRI)

16. What findings on skull radiographs suggest sinusitis? When should skull radiographs be used in the management of sinusitis?

Radiographic findings suggestive of sinusitis include diffuse opacification, mucosal thickening of at least 4 mm, or an air-fluid level. Plain sinus radiographs are abnormal in approximately 30% of children without clinical or CT evidence of sinus disease. The ethmoid sinuses are poorly visualized by radiography. Coronal sinus CT has replaced radiography for evaluating sinus disease.

17. When are CT scans indicated in the management of children with sinusitis?

CT scans are indicated in children who (1) present with complications of acute bacterial sinus infection; (2) have highly persistent or recurrent infections that are not responsive to medical management; or (3) may require surgical management of sinus disease. Any patient who has proptosis, impaired vision, limited extraocular movements, severe facial pain, notable swelling of the forehead or face, deep-seated headaches, or toxic appearance should receive a CT scan.

18. What are the limitations of CT scans in the management of sinusitis?

CT scan cannot distinguish between mucosal abnormalities due to viral infection and those due to acute bacterial sinusitis. CT reveals soft tissue changes in most children with a recent (within 2 weeks) upper respiratory tract infection even in the absence of clinical sinus disease.

19. When is MRI indicated in the management of children with sinusitis?

MRI is helpful in diagnosing orbital and intracranial complications of sinusitis. Because of cost, limited availability, and long scan times that require frequent use of sedation, MRI should not be used in the management of uncomplicated acute sinusitis.

20. List the indications for sinus aspiration.

Sinus aspiration is not routinely recommended. Indications for sinus aspiration include: (1) failure to respond to multiple courses of antibiotics, (2) severe facial pain, (3) orbital or intracranial complications, and (4) evaluation of an immunocompromised host. Aspirated material should be sent for aerobic and anaerobic culture, Gram stain, and fungal stain and cultures.

21. What percent of children with acute bacterial sinusitis recover spontaneously?

Overall, approximately 50% of children with acute bacterial sinusitis recover spontaneously. Extrapolating from data derived from patients with acute otitis media, 15% of children with acute bacterial sinusitis caused by *S. pneumoniae* recover spontaneously; 50% of children with acute bacterial sinusitis caused by *H. influenzae* and 50–75% of children infected with *M. catarrhalis* also recover spontaneously.

22. What is the appropriate first-line therapy for acute bacterial sinusitis? Why?

Amoxicillin (45 mg/kg/day) is considered first-line therapy because of its effectiveness, safety, tolerability, low cost, and narrow spectrum.

23. If the patient is allergic to amoxicillin, what are the appropriate antibiotics to use?

The amoxicillin-allergic patient should receive either cefdinir, cefuroxime, or cefpodoxime if the allergic reaction was not a type 1 hypersensitivity reaction. In cases of serious allergic reactions, clarithromycin or azithromycin can be used in an effort to select an antimicrobial of an entirely different class. The Food and Drug Administration had not yet approved azithromycin for treatment of sinusitis, but clindamycin is a reasonable alternative for the penicillin- or amoxicillin-allergic patient infected with penicillin-resistant *S. pneumoniae*.

24. What is the appropriate duration of treatment for sinusitis?

The duration of therapy is unknown. Typically, a course of 10–14 days is prescribed. Patients with longstanding symptoms may require longer courses.

25. What percent of children with acute bacterial sinusitis respond to treatment with amoxicillin?

Taking into account the rate of spontaneous resolution, approximately 80% of children with acute bacterial sinusitis respond to treatment with standard doses of amoxicillin (45 mg/kg/day).

Likelihood that a Child with Acute Bacterial Sinusitis Will Fail Treatment with Amoxicillin

BACTERIA	PREVALENCE (%)	SPONTANEOUS CURE (%)	PREVALENCE OF RESISTANCE (%)	FAILURE TO AMOXICILLIN* (%)
S. pneumoniae	30	15	25	3
H. influenzae	20	50	50	5
M. catarrhalis	20	50–75	100	5–10

* Consider that 50% of resistant strains are highly resistant to penicillin, and only highly resistant isolates will fail to respond to standard doses of amoxicillin (45 mg/kg/day); minimum inhibitory concentration (MIC) of susceptible *S. pneumoniae* < 0.1 µg/ml; MIC of moderately resistant *S. pneumoniae* = 0.1–1.0 µg/ml; MIC of highly resistant *S. pneumoniae* > 2.0 µg/ml.
From Clinical Practice Guideline: Management of sinusitis. Pediatrics 108:798–808, 2001, with permission.

26. List the main risk factors for sinus infection by bacterial species that are resistant to amoxicillin.
- Attendance in day care
- Recent receipt (< 90 days) of antibiotics
- Age less than 2 years

27. When should antibiotics other than amoxicillin be considered in the treatment of acute bacterial sinusitis? What other antibiotics should be used?

Other antibiotics should be considered if patients (1) do not improve while receiving the usual dose of amoxicillin (45 mg/kg/day), (2) have recently been treated with an antimicrobial, (3) have moderate or severe illness, (4) present with protracted symptoms (> 30 days), or (5) attend day care. In these situations, initiate therapy with high-dose amoxicillin-clavulanate (80–90 mg/kg/day of amoxicillin, with 6.4 mg/kg/day of clavulanate in 2 divided doses). This dose of amoxicillin will yield sinus fluid levels that exceed the minimum inhibitory concentration of all *S. pneumoniae* that are intermediate in resistance to penicillin and most, but not all, highly resistant *S. pneumoniae*. The dose of potassium clavulanate is sufficient to inhibit all beta-lactamase producing *H. influenzae* and *M. catarrhalis*.

Alternate therapies include cefdinir, cefuroxime, or cefpodoxime. Antibiotic selection should be guided by susceptibility results, when available.

28. How quickly does a patient treated for sinusitis improve?

Most patients with acute bacterial sinusitis who are treated with an appropriate antimicrobial agent respond within 48–72 hours with a diminution of respiratory symptoms (reduction of nasal discharge and cough) and an improvement in general well-being. If a patient fails to improve, either the antimicrobial is ineffective, or the diagnosis of sinusitis is not correct.

29. Name the adjuvant therapies commonly used to supplement the effect of antimicrobials in the treatment of acute bacterial sinusitis.

Adjuvant therapies include saline nasal irrigation (hypertonic or normal saline), antihistamines, decongestants (topical or systemic), topical intranasal steroids, and mucolytic agents.

30. Are these adjuvant therapies beneficial in the treatment of acute bacterial sinusitis?

Adjuvant therapies used to supplement the effect of antimicrobials have not been studied extensively.
- Saline nose drops and sprays may help by liquefying secretions and facilitating nasal drainage without affecting mucociliary activity. Saline also may act as a mild vasoconstrictor of nasal blood flow. Saline irrigation is inexpensive, readily available, and devoid of serious side effects.
- Topical decongestants shrink nasal mucous membranes, improve ostial drainage, and provide symptomatic improvement. However, they cause ciliary stasis, delaying clearance of infected material. By decreasing local blood flow to the mucosa, topical decongestants also may impair diffusion of antimicrobial drugs into the sinuses.
- H_1 antihistamines do not hasten clinical or radiographic resolution.
- Intranasal budesonide may decrease nasal discharge during the second week of therapy. Because most patients with acute bacterial sinusitis improve within the first 48–72 hours, intranasal steroids are not routinely recommended for the management of acute bacterial sinusitis. They may be helpful if the child has underlying allergic rhinitis.
- Mucolytics have not been studied in previously healthy children.

31. What is Pott's puffy tumor?

Pott's puffy tumor is an anterior extension of a frontal sinus infection that results in frontal bone osteomyelitis and subperiosteal abscess. Do you know the difference between Pott's disease and Pott's puffy tumor?

32. What are other major complications of bacterial sinusitis?

- Meningitis
- Brain abscess
- Epidural/subdural empyema
- Orbital cellulitis
- Cavernous/sagittal sinus thrombosis
- Cranial osteomyelitis

33. Name the most common pathogens responsible for sinusitis in immunocompromised children.

Immunocompromised children, including those with neutropenia, are at risk for sinus infection with *S. pneumoniae*, *H. influenzae*, and *M. catarrhalis* as well as *Pseudomonas aeruginosa* and anaerobes. Fungal sinusitis also has been increasingly recognized as a cause of morbidity and mortality in immunocompromised children. *Aspergillus* species are most commonly isolated. Other causes of fungal sinusitis include *Fusarium* species, *Pseudallescheria boydii*, *Bipolaris* species, *Rhizopus arrhizus*, and *Mucor* species. Do not be alarmed; most of you will not see anything like this in your career.

34. Describe the most appropriate initial management of the immunocompromised child with sinusitis.

Appropriate management includes initiation of empiric broad-spectrum antibiotic therapy using agents with activity against gram-positive, gram-negative, and anaerobic bacteria. If the child fails to improve within 72 hours, endoscopic sampling, aspiration of sinus contents, or biopsy of the sinus mucosa is indicated.

35. Describe the classification of fungal sinusitis.

Acute fulminant invasive sinusitis. Sinus infection with rapid progression from sinus air space into adjacent structures. Patients are immunosuppressed. Treatment is discussed below.

Chronic indolent invasive sinusitis. Slow progression but ultimately causes bony destruction if untreated. Patients are usually immunologically normal. Treatment is discussed below.

Fungal ball sinusitis (sinus aspergilloma). Benign mass of hyphae (usually *Aspergillus* sp.) obstructing the sinus. Maxillary and ethmoid sinuses are most commonly affected. Mucosal invasion is rare. Surgical drainage is curative. Antifungal treatment is not necessary in the absence of mucosal or bony erosion.

Allergic fungal sinusitis. Patients have hypersensitivity to fungus (usually *Aspergillus* sp.) colonizing the sinuses. Sinuses are filled with eosinophil-rich mucin that often contains Charcot-Leyden crystals. Management consists of aeration of the affected sinus. Antifungal agents are not necessary. Patients usually have a history of allergic rhinitis and nasal polyps.

36. List the risk factors for invasive Aspergillus sinusitis.

Invasive *Aspergillus* sinusitis is characterized by vascular invasion, vessel thrombosis, and tissue necrosis. Risk factors include prolonged neutropenia, defects in phagocytosis (e.g., chronic granulomatous disease), hematologic malignancies, use of chemotherapy to treat malignancies, and use of immunosuppressive medications for organ transplant patients. Risk factors in HIV-infected children include CD4$^+$ T lymphocyte counts < 50 cells/mm^3.

37. Describe the clinical presentation of fungal sinusitis in the immunocompromised child.

Clinically, the child may be asymptomatic or present with facial pain, swelling, headache, and erythema. Infections with fungal organisms can begin with crusting and eschar formation of the anterior nares, turbinates, or hard palate. This finding can be accompanied by destructive and erosive extension into the orbit, cavernous sinus, and brain (rhinocerebral syndrome).

38. What is the appropriate diagnostic evaluation in a child with suspected fungal sinusitis?

A careful radiographic evaluation, including CT or MRI of the brain, orbits, and sinuses, is needed to assess the anatomic extent of suspected fungal sinusitis and to guide diagnostic biopsies.

39. What is the appropriate initial therapy for suspected fungal sinusitis?

Invasive fungal sinusitis can be devastating and requires aggressive antifungal therapy with high doses of conventional amphotericin B (1.0–1.5 mg/kg/day) or one of the lipid formulations of amphotericin B (starting dosage 3.0–5.0 mg/kg/day). New antifungals agents include voriconazole (a new azole like fluconazole) and caspofungin (an echinocandin class drug). Extensive surgical debridement may be required for progressively invasive disease that proves refractory to medical management. Restoration of host defenses, always a prerequisite for successful outcome, includes reversal of neutropenia and discontinuation of corticosteroids, if feasible. Take home message: white blood cells are your friend.

BIBLIOGRAPHY

1. American Academy of Pediatrics: Clinical practice guideline: Management of sinusitis. Pediatrics 108:798–808, 2001.
2. Lee BCP: Radiology of the paranasal sinuses. In Wetmore RF, Muntz HR, McGill TJ (eds): Pediatric Otolaryngology. New York, Thieme Medical Publishers, 2000, pp 423–437.
3. Williams JW Jr, Simel DL: Does this patient have sinusitis? Diagnosing acute sinusitis by history and physical examination. JAMA 270:1242–1246, 1993.

7. OTITIS

Samir S. Shah, M.D.

1. How is otitis media classified?

The term *otitis media* refers to inflammation of the mucoperiosteal lining of the middle ear. It may be classified as acute otitis media, otitis media with effusion, chronic otitis media with effusion, or chronic suppurative otitis media.

2. Define acute otitis media.

Acute otitis media is defined by the presence of fluid in the middle ear in conjunction with signs or symptoms of acute local or systemic illness. Accompanying signs and symptoms may be specific for acute otitis media, such as otalgia or otorrhea, or nonspecific, such as fever.

3. When is a child considered to have recurrent acute otitis media?

A child who has more than three episodes in 6 months or more than 4 episodes in 1 year is said to experience recurrent acute otitis media.

4. What is the difference between otitis media with effusion and chronic otitis media with effusion?

Otitis media with effusion is defined by the presence of fluid in the middle ear in the absence of signs or symptoms of acute infection. Chronic otitis media with effusion refers to persistence of middle ear effusion for more than 3 months. If still interested in otitis media, proceed to question 5 at your own risk.

5. How common is otitis media?

Very common. Acute otitis media accounts for 15–20% of all ambulatory care visits among preschool children. By three years of age, 80% of all children in the U.S. have had at least one episode of otitis media, and 50% have had at least three episodes. Recurrent acute otitis media occurs in 20–30% of the pediatric population.

6. Describe a normal tympanic membrane.

Position: slightly convex.

Appearance and color: translucent and pearly gray.

Integrity of the membrane: all four quadrants of the tympanic membrane are intact.

Mobility: rapid excursion of the membrane with positive and negative pressures applied by pneumatic otoscopy.

The presence of cerumen requires imagination to visualize the tympanic membrane.

7. Describe the otoscopic findings in a child with acute otitis media.

- Bulging tympanic membrane
- Thickened appearance
- Red or yellow color
- Aberrant light reflex
- Perforation with drainage
- Decreased mobility by pneumatic otoscopy

8. Name the most common bacterial pathogens responsible for acute otitis media.

S. pneumoniae causes 40–50% of cases of acute otitis media, *H. influenzae* causes 20–30%, and *M. catarrhalis* causes 10–15%.

9. What is role of Mycoplasma pneumoniae in the etiology of acute otitis media?

A role for *M. pneumoniae* as a cause of acute otitis media was suggested by the observation of bullous myringitis in nonimmune adults inoculated with this organism. In a subsequent study by Klein and Teele, the organism was isolated from the middle ear fluid in only 1 of 771 patients with otitis media. In a study by Palmu et al. of 82 children with bullous myringitis, the most common pathogens were S. pneumoniae, *H. influenzae*, and *M. catarrhalis*. *M. pneumoniae* was not isolated. These data suggest that *M. pneumoniae* is an infrequent cause of acute otitis media and bullous myringitis. However, some patients with lower respiratory tract infection due to *M. pneumoniae* may have associated otitis media.

10. Are antimicrobials beneficial in the treatment of acute otitis media?

Approximately 80% of untreated children have clinical resolution by 7–14 days, compared with 95% of those treated with antimicrobials. Although acute otitis media is often a mild, self-limiting infection, most clinicians recommend use of antibiotics to avoid suppurative complications, prevent progression to chronic otitis media, and reduce the risk of rare but serious sequelae, including meningitis, mastoiditis, and bacteremia.

11. What is the best initial antimicrobial agent for treating acute otitis media?

Amoxicillin (45 mg/kg/day) is considered first-line therapy. Children younger than 2 years and children who have received antimicrobial therapy in the preceding 3 months or attend day care should receive high-dose amoxicillin (80–90 mg/kg/day).

12. What is the appropriate duration of antimicrobial therapy for uncomplicated acute otitis media?

Children older than 2 years with uncomplicated acute otitis media can be treated for 5 days. Children younger than 2 years and children with underlying medical conditions, chronic or recurrent otitis media, or tympanic membrane perforation are at higher risk for treatment failure and should receive a 10-day course of antibiotics.

13. What does the abbreviation MIC represent? How do the MICs for S. *pneumoniae* affect the approach to otitis media?

The MIC, or minimum inhibitory concentration, is the lowest concentration of the antimicrobial agent that prevents visible bacterial growth after an 18- to 24-hour incubation period. Effective bacterial killing occurs when free antibiotic concentration at the infection site exceeds the MIC for the organism for 40–50% of the dosing interval. Maximum killing occurs when the antibiotic concentration exceeds the MIC for 60–70% of the dosing interval.

Antibiotic activity against S. *pneumoniae* is affected by alterations in the penicillin-binding proteins. As these alterations occur, the MIC of the organism increases. Thus, as MICs increase for S. *pneumoniae*, concentrations of antibiotics in the middle ear fluid must also increase to allow adequate time above the MIC for effective bacterial killing. This is the basis for recommending increased antibiotic dosages (80–90 mg/kg/day of amoxicillin) to treat acute otitis media in children likely to be infected with penicillin-resistant S. *pneumoniae*. The MIC is the key to the cure for otitis media.

14. Compare middle ear fluid and blood levels for the antibiotics commonly used to treat acute otitis media.

Antibiotics in middle ear fluid reach 20–50% of their blood levels. Peak plasma concentrations of amoxicillin occur 1–1.5 hours after ingestion, and peak middle ear fluid concentrations occur approximately 3 hours after ingestion.

15. When should antibiotics other than amoxicillin be considered in the treatment of acute otitis media? What other antibiotics should be used?

Other antibiotics should be considered in cases of treatment failure. Other antibiotics also are indicated if the patient is allergic to amoxicillin or is not able to tolerate oral medications.

In cases of documented treatment failure, unless the etiologic agent is identified by tympanocentesis or a culture of middle ear fluid drainage, use an antibiotic with activity against beta-lactamase–producing pathogens and penicillin-resistant S. *pneumoniae*. Appropriate antibiotics include amoxicillin-clavulanate (using 80–90 mg/kg/day of the amoxicillin component), cefuroxime axetil, cefdinir, clindamycin, and ceftriaxone. Azithromycin has been shown to be effective for the treatment of otitis media and has the advantage of a single dose.

16. How many doses of ceftriaxone are needed to treat acute otitis media?

Ceftriaxone is effective but painful and expensive and may alter microflora, leading to resistance. A single dose of ceftriaxone (50 mg/kg/day) leads to almost 100% success when the infection is caused by *H. influenzae* or penicillin-susceptible *S. pneumoniae*. When penicillin-nonsusceptible *S. pneumoniae* (penicillin MIC > 1.0 µg/ml) are isolated, bacteriologic cure is accomplished in 52% of cases after 1 dose of ceftriaxone and in 97% of cases after 3 doses of ceftriaxone. Rather than recommending a fixed schedule of either a single dose or three daily doses of ceftriaxone, most specialists administer a single injection and then determine the need for subsequent injections on the basis of clinical response at follow-up during the next 2 days.

17. When can a child with acute otitis media be considered a treatment failure?

Treatment failure can be defined by a lack of clinical improvement in signs and symptoms such as ear pain, fever, and tympanic membrane findings of bulging or otorrhea after 3 days of therapy. Children with signs or symptoms that are not specific to acute otitis media, such as persistent middle ear effusion, coryza, cough, or other symptoms of viral respiratory tract infection, should not be considered treatment failures.

18. What percentage of children with acute otitis media have a middle ear effusion at the completion of antimicrobial treatment? How quickly does the effusion resolve?

Approximately 50–60% of children with acute otitis media have a middle ear effusion after 10 days of therapy. Without further treatment, 30–40% have an effusion at 1 month, 20% at 2 months, and < 10% at 3 months.

19. Are antibiotics indicated when a child has persistent middle ear effusion after therapy for acute otitis media?

The natural history of appropriately treated acute otitis media includes persistence of middle ear effusion for weeks to months. Additional antibiotic therapy increases the risk for both colonization and invasive disease with penicillin-resistant *S. pneumoniae* and does not hasten resolution of the effusion. Thus, when middle ear fluid is detected in asymptomatic children at follow-up visits for acute otitis media, administering additional courses of antimicrobials is generally unnecessary.

20. What is tympanometry?

Tympanometry measures the compliance of the tympanic membrane and can be used to confirm the presence of a middle ear effusion when pneumatic otoscopy cannot be performed adequately. Abnormal tympanograms obtained in the presence of fluid in the middle ear are characterized by reduced height of the curve (reduced compliance of the tympanic membrane) or a flat curve without a definite peak (see figure at top of following page).

21. When should tympanocentesis be considered?

Tympanocentesis (needle aspiration of middle ear fluid) is the only reliable means to confirm the etiology of otitis media. This procedure is used to relieve severe pain; to confirm pathogens in neonates, immunocompromised children, or children who fail antibiotic therapy; and to treat complications such as mastoiditis.

22. What is the recurrence rate of acute otitis media after antimicrobial treatment?

Approximately 50% of children develop one or more new episodes of otitis media during the next 3 months. The rate varies depending on the age of the child.

Recurrence of Otitis Media after Antimicrobial Treatment

AGE	RECURRENCE WITHIN 3 MONTHS(%)
< 2 years	55
2–5 years	25
> 5 years	10

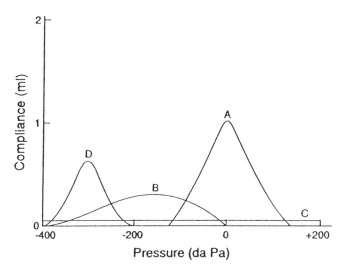

Tympanogram tracings. *A*, Normal; *B*, Middle ear effusion; *C*, Middle ear effusion or tympanic membrane perforation; *D*, Eustachian tube dysfunction.

23. List the risk factors for recurrent acute otitis media.
- Male gender
- Recurrent acute otitis media in parents or siblings
- Very low birth weight (< 1500 gm) or gestational age (< 33 weeks)
- Episode of otitis media at or before 6 months of age
- Prone sleeping position
- Pacifier use
- Absence of breast-feeding
- Group child care
- Exposure to cigarette smoke
- Congenital or acquired immune deficiency

24. Name the most common bacterial pathogens responsible for recurrent acute otitis media.
S. pneumoniae is the predominant bacterial pathogen associated with recurrent otitis media. Other pathogens to consider include *H. influenzae*, *M. catarrhalis*, *Streptococcus pyogenes*, *S. aureus*, and mixed infections with these species. Penicillin-resistant *S. pneumoniae* or beta-lactamase-producing strains of *H. influenzae* or *M. catarrhalis* are present in approximately 50% of cases.

25. When should antibiotic prophylaxis be considered for the prevention of acute otitis media?
Antibiotic prophylaxis reduces episodes of recurrent acute otitis media among children with ≥ 3 well-documented and separate episodes in the preceding 6 months or ≥ 4 episodes in the preceding 12 months.

26. Which antibiotics should be used for prophylaxis against recurrent acute otitis media?
Either sulfisoxazole or amoxicillin should be used; cephalosporins are not effective as prophylaxis. Sulfisoxazole has been used in the majority of controlled trials of prophylaxis, appears to be more efficacious at preventing recurrences than other agents, and may be less likely than amoxicillin to promote colonization with beta-lactamase–producing bacteria or penicillin-resistant *S. pneumoniae*.

27. How long should antibiotic prophylaxis for recurrent acute otitis media continue?

The duration of prophylactic therapy should be no more than 6 months, because longer courses are less effective and may be more likely to promote colonization with resistant bacteria.

28. Explain the rationale for tympanostomy tube placement.

Tympanostomy tube placement (1) equalizes middle ear pressure with atmospheric pressure, (2) provides prolonged ventilation, and (3) promotes drainage and clearance of the middle ear.

29. List the indications for tympanostomy tube placement.

• Chronic otitis media with effusion and associated conductive hearing loss > 15 dB
• Failed chemoprophylaxis for recurrent acute otitis media
• Tympanic membrane retraction with ossicular erosion or cholesteatoma formation

30. What other interventions may decrease the incidence of recurrent acute otitis media?

In addition to prophylactic antibiotic therapy and tympanostomy tube placement, interventions that may decrease the incidence of recurrent acute otitis media include eliminating smoking in the home, reducing day care attendance, eliminating pacifiers, and giving influenza vaccine.

31. How effective is the current heptavalent pneumococcal conjugate vaccine in preventing otitis media?

In addition to their immunogenicity and efficacy in preventing invasive disease, pneumococcal conjugate vaccines reduce both the nasopharyngeal carriage of pneumococci and the frequency of otitis media.

Efficacy of the Heptavalent Pneumococcal Conjugate Vaccine in Preventing Otitis Media

	PERCENT REDUCTION IN INCIDENCE COMPARED WITH CONTROLS	
OUTCOME	UNITED STATES*	FINLAND[†]
All otitis media	7.0	6.0
Frequent otitis media[‡]	22.8	N/A
Pneumococcal otitis media	N/A	34.0
Otitis media caused by pneumococcal serotypes contained in the vaccine	64.7	57.0
Tympanostomy tube placement	20.1	N/A

N/A = not available.
* Black S, Shinefield H, Fireman B, et al: Efficacy, safety and immunogenicity of heptavalent pneumococcal conjugate vaccine in children. Pediatr Infect Dis J 19:187-195, 2000.
[†] Eskola J, Kilpi T, Palmu A, et al: Efficacy of a pneumococcal conjugate vaccine against acute otitis media. N Engl J Med 344:403-409, 2001.
[‡] Frequent otitis media is defined as 5 episodes in 6 months or 6 episodes in 1 year.

32. Do other vaccines help prevent otitis media?

During a community outbreak of influenza, use of an influenza virus vaccine resulted in a 36% decline in otitis media in children attending a day-care center. A similar reduction in episodes of febrile otitis media also was reported in children after administration of live attenuated cold-adapted intranasal influenza vaccine.

33. How long does a perforated tympanic membrane take to heal?

The perforation is usually not apparent within 24–72 hours.

34. Define chronic suppurative otitis media.

Chronic suppurative otitis media refers to an infection of the middle ear that is defined by three elements: (1) perforation of the tympanic membrane, (2) purulent drainage from the middle ear (otorrhea), and (3) prolonged duration (> 4 weeks).

35. What bacteria are responsible for chronic suppurative otitis media?

Perforation makes the middle ear vulnerable to invasion from organisms in the external ear canal. *Pseudomonas aeruginosa* (approximately 50% of cases) and *S. aureus* (approximately 30% of cases) are most commonly isolated. *S. pneumoniae, H. influenzae,* anaerobic bacteria, and enteric gram-negative bacilli are occasionally responsible. *Mycobacterium tuberculosis* is a rare cause of chronic suppurative otitis media.

36. How should chronic suppurative otitis media be treated?

Initial management includes 7–14 days of ototopical antibiotics with or without oral antimicrobial agents. Currently available ototopical drugs include (1) colistin-neomycin thonzonium bromide with hydrocortisone; (2) neomycin and polymyxin B with hydrocortisone; (3) ciprofloxacin hydrochloride with hydrocortisone; and (4) ofloxacin otic solution 0.3%. Many clinicians include an oral antimicrobial agent effective for acute otitis media. Surgery and parenteral therapy with an antipseudomonal penicillin are occasionally required.

37. What are the complications of acute otitis media?

SITE	COMPLICATION
Middle ear	Cholesteatoma
	Conductive hearing loss
	Facial nerve paralysis
	Ossicular damage
	Tympanic membrane perforation
Inner ear	Labyrinthitis
	Sensorineural hearing loss
Bone	Mastoiditis
	Petrositis
Intracranial	Meningitis
	Brain abscess
	Epidural/subdural abscess
	Lateral sinus thrombosis
	Otic hydrocephalus

38. What is the significance of Griesinger's sign?

Griesinger's sign, edema over the posterior mastoid, signifies mastoid emissary vein thrombosis complicating otitis media or mastoiditis. If you study hard, someday you will have a disease or sign named after you.

39. Describe the pathogenesis of intratemporal and intracranial complications of acute otitis media.

Intratemporal and intracranial complications of otitis media occur by one of three mechanisms: (1) direct extension of infection through bone weakened by osteomyelitis or cholesteatoma; (2) retrograde spread of infection by thrombophlebitis; or (3) extension of infection along preformed pathways, such as the round or oval windows or through dehiscences that are the result of congenital malformations.

40. Describe the clinical presentation of the child with mastoiditis.

Children with mastoiditis develop fever and otalgia. Auricular displacement and retroauricular tenderness, swelling, and erythema are present. In addition, patients have otorrhea or a bulging, immobile, and opaque tympanic membrane.

41. How does the clinical presentation of mastoiditis differ in younger and older children?

Infant: auricle is displaced downward and outward.
Older child: auricle is displaced upward and outward.

42. Name the most common bacterial pathogens responsible for mastoiditis.

S. pneumoniae, *S. aureus*, and group A *Streptococcus* are the most frequently isolated pathogens. *H. influenzae*, a common cause of acute otitis media, is rarely found in mastoiditis.

43. Describe the management of the child with mastoiditis.

1. Empiric parenteral antibiotics
2. Myringotomy to provide drainage of the middle ear and mastoid and to obtain culture data.
3. If the infection progresses or if fever and otalgia persist over the next 24 to 48 hours, mastoidectomy is indicated to prevent spread of the infection to adjacent structures.
4. Continue parenteral antibiotics until the signs and symptoms of infection have subsided (usually 5–10 days). Antibiotic therapy should continue orally for at least 7 days after resolution of infection (typical total antibiotic course = 2–4 weeks). Longer antibiotic courses are required for complicating osteomyelitis.

44. What is Bezold's abscess?

Erosion of a mastoid infection through the medial aspect of the mastoid tip results in a neck abscess (Bezold's abscess) beneath the attachment of the sternocleidomastoid and digastric muscles. This route of spread occurs in older children and adults in whom the mastoid tip is pneumatized.

45. List the complications of mastoiditis.

- Bezold abscess
- Subperiosteal abscess
- Osteomyelitis
- Petrositis
- Deafness
- Labyrinthitis
- Facial nerve paralysis
- Meningitis
- Temporal lobe or cerebellar abscess
- Epidural or subdural empyema
- Venous sinus thrombosis

46. What is petrositis? How is it related to Gradenigo's syndrome?

Petrositis, a rare complication of otitis media and mastoiditis, develops when mastoid infection extends into the petrous portion of the temporal bone. Gradenigo's syndrome consists of the triad of severe retrobulbar (behind the eye) pain, persistent purulent otorrhea, and ipsilateral abducens (sixth cranial) nerve palsy seen with petrositis. Occasionally, patients have associated facial palsy, disequilibrium, and fever. If left untreated, the petrous infection may extend intracranially.

47. Name the pathogens commonly responsible for otitis externa.

Otitis externa (infection of the external auditory canal) is caused by normal skin flora, including *Staphylococcus epidermidis*, *S. aureus*, *S. pyogenes*, and, to a lesser extent, *Propionibacterium acnes*. *P. aeruginosa* is also a relatively common cause of otitis externa. Fungi cause < 10% of auditory canal infections.

48. What is swimmer's ear?

Swimmer's ear (acute diffuse otitis externa) occurs in hot, humid weather. The ear canal is pruritic, erythematous, edematous, and painful. *P. aeruginosa* is the most common cause.

49. List a differential diagnosis for otitis externa.

- Furunculosis
- Foreign body
- Suppurative/nonsuppurative otitis media
- Bullous myringitis
- Herpes zoster oticus (Ramsay Hunt syndrome)
- Mastoiditis
- Benign necrotizing otitis externa
- Malignant otitis externa
- Various malignancies (squamous cell carcinoma, basal cell carcinoma, metastatic lymphoma)

50. What factors predispose to otitis externa?

Traumatic removal of cerumen, increase in pH, trauma, or moisture predispose to otitis externa. Common predisposing factors include:

- Compromised host (e.g., diabetes mellitus, mucocutaneous candidiasis)
- Chronic suppurative otitis media
- Dermatologic disorders (e.g., eczema, seborrhea, psoriasis)
- Contiguous neoplasm (e.g., Langerhans cell histiocytosis)
- Swimming
- Trauma/excessive cleaning

51. What is the treatment for otitis externa?

1. Cleanse the ear with hypertonic saline (3%), 2% acetic acid, or mixtures of acetic acid and alcohol.

2. Apply ototopical drops of neomycin-polymyxin or a quinolone combined with topical hydrocortisone to diminish local inflammation and infection.

3. If treatment fails, culture the exudate and consider empiric topical antifungal therapy.

52. Describe the management of "malignant" otitis externa.

Invasive or malignant otitis externa is a severe, necrotizing infection that spreads from the squamous epithelium of the ear canal to adjacent areas of soft tissue, blood vessels, cartilage, and bone. This infection, commonly occurring in immunocompromised patients, should be managed aggressively with surgical debridement and 4–6 weeks of antibiotic therapy that includes coverage against *P. aeruginosa*.

BIBLIOGRAPHY

1. Dowell SF, Butler JC, Giebink GS, et al: Acute otitis media: Management and surveillance in an era of pneumococcal resistance—a report from the Drug-resistant *Streptococcus pneumoniae* Therapeutic Working Group. Pediatr Infect Dis J 18:1–9, 1999.
2. Dowell SF, Marcy SM, Phillips WR, et al: Otitis media: Principles of judicious use of antimicrobial agents. Pediatrics 101:165–171, 1998.
3. Giebink GS: The prevention of pneumococcal disease in children. N Engl J Med 345:1177–1183, 2001.
4. Pichichero ME: Recurrent and persistent otitis media. Pediatr Infect Dis J 19:11–16, 2000.
5. Wetmore RF: Complications of otitis media. Pediatr Ann 29:637–646, 2000.

8. CROUP SYNDROME AND EPIGLOTTITIS

John Donnelly, M.D., and Keith J. Mann, M.D.

1. What disease entities are included in the term *croup syndrome*?

The term *croup syndrome* defines a group of diseases or a syndrome identifiable by a constellation of symptoms, including a bark-like cough, hoarseness, stridor, and varying degrees of respiratory distress. **Viral laryngotracheitis** (classic croup) and **spasmodic croup** account for most cases of croup syndrome. **Laryngotracheobronchitis** and **laryngotracheobronchopneumonia** occur further down the respiratory tract and may be caused by viral or bacterial agents. **Bacterial tracheitis** refers to a bacterial infection of the trachea.

2. How do classic croup and spasmodic croup differ?

Viral laryngotracheitis (classic croup) affects children most commonly between the ages of 6 months and 3 years with a peak incidence at 2 years of age, when it affects 5 of 100 children. Patients typically have an upper respiratory prodrome (cough, rhinorrhea, pharyngitis) for 1–3 days, followed by a loud, barking cough and hoarseness. As the airway becomes more occluded, stridor becomes more evident. The stridor is usually inspiratory but may be biphasic. Patients may be febrile but rarely have a temperature that reaches 39–40°C. Symptoms are typically worse at night and when patients become agitated. Children often sit upright with the neck extended to relieve the obstruction. The illness usually lasts 3–7 days. In more severe cases, symptoms may persist for weeks.

Spasmodic croup presents with a loud, barking cough usually without an associated viral prodrome. The symptoms usually begin suddenly in the middle of the night; the child awakens with a hoarse voice, barking cough, and inspiratory stridor. Fever is not present. Moist, cold air may alleviate the symptoms, but recurrences are common. The cause of spasmodic croup is unclear, but subglottic edema with pale mucosa is often seen on endoscopy.

3. What else should be considered in the differential diagnosis of acute viral laryngotracheitis?

Bacterial tracheitis is caused most commonly by *Staphylococcus aureus*. It can occur in children 6 months to 8 years of age but is more common between the ages of 4 and 6 years. It frequently is a complication of viral laryngotracheitis, presenting with a rapid onset of high fever, worsening croup symptoms, and respiratory distress several days into a course of seemingly typical croup. Other causes include *Moraxella catarrhalis*, *Streptococcus pneumoniae* and group A streptococci.

Epiglottitis is usually caused by *Haemophilus influenzae* type B (HIB). The incidence of epiglottitis decreased with the advent of the HIB vaccine in the 1980s. Isolated cases caused by group-A streptococci, *S. aureus*, pneumococci, and *Klebsiella*, *Candida*, and *Pseudomonas* spp. have been reported. Epiglottitis remains an airway emergency despite the changing epidemiology. Patients present with symptoms of high fever and a worsening sore throat, leading to odynophagia and drooling. Stridor is not a prominent feature. Patients progress to dyspnea and respiratory distress as edema of the epiglottis and supraglottic area leads to airway occlusion. Patients often assume the tripod position to open the edematous airway. Epiglottitis most commonly affects children age 2–6 years.

Foreign body aspiration should be considered in a patient of the appropriate age group with new-onset stridor, cough, respiratory distress, or wheezing.

Retropharyngeal abscess can present with fever, stridor, drooling, sore throat, and a muffled voice. Affected children are usually under the age of 5 years; most cases occur in children under 2 years.

Angioedema can present with stridor and respiratory distress but is usually associated with facial edema as well.

Laryngomalacia, tracheomalacia, laryngeal papillomatosis, unilateral vocal cord paralysis, and vascular rings can present with stridor and are often initially misdiagnosed as croup.

4. What are the most common causes of classic croup?

Approximately 75% of viral causes of croup can be attributed to parainfluenza viruses. Respiratory syncytial virus, influenza, and adenoviruses cause the remainder of cases. *Mycoplasma pneumoniae* has been implicated as an atypical cause.

5. What is the croup score?

The croup score is used as an indicator of severity. The most commonly used scoring system is the Westley score:

	0	1	2	3	4	5
Stridor	None or only when agitated	Audible at rest only with a stethoscope	Audible at rest without a stethoscope			
Retractions	None	Mild	Moderate	Severe		
Air entry	Normal	Decreased	Severely decreased			
Cyanosis	None				With agitation	At rest
Level of consciousness	None					Altered or depressed

A score of 0–3 indicates mild disease; 4–6, moderate disease; and > 6, severe disease.

6. Which is the classic radiographic finding in viral laryngotracheitis: (1) thumbprint sign, (2) subglottic narrowing (steeple sign), (3) widening of the soft tissue shadow between the vertebral body and airway, or (4) a shaggy-appearing trachea?

The classic finding in viral laryngotracheitis is the steeple sign or narrowing of the subglottic airway (see Fig. 1 below). The thumbprint sign indicates posterior displacement and edema of the epiglottis (epiglottitis). Widening of the prevertebral soft tissue space occurs with a retropharyngeal abscess (see Fig. 2 on following page). A shaggy-appearing trachea may be seen in bacterial tracheitis.

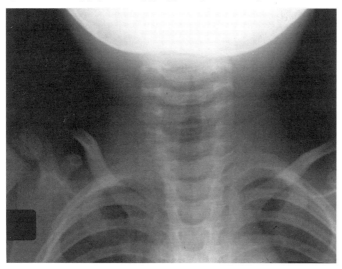

FIGURE 1.   Steeple sign.

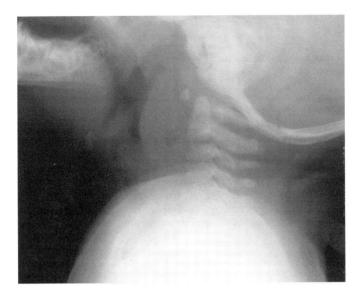

FIGURE 2.   Retropharyngeal abscess.

7. Define the rebound effect.

In the rebound effect, which occurs within 2 hours of treatment with racemic epinephrine, patients may return to their previous level of illness or appear clinically worse after initial improvement. Treatment with dexamethasone, followed by a 3- to 4-hour waiting period, is sufficient if clinical symptoms allow discharge.

8. What scientific evidence supports the use of steroids in viral laryngotracheitis?

Studies have shown that a single dose of dexamethasone, 0.6 mg/kg intramuscularly or orally, improves symptoms, decreases the rate of admission, and decreases the need for further treatment after discharge. Once admitted to the hospital, one intramuscular or oral dose of dexamethasone also decreases the length of stay and rate of intubation. Steroids appear to decrease submucosal edema by decreasing capillary permeability, but the exact mechanism by which they improve symptoms in croup is unclear.

9. Should you treat every patient suspected of having viral croup with dexamethasone?

No absolute criteria determine when to use steroids in the treatment of croup. Patients with mild disease (no stridor at rest, no retractions, normal air movement) can be managed without dexamethasone.

10. What evidence supports the use of nebulized steroids in viral laryngotracheitis?

Evidence indicates that the use of nebulized budesonide improves symptoms and decreases admission rates, length of hospital stay for patients already admitted, and relapse rates. The optimal dose is not yet established. No data support the use of inhaled or nebulized dexamethasone. There appears to be no significant difference between inhaled budesonide and systemic dexamethasone, although one retrospective controlled trial found slightly decreased admission rates with oral dexamethasone compared with nebulized budesonide.

11. What evidence supports the use of nebulized racemic epinephrine in the treatment of viral laryngotracheitis?

The alpha-agonistic activity of racemic epinephrine improves symptoms by vasoconstriction of vessels and a subsequent decrease in edema of the subglottic area. In addition, the beta$_2$ effect of racemic epinephrine may relax bronchial smooth muscles. Retrospective controlled trials have shown that nebulized racemic epinephrine significantly improves symptoms and croup score 30 minutes after treatment. About one-third of children may experience a rebound effect within 2 hours of treatment.

12. How many doses of racemic epinephrine can be given? Are there any significant side effects?

The maximal number of doses that can be given safely has not been determined. There are case reports of myocardial infarction after repeated doses of racemic epinephrine. The drug should be given with caution in patients with ventricular outflow obstruction.

13. What evidence suggests that humidified air improves viral laryngotracheitis?

None. Despite widespread use by parents, nurses, and physicians, no systematic reviews or prospective trials have evaluated the efficacy of humidified air in croup. You may do more harm than good in a child who becomes agitated after placement in the croup tent; symptoms may be exacerbated.

14. When is bronchoscopy indicated for children with croup syndrome?

Bronchoscopy should be considered when suspected viral laryngotracheitis does not follow a typical course. Recurrent stridor, prolonged symptoms, severe symptoms, age < 6 months or > 5 years, failed extubation, and traumatic intubation are possible indications for bronchoscopy. Laryngomalacia, laryngeal papillomatosis, vascular rings, hemangiomas, vocal cord paralysis, bacterial tracheitis, and epiglottis can be identified or ruled out via bronchoscopy.

15. When should you suspect bacterial tracheitis?

Bacterial tracheitis is a secondary bacterial infection that complicates viral laryngotracheitis. Patients present with a high fever, respiratory distress, stridor, and a toxic appearance several days after the initial symptoms of croup appear. If the infection is contiguous with the lower airway, it is called laryngotracheobronchopneumonia. The incidence peaks in the fall and winter; the peak age is 5 years.

16. How is bacterial tracheitis diagnosed?

Bacterial tracheitis, like viral laryngotracheitis, is largely a clinical diagnosis. Patients often have laboratory manifestations of a bacterial infection (i.e., leukocytosis and elevation of acute-phase reactants). As in laryngotracheitis, the anteroposterior neck film may show the steeple sign. A lateral neck film may be more useful, demonstrating a shaggy appearance to the airway. Bronchoscopy is the diagnostic gold standard. Typical findings include thick secretions and pseudomembrane formation in the trachea and subglottic edema. Secretions should be suctioned, and specimens should be sent for Gram stain, culture, and sensitivity.

17. Which antibiotics should be used to treat bacterial tracheitis?

S. aureus has always been the most commonly implicated organism, but a recent study suggests that *M. catarrhalis* may cause many cases. Isolated cases are also caused by *H. influenzae* and *Streptococcus* species. Antibiotic therapy, therefore, should have broad-spectrum coverage against both gram-positive and gram-negative organisms. A semisynthetic penicillin, such as nafcillin, combined with a third-generation cephalosporin, such as ceftriaxone, is appropriate initial therapy. Clindamycin can be substituted in patients allergic to penicillin. The antibiotic regimen ultimately should be determined by the culture and sensitivity of the organism.

18. What other treatments or supportive measures may be required for patients with bacterial tracheitis?

Most patients with bacterial tracheitis require tracheal intubation and mechanical ventilation. Studies have quoted intubation rates ranging from 57% to over 80%. Patients often remain intubated for several days. Extubation can be attempted when signs of clinical improvement, decreased secretions, and lack of fever are noted. Patients with both laryngotracheitis and bacterial tracheitis often have an air leak around the endotracheal tube as the submucosal edema resolves and the airway increases in diameter around a small endotracheal tube. This air leak is an indicator of clinical improvement and can help guide the decision to extubate.

19. What happened to all of the cases of epiglottitis?

The advent of the HIB vaccination in the 1980s has markedly decreased the incidence of epiglottitis. The annual incidence is now approximately 60 per million children. In addition to *H. influenzae*, isolated cases caused by group-A streptococci, *S. aureus*, pneumococci, and *Klebsiella*, *Candida*, and *Pseudomonas* spp. have been reported.

20. List the classic symptoms of epiglottitis.

- Lack of a viral prodrome
- Sore throat
- Fever
- Odynophagia
- Drooling
- Fearful patient
- Tripod position to open the airway

Respiratory distress, cyanosis, and shock can ensue. The typical age is 2 years to 7 years, with a peak incidence at 3.5 years. Typically there are no ill contacts in the family.

21. If you suspect epiglottitis, should you use a tongue depressor to perform an oropharyngeal examination?

No—put it away! The risk of precipitating respiratory failure with manipulation of the oropharynx and reflex laryngospasm (or provocation of anxiety in the child) mandates that the oropharynx and epiglottis be visualized under general anesthesia in the operating room.

22. If you strongly suspect epiglottitis, should you order a lateral neck film?

No. When you strongly suspect epiglottitis, any delay in treatment could worsen the clinical outcome. Transport of any child with suspected epiglottitis, other than to the operating room, should be avoided. As stated above, any unnecessary manipulation of the child (including extension of the neck for a lateral film) can precipitate respiratory failure. Lastly, in approximately 30–50% of cases, the lateral neck radiograph appears normal. It may be helpful when you are unsure of the diagnosis.

23. Are arterial blood gas measurements indicated in the evaluation of epiglottitis?

No. Again, any unnecessary manipulation of a child with suspected epiglottitis should be avoided.

24. How is epiglottitis diagnosed?

Lateral neck radiographs may show a thumbprint sign, indicating posterior displacement and edema of the epiglottis. The best way to confirm diagnosis, however, is by direct visualization of a large, swollen, erythematous epiglottis via laryngoscopy.

25. How is epiglottitis treated?

Intubation is required to stabilize the airway and should be done at the time of direct visualization of the epiglottitis and confirmation of the diagnosis. Parenteral antibiotic treatment against beta-lactamase–producing gram-negative rods should be instituted; appropriate drugs include ceftriaxone, cefotaxime, or ampicillin/sulbactam.

26. Why are children more likely than adults to require tracheal intubation for epiglottitis?

The anatomy of the pediatric airway renders children more susceptible than adults to respiratory failure from airway compromise. The pediatric airway obviously is smaller than the adult airway. In addition, the pediatric airway is narrowest at the subglottis, which is surrounded by rigid cricoid cartilage. The adult airway is narrowest at the flexible glottis. The cross-sectional area of a cylinder is proportional to the radius squared; in other words, the smaller pediatric airway has a greater proportional reduction compared with the larger adult airway with the same increment of change. Lastly, many pediatric patients have congenital anomalies (laryngomalacia, tracheomalacia, subglottic stenosis) that already compromise the airway. All of these factors lead to a higher intubation rate in pediatric patients with epiglottitis.

27. When can you safely extubate a patient with resolving epiglottitis?

Tracheal extubation may be safely accomplished when the child is afebrile, alert, and clinically improved—usually after 24–72 hours of therapy. Flexible laryngoscopy can be performed through the endotracheal tube to document decreased epiglottic swelling and erythema. Patients with epiglottitis are often bacteremic. Systemic manifestations of sepsis may lengthen the course of illness and prolong endotracheal intubation.

28. Do close contacts of patients with epiglottitis need prophylaxis?

Oral rifampin prophylaxis is given to all household contacts of patients infected with HIB.

BIBLIOGRAPHY

1. Bernstein T, Brilli R, Jacobs B: Is bacterial tracheitis changing? A 14-month experience in a pediatric intensive care unit. Clin Infect Dis 27:458–462; 1998.
2. Butte MJ, Nguyen BX, Hutchinson JJ, et al: Pediatric myocardial infarction after racemic epinephrine administration. Pediatrics 104:9, 1999.
3. Cressman WR, Myer CM III: Diagnosis and Management of Croup and Epiglottitis. Pediatr Clin North Am 41:265–275, 1994.
4. Gradon JD: Space-occupying and life-threatening infections of the head, neck, and thorax. Infect Dis Clin North Am 10:857–878, 1996.
5. Kaditis AG, Wald ER: Viral croup: Current diagnosis and treatment. Pediatr Infect Dis J 17:827–834; 1998.
6. Klassen TP: Croup: A current perspective. Pediatr Clin North Am 46:1167–1177, 1999.
7. Leung AKC, Cho H: Diagnosis of stridor in children. Am Fam Physician 60:2289–2296, 1999.
8. Malhotra A, Krilov LR: Viral croup. Pediatr Rev 22:5–12, 2001.
9. Middleton DB: Community acquired respiratory infections in children. Prim Care Clin Off Pediatr 23:719–739, 1996.
10. Osmond M: Croup. Br J Med Clin Evid 6:268–276. 2001.
11. Stroud RH, Friedman NR: An update on inflammatory disorders of the pediatric airway: Epiglottitis, croup, and tracheitis. Am J Otolaryngol 22:268–785, 2001.

9. PHARYNGITIS AND STOMATITIS

John Donnelly, M.D., and Keith J. Mann, M.D.

1. What is the most common virus implicated in pharyngitis?

Rhinoviruses (100 types) are implicated in approximately 20% of all cases of pharyngitis. Adenovirus, Epstein-Barr virus (EBV), coronavirus, parainfluenza, influenza A and B, and herpes simplex virus (HSV) are less common (2–5% each). Enterovirus, respiratory syncytial virus (RSV), cytomegalovirus (CMV), human immunodeficiency virus (HIV), and rubella and measles viruses are rare causes of pharyngitis (< 1% each).

2. What percentage of all cases of pharyngitis are caused by group A beta-hemolytic streptococcus?

Streptococcus pyogenes accounts for 15–30% of all cases of pharyngitis. Other bacteria implicated include group C and G beta-hemolytic streptococci, *Mycoplasma pneumoniae*, *Chlamydia pneumoniae*, *Neisseria gonorrhoeae*, *Arcanobacterium haemolyticum* (reported to be an important cause of pharyngitis in Scandinavia and the United Kingdom, especially in adolescents), *Yersinia pestis*, *Yersinia enterocolitica*, *Francisella tularensis*, and *Corynebacterium diphtheriae*.

3. Describe the classic features of group A beta-hemolytic streptococcal (GABHS) pharyngitis.

Patients are usually between 5 and 15 years of age. The disorder occurs most commonly in the winter and early spring in temperate climates. Common symptoms include the abrupt onset of a sore throat with fever and pain on swallowing. Associated symptoms include headache, nausea, vomiting, and abdominal pain. Physical exam reveals tonsillar erythema with or without exudates, pharyngeal erythema, and tender anterior cervical lymphadenopathy. Other possible exam findings include pharyngeal petechiae, scarlatiniform rash, and an erythematous uvula.

4. List five suppurative complications of GABHS pharyngitis.
1. Cervical lymphadenitis
2. Retropharyngeal abscess
3. Peritonsillar abscess
4. Otitis media
5. Sinusitis

5. Name three nonsuppurative complications specific to GABHS pharyngitis.
1. Acute rheumatic fever
2. Poststreptococcal glomerulonephritis
3. Toxin-mediated disease

6. What is the antibiotic treatment of choice for streptococcal pharyngitis?

Ten days of penicillin V or amoxicillin. One intramuscular dose of benzathine penicillin G can be used for patients unable to take oral medication and patients in whom compliance is a problem. Erythromycin can be used in penicillin-allergic patients.

7. How many swabs should you use when culturing a patient's throat?

Always use two culture swabs: one for the rapid streptococcal test and one for the throat culture. Some rapid streptococcal detection tests have a reported sensitivity as low as 60%. Within one institution, the sensitivity of a single kit varied by up to 20%. A good screening test should have at least 95% sensitivity to detect the maximal number of patients who are infected. Because of low sensitivity, a negative test should be followed by a throat culture (the second swab). Most rapid diagnostic tests have a better specificity, approaching 95%. Thus, a positive test confirms the presence of streptococcal infection. Patients with a positive test should be treated as outlined above.

8. What is the proper procedure for obtaining a throat culture?
The specimen should be obtained by swabbing both tonsils or tonsillar fossae and the posterior pharyngeal wall. Be careful not to contaminate the swab on the oral mucosa before or after the specimen is obtained (on the way in and out of the mouth). *Try this procedure in a 2-year-old child.* The culture should be taken to the laboratory and plated on a sheep blood agar plate. A single swab, collected and plated correctly, has a 90–95% sensitivity in detecting the presence of GABHS.

9. How does the laboratory detect the difference between group A and other beta-hemolytic streptococci?
The bacitracin disc test is the most commonly used method of differentiation. In more than 95% of cases, GABHS shows a ring or zone of inhibition surrounding the disc. Non-group A streptococci show this zone of inhibition in only 5–15% of cases. Another more expensive and less commonly used mechanism is to show the group specific cell-wall carbohydrate antigen.

10. Should you screen asymptomatic family members or close contacts of a child with documented GABHS pharyngitis?
No. Between 5% and 20% of healthy people are carriers for group A streptococci. Carriers need no further antibiotic therapy because they demonstrate no immunologic reaction to the organism. They are also at low risk for developing suppurative complications of GABHS pharyngitis. Infectivity to others is inversely related to the duration of the carrier state. Thus routine screening is no longer advised.

11. Is there any benefit to obtaining a throat culture after completing therapy for GABHS pharyngitis?
No. There is no need to document clearance of the organism. Treatment failure is very uncommon. If a patient returns for a recurrent episode of pharyngitis, however, a throat culture is indicated. A GABHS-positive culture after successful treatment and recurrence of disease can mean any of the following: (1) the patient is a carrier and has an intercurrent viral illness; (2) the patient was noncompliant; or (3) the patient has a new case of GABHS pharyngitis.

12. What laboratory data other than a throat culture help to differentiate between causes of pharyngitis?
In patients with culture-negative pharyngitis, laboratory evidence of specific viral infections may be helpful. EBV mononucleosis often has a positive heterophile antibody or monospot test (unreliable before the age of 4 years). The complete blood count (CBC) often shows an atypical lymphocytosis. IgM and IgG antibodies against the viral capsid antigens are positive. A nasopharyngeal wash can be done to detect RSV, adenovirus, influenza, rhinovirus, or parainfluenza. Rapid antigen testing is also available for influenza A and RSV at many hospitals.

13. Which organism causes pharyngoconjunctival fever?
Adenovirus can cause typical pharyngitis or pharyngitis associated with conjuctivitis (usually adenovirus type 3). Patients with pharyngoconjunctival fever present with a sore throat, high fever, rhinorrhea, and nonpurulent unilateral or bilateral conjunctivitis. The fever and pharyngitis typically last 4–5 days, but the conjunctivitis may last longer. Headache, malaise, lethargy, and weakness are also common symptoms.

14. When should steroids be used to treat EBV mononucleosis?
Glucocorticoids generally are indicated only for patients who exhibit symptoms of life-threatening upper airway obstruction.

15. Match the following presentations of sore throat with the likely etiologic agent:

1. A 2-year-old boy presents with fever, sore sore throat, and decreased oral intake. You notice small ulcers on his soft palate, hands, and feet.

    a. Epstein-Barr virus

2. A 15-year-old adolescent presents with fever and sore throat. On exam you notice posterior cervical lymph nodes; large, erythematous, and exudative tonsils; and splenomegaly.

    b. Coxsackie virus

3. A 5-year-old child presents with fever, sore throat, headache, nausea, and vague abdominal pain but has no cough, rhinorrhea, or conjunctival involvement. On exam you note submandibular lymphadenopathy, enlarged and erythematous tonsils with exudates, and a fine, generalized, sandpaper-like rash.

    c. Human immunodeficiency virus

4. A 14-year-old adolescent presents with fatigue, fever, myalgias, and sore throat. On exam you note an erythematous pharynx without tonsillar enlargement or exudate, a diffuse maculopapular rash, and track marks on the extremities.

    d. Group A beta-hemolytic streptococci

Answers:

1, b (coxsackie virus causing hand-foot-mouth syndrome)
2, a (EBV causing acute mononucleosis)
3, d (GABHS causing scarlet fever)
4, c (HIV causing acute retroviral syndrome)

Although no one presenting symptom or clinical finding can absolutely identify various causes of pharyngitis, a good clinical history and focused exam can help narrow the options.

16. What is Lemierre's syndrome?

Lemierre's syndrome is septic thrombophlebitis of the jugular vein occurring as a complication of acute pharyngitis. Metastatic septic emboli, most commonly to the lungs, can develop without treatment. This complication should be considered in patients with unresolving pharyngitis complicated by headache, neck swelling, pulmonary symptoms, or sepsis. Most cases are caused by *Fusobacterium necrophorum*, a gram-negative anaerobic bacillus that is part of normal flora. Treatment is with antibiotic therapy. In some case reports, the syndrome has resolved without anticoagulation; other authorities recommend variable periods of anticoagulation.

17. How long after untreated GABHS pharyngitis do symptoms of rheumatic fever develop?

GABHS pharyngitis precedes acute rheumatic fever (ARF) by 2–5 weeks.

18. Can a child develop ARF after a streptococcal skin infection?

No—otherwise all of this information would be found in a different chapter. Patients can develop poststreptococcal glomerulonephritis, however, after either GABHS pharyngitis or skin infection.

19. What are the Jones Criteria for ARF?

MAJOR CRITERIA	MINOR CRITERIA
Arthritis, usually migratory with two or more large joints involved; occurs in approximately 70% of patients.	Arthralgia (in the absence of arthritis)

(Continued. on next page.)

MAJOR CRITERIA	MINOR CRITERIA
Cardiac involvement, which ranges from valvulitis to pancarditis with associated valvular involvement. The mitral valve is most commonly involved; occurs in approximately 50% of patients.	Fever
Subcutaneous nodules, which usually manifest as painful nodules over the extensor surfaces of large joints; occurs in approximately 5% of patients.	Prolongation of PR interval
Erythema marginatum, a light pink, evanescent rash with serpiginous borders; Occurs in approximately 10% of patients.	Elevation of acute-phase reactants (erythrocyte sedimentation rate, C-reactive protein)
Sydenham chorea, characterized by involuntary, purposeless, random, uncoordinated movements often associated with bizarre or abnormal behavior; occurs in approximately 10–15% of patients.	

To make the diagnosis of ARF, you must have supporting evidence of an antecedent group A streptococcal infection. Such evidence may include an elevated or rising ASO titer, a positive rapid streptococcal test, or culture-positive pharyngitis. Along with evidence of a recent group A streptococcal infection, two major criteria or one major and two minor criteria are needed to make the diagnosis. If you have evidence of a recent infection and chorea alone, recurrent rheumatic fever, or indolent carditis, ARF can be diagnosed without the Jones criteria.

20. Name five noninfectious causes of pharyngitis.
- Kawasaki's disease
- Behçet's syndrome
- Stevens-Johnson syndrome
- Tobacco smoke irritation
- Allergic postnasal drip

21. A 3-year-old boy presents with a 5-day history of spiking fevers, sore throat, and a mass in his left neck. He developed dry, cracked lips and bilateral, nonexudative conjunctivitis on the day before presentation. On exam his temperature is 39.3°C. He appears ill but is in no respiratory distress. He has bilateral bulbar conjunctival injection, cracked lips, and a red tongue. His pharynx is erythematous without exudates. He has a left-sided, tender, warm anterior cervical lymph node that measures 2 × 3 cm. The lungs are clear, the heart is regular but tachycardic, and the abdomen is benign. He has swollen palms and soles and a diffuse macular rash. What is the likely diagnosis?

The patient probably has Kawasaki's disease, which is diagnosed by the following criteria:
Fever of at least 5 days' duration and four of the following five criteria
1. Mucus membrane involvement (dry, cracked lips or strawberry tongue).
2. Bilateral, nonpurulent conjunctival injection
3. Unilateral cervical lymphadenopathy
4. Swelling and erythema of the hands and feet (periungal and palmar desquamation occur later)
5. Diffuse, generalized, polymorphous rash

The initial treatment, intended to reduce the incidence of coronary artery aneurysms by controlling the vasculitis, includes intravenous immunoglobulin (2 gm/kg) and high-dose aspirin (100 mg/kg divided into 4 doses/day).

22. What is Vincent's angina?

Vincent's angina is an acute exudative anaerobic infection of the pharynx or tonsils caused by a combination of anaerobic oral bacteria and spirochetes. It is more common in adults but may be seen in children with poor dentition. In the setting of physiologic stress, poor oral hygiene, and malnutrition, *Bacteroides* spp. and *Fusobacterium* spp. act synergistically to cause oral soft tissue breakdown. Symptoms often arise abruptly and include throat and neck pain, halitosis, and gingival or tonsillar bleeding. The disease may be complicated by secondary bacteremia and sepsis. Treatment consists of adequate dental or surgical debridement and combination therapy with penicillin and metronidazole.

Editor's note: Brush your teeth.

23. Match the suppurative complication of GABHS pharyngitis with the appropriate presentation.

1. A 13-year-old adolescent presents with high fever, dyspnea, dysphagia, and odynophagia. No drooling is seen. On exam you note symmetrically enlarged, erythematous tonsils and a midline uvula.	a. Retropharyngeal abscess
2. A 2-year-old boy presents with high fever, dysphagia, drooling, and neck stiffness. He appears toxic and is sitting in the tripod position. His tonsils are symmetrically enlarged and erythematous. His uvula is midline. You note unilateral posterior pharyngeal fullness on the left.	b. Peritonsilar abscess
3. A 12-year-old child presents with high fever, muffled voice, trismus, throat pain, and dysphagia. On exam you note an erythematous pharynx with unilateral tonsillar enlargement and a deviated uvula away from the affected side.	c. Lateral pharyngeal abscess

Answer: 1, c; 2, a; 3, b.

The treatment for all three is hospitalization, intravenous antibiotics, and surgical drainage.

24. What is diphtheria?

Diphtheria is a potentially life-threatening pharyngitis caused by *Corynebacterium diphtheriae* and associated with pseudomembrane formation. The membrane is gray, sharply demarcated, and adherent to the underlying mucosa. It is often localized only to the nose or larynx. Diphtheria associated with a toxin may lead to myocardial damage and nervous system dysfunction. The systemic manifestations are preventable by toxoid vaccination.

25. When does pharyngitis lead to tonsillectomy?

- Tonsillar hemorrhage during acute tonsillitis is an indication for a tonsillectomy.
- Recurrent throat infections are generally accepted as an indication for tonsillectomy, adenoidectomy, or both. There is no absolute consensus, however, about how many infections constitute too many infections. The American Academy of Pediatrics (AAP) recommends surgery as a reasonable option for children with "many severe sore throats."
- Chronic tonsillitis, persisting for at least 3 months, is a relative indication for surgery.
- Peritonsillar abscess is a relative indication for tonsillectomy. Some surgeons prefer to perform the tonsillectomy while draining the abscess, whereas others wait for the infection to subside. Recurrent peritonsillar abscess is a more definitive indication for tonsillectomy.
- Asymptomatic carriers of GABHS do not require tonsillectomy.

26. Name the two most common viral causes of stomatitis in children.

Herpes simplex virus and coxsackie virus.

27. Describe the usual course of primary herpes gingivostomatitis.

Fever, malaise, irritability, and headache usually precede the primary illness. The oral mucosa is erythematous, and small vesicles appear on the gingiva, tongue, lips, palate, and buccal mucosa. The lesions are often clustered and coalesce. Once the vesicles rupture, a shallow ulcer with pale yellow base is left. New lesions usually develop for the first 5 days of the illness. Complete resolution takes 2 weeks.

28. What age groups are usually affected by primary herpes gingivostomatitis?

Traditionally, children between the ages of 10 months and 3 years are the most likely to be infected with primary herpes gingivostomatitis. A recent small Icelandic study, however, suggests that primary infection in adolescents may be more common than previously appreciated.

29. At what time of the year does primary herpes stomatitis most commonly occur?

Fall and winter.

30. The mother of a 2-year-old girl with herpes stomatitis calls 1 week into the illness. She wants to know how long her daughter will have mouth pain. What should you tell her?

Although viral shedding and infectivity usually last for only 5–7 days, children generally have lesions and pain for 10 days.

31. What should you tell the mother in question 30 about the risk of recurrent lesions?

Recurrence is common.

32. How does recurrent stomatitis differ from the primary disease?

The prodrome for recurrence is usually limited to burning, itching, and mild generalized pain. Vesicles appear in clusters on the hard palate and gingiva during the first 2 days of illness. The vesicles rupture, leaving a 1- to 3-mm shallow ulcer. Most lesions heal in 7–10 days. Pain is usually much less severe with recurrences than with primary infection.

33. Which drug has been proved to ameliorate herpes gingivostomatitis?

Acyclovir in a dose of 15 mg/kg 5 times/day has shown some benefit in reducing symptom duration and viral shedding, although is not recommended for immunocompetent children. An alternative therapy is popsicles.

34. What medical complications cause children with herpes stomatitis to be admitted to the hospital?

The most serious complication of stomatitis is dehydration caused by pain and decreased oral intake. Occasionally, children need to be admitted to the hospital for intravenous rehydration.

35. A 3-year-old boy with primary herpes gingivostomatitis presents with high fever and a painful, swollen, warm right knee. What bacterial cause of septic arthritis has been associated with herpes stomatitis?

In case reports bacteremia with *Kingella kingae* has been associated with herpes stomatitis. This bacteremia can result in septic arthritis, osteomyelitis, or endocarditis.

36. Which topical drug regimen is most effective for treating the pain of herpes stomatitis?

A 10% benzocaine ointment can be used for spot treatment of severe lesions, but its application should be limited. A 2% solution of viscous lidocaine can be helpful as a mouth rinse. The most effective regimen is a solution of equal parts of 2% viscous lidocaine, diphenhydramine hydrochloride, and Maalox. Care should be taken to avoid swallowing the solution. Over-anesthetizing the posterior pharynx can result in aspiration.

37. A 4-year-old girl undergoing treatment for leukemia presents with severe mouth pain that began on the previous day. Clustered vesicles and ulcers are seen along the gingival surface and on the hard palate. She appears stable but has decreased oral intake. What is the next step in management?

Aggressive therapy is often needed for gingivostomatitis in an immunocompromised host. Again, supportive care is vital to maintain hydration. Topical medications can be used for pain control. Parenteral antivirals such as acyclovir have been shown to improve morbidity associated with herpes gingivostomatitis in immunocompromised hosts.

38. Can herpes infection be spread to other parts of the body from herpes stomatitis?
Yes—particularly to the eyes and genitals.

39. What is a herpetic whitlow?
Children who have a tendency to put their fingers in their mouth can spread vesicles to their digits. Clustered vesicles on a finger are called a herpetic whitlow. This sign is common in thumb-suckers.

40. A local day-care center asks when a 4-year-old child with herpetic gingivostomatitis should be allowed to return. How should you respond?
Daycare exclusion may be limited to children who do not have control of their oral secretions. A 4-year-old child probably does not need to stay home. Younger day-care attendees are considered no longer infective 5 days after the first vesicles appear, if no new lesions erupt.

41. Name the virus and serotype responsible for causing hand-foot-mouth (HFM) disease in humans.
Coxsackie virus is the most common cause of HFM disease. The most common subtypes associated with HFM are A5, A9, A10, A16, B1, and B3. A16 is responsible for most of the cases. Some cases are caused by enterovirus 71.

42. What time of year is HFM most prevalent?
Like other enterovirus infections, it is most common in the summer and fall.

43. Can humans get HFM disease from livestock?
No. The two diseases are quite distinct.

44. What age groups are most often affected by HFM?
The disease can effect patients of all ages, but it is most commonly seen in children under the age of 10 years.

45. Where is the rash of HFM disease most commonly located?
Recognizing the rash of HFM disease is essential for the diagnosis. Vesicles measuring 3–7 mm are found on the hands and feet, including the palms, soles, and sides of the feet. Despite the misleading name, the rash also may be located on the arms, legs, buttocks, and perineum. The buttock rash may not turn into true vesicles.

46. How is HFM disease different in adolescents and adults?
It is usually less severe, and often the skin rash is absent.

47. How is HFM disease spread?
Like other enteroviruses, HFM disease is most commonly spread by the fecal-oral route. Some evidence indicates that it also may be transmitted by large droplets via the respiratory route.

48. The father of a 10-month-old boy with HFM disease asks how he can prevent the other children in the family from getting the disease. What should you tell him?
Handwashing is a must. Encourage personal hygiene, and use caution with diaper changes.

49. Describe the usual course of HFM disease in children.
The incubation period is generally 3 or 4 days. A prodrome of sore throat, fever, and fatigue is often present. The rash starts as a papular rash on the hands and feet. Often the arms, legs, buttocks, and perineum are effected. Small vesicles develop and rupture, leaving a slightly painful ulcer. Painful mouth lesions develop as isolated vesicles on the palate, tongue, and posterior pharynx. The mouth lesions are 4–8 mm in size and often rupture, leaving a small painful ulcer. The disease lasts for 1 week, but viral shedding can continue in the stool for many weeks.

50. What treatment can be used to improve the course of HFM disease?
For severe mouth pain, topical treatment is identical to that for herpes stomatitis.

51. What is herpangina?
Herpangina is also a vesicular/ulcerative process of the mouth caused by coxsackie virus or echovirus. It occurs most commonly in the summer.

52. How does herpangina differ from HFM disease and herpes gingivostomatitis?
Patients with herpangina usually have only 5 or 6 oral ulcers at a time, but they are extremely painful. Unlike herpes gingivostomatitis, the mouth lesions are predominantly in the posterior pharynx. Unlike HFM disease, no skin rash is associated with herpangina.

53. Describe the lesions of herpangina.
The mouth lesions are small at first appearance but increase in size over the first 3–4 days of illness. As the vesicles ulcerate, there is usually a surrounding ring of erythema that may be many centimeters in diameter. The lesions have a similar distribution as HFM disease; the most common locations are the soft palate, tonsillar pillars, uvula, and posterior pharynx.

54. What systemic symptoms often accompany herpangina?
Systemic symptoms are often variable. Fever, malaise, and headache are fairly common. Herpangina also may be seen in conjunction with aseptic meningitis caused by enteroviruses.

55. What is the best treatment for herpangina?
No antiviral therapy is available. Supportive care and pain control are the mainstays of treatment.

56. Which viruses other than enterovirus and HSV have been associated with stomatitis?
Mucous membrane involvement is not unusual with varicella-zoster and EBV infections. The other manifestations of these diseases usually make it easy to differentiate them from other causes of viral stomatitis. HIV is also associated with multiple causes of stomatitis.

57. List the systemic diseases that should be included in the differential diagnosis of mouth ulcers.
  • Systemic lupus erythematosus
  • Crohn's disease
  • Behçet's disease
  • Stevens-Johnson syndrome

58. A 7-year-old boy with Crohn's disease presents with mouth pain. Physical exam shows oral ulcers and small oral pustules. What is the most likely diagnosis?
Pyostomatitis vegetans is a noninfectious stomatitis associated with inflammatory bowel disease. It is characterized by small pustules, ulcers, erythema, and vegetations of the labial, gingival, and buccal mucosa. It is rare in children but can be seen in patients who also have pyoderma gangrenosum.

59. What infection is most commonly associated with Stevens-Johnson syndrome?
Mycoplasma pneumoniae.

60. List the oral manifestations of HIV in children.

Mucocutaneous candidiasis	Parotid enlargement
Gingivitis	Hairy leukoplakia
Herpes stomatitis	

61. What are the basic characteristics of aphthous ulcers?

	APHTHOUS MAJOR	APHTHOUS MINOR	HERPETIFORM
Size	< 5 mm	> 5 mm	< 5 mm
Distribution	Isolated	Isolated	Clustered
Duration	10-14 days	14-28 days	7-10 days
Scarring	No	Yes	No

62. How are idiopathic aphthous ulcers treated?
Treatment may be quite variable. systemic steroids, cimetidine, colchicine, cyclosporine, and thalidomide have been tried. Thalidomide is a known teratogen, and its use is restricted.

63. What is PFAPA syndrome?
Periodic fever, aphthous stomatitis, pharyngitis, and adenitis. Onset is usually before age 5 years. The fever may be as high as 40°C and occurs at a fixed interval of 2–8 weeks. Fever usually lasts 4 days and resolves spontaneously, but oral ulcers may last longer. Seventy percent of patients have aphthous ulcers, 72% have pharyngitis, and 88% have cervical adenitis. No lab abnormalities can be found, and no familial tendency has been identified.

64. Patients with PFAPA respond quickly to what medication?
Symptoms can be aborted with one or two doses of prednisone.

65. How does PFAPA syndrome differ from cyclic neutropenia?

	PFAPA	CYCLIC NEUTROPENIA
Age of onset	< 5 years old	< 1 year old
Oral ulcers	Yes	Yes
Fever interval	4-8 weeks	3 weeks
Inherited	No	Yes
Lab abnormalities	None	Neutropenia

BIBLIOGRAPHY

1. Al-Rimawi HS, Hammad MM, Raweily EA, Hammad HM: Pyostomatitis vegetans in childhood. Eur J Pediatr 157:402–405, 1998.
2. Amir J, Harel L, Smetana Z, Varsano I: Treatment of herpes simplex gingivostomatitis with acyclovir in children: A randomized double blind placebo controlled study. Br Med J 314:1800–1803, 1997.
3. Amir J, Yagupsky P: Invasive Kingella kingae infection associated with stomatitis in children. Pediatr Infect Dis J 17:757–758, 1998.
4. Attia MW, Zaoutis TK: Pharyngitis in children. Del Med J 71:459–465, 1999.
5. Bisno AL, Gerber MA, Gwaltney JM, et al: Diagnosis and management of group A streptococcal pharyngitis: A practice guideline. Clin Infect Dis 25:574–583, 1997.
6. Bisno AL: Primary care: Acute pharyngitis. N Engl J Med 344:205–211, 2001.
7. Deutsch ES: Tonsillectomy and adenoidectomy: Changing indications. Pediatr Clin North Am 43:1319–1338; 1996.
8. Feder HM: Periodic fever, aphthous stomatitis, pharyngitis, adenitis: A clinical review of a new syndrome. Curr Opin Pediatr 12:253–256, 2000.
9. Fiesseler FW: Pharyngitis followed by hypoxia and sepsis: Lemierre syndrome. Am J Emerg Med 19:320–332, 2001.
10. Holbrook WP, Gudmundsson GT, Ragnarsson KT: Herpetic gingivostomatitis in otherwise healthy adolescents and young adults. Acta Odontol Scand 59(3):113–115, 2001.
11. Peter JR, Haney HM: Infections of the oral cavity. Pediatr Ann 25:572–576, 1996.
12. Peterson LR, Thomson RB Jr: Oral infection: Use of the clinical laboratory for the diagnosis and management of infectious diseases related to the oral cavity. Infect Dis Clin North Am 13:775–795, 1999.

10. THE COMMON COLD

John Donnelly, M.D, and Keith J. Mann, M.D.

1. Describe the clinical features of the common cold.

Symptoms usually include coryza. A characteristic scratchy or sore throat is not unusual early in the illness. Nasal congestion, rhinorrhea, sneezing, headache, and cough are the most common symptoms. Fever is more common in children than in adults. Fever height can be variable.

2. Name the viruses most commonly associated with the common cold.

Many viruses can cause cold symptoms. Rhinoviruses probably cause about 50% of colds worldwide. Other viruses include enterovirus (particularly coxsackie A21), coronavirus, respiratory syncytial virus (RSV), adenovirus, and influenza virus. However, RSV and influenza generally cause associated lower respiratory tract symptoms in addition to upper respiratory symptoms. In addition, enteroviruses and adenovirus often are associated with systemic symptoms.

3. Describe the usual course of an upper respiratory infection (URI).

The incubation period is usually 12 hours to 3 days. A sore throat is often the first symptom and considered the most prominent complaint on the first day of illness. Nasal congestion quickly follows and is usually the primary symptom by the second day of illness. Cough is present in about 30% of cases. Symptoms often resolve in 5–7 days. Some symptoms can linger for 2 weeks, particularly the cough.

4. Describe the pathophysiology of rhinovirus infection.

Rhinovirus infection actually causes little mucosal damage. Infection of the nasal mucosa causes a cytokine response that produces the symptoms of the common cold. When healthy volunteers are subjected to intranasal bradykinin, symptoms of nasal congestion and sore throat are reproduced. However, therapy designed to block kinins has not been found to be effective. Other research has shown that interleukins probably plays a role in the pathophysiology. There also appears to be an important neurologic role in symptom development. Nasal congestion is clearly under the influence of cholinergic tone.

5. Why do patients with colds cough?

Much of the cough is caused by postnasal drip and nasal congestion and should respond to decongestant or antihistamine treatment.

6. List the complications associated with rhinovirus infection.
- Asthma exacerbation
- Otitis media
- Sinusitis
- Pneumonia
- Cystic fibrosis exacerbation

7. A 4-year-old child with a history of reactive airway disease presents with symptoms of URI. What should you tell the family about the possibility of an asthma exacerbation?

Although not all colds result in asthma exacerbation, about 80% of exacerbations of reactive airway disease in children occur in the setting of acute viral URI. Families should watch for wheezing or respiratory distress if the child has a history of reactive airway disease.

8. If URIs are by definition *upper* respiratory infections, why should they cause exacerbations of asthma?

The most likely cause of asthma exacerbation is the systemic inflammatory response secondary to the cytokine and interleukin response to viral infection. Recent studies, however, have shown viral replication of rhinovirus in the bronchial epithelium. Although the significance of this infection of the lower respiratory tract is uncertain, it may be assumed that even minor inflammation of the bronchial tree can result in significant compromise in patients with reactive airway disease. This same process also may result in exacerbations of other lower airway disease, such as cystic fibrosis and bronchopulmonary dysplasia.

9. What is the association between cold viruses and otitis media?

Otitis media is more common in the setting of viral URI. In studies using polymerase chain reaction (PCR), common cold viruses were found in 75% of children presenting with otitis media. The viruses most frequently associated with otitis media are rhinovirus and RSV; coronavirus is rare. Most patients with virus in the middle ear fluid also have a bacterial coinfection. It is unknown how the presence of virus affects the outcome of bacterial otitis media.

10. How do URI viruses predispose to otitis media?

Viral inflammation of the middle ear probably causes effusion and an opportunity for bacterial replication and infection. Viruses also cause inflammation of the nasal mucosa and subsequent eustachian tube dysfunction.

11. How is rhinovirus associated with acute sinusitis?

Rhinovirus infection is actually rhinosinusitis; 85% of patients show some evidence of sinus inflammation during the acute infection. However, in looking at patients with suspected acute bacterial sinusitis, researchers using PCR technology have been able to isolate rhinovirus in sinus aspirates in up to 40% of patients.

12. An 8-year-old child presents with headache, nasal congestion, rhinorrhea, sore throat, cough, and fatigue. You explain to the mother that the child has a URI. She asks how you know that it is not anthrax. What should you tell her?

The public has been concerned since the anthrax-related deaths in the fall of 2001. Although anthrax can present as a flu-like illness, it is not associated with coryza. The presence of significant nasal congestion makes anthrax very unlikely.

13. How much money is spent each year in the United States on over-the-counter cold therapies: (a) more than the gross national product of France, (b) 1 million dollars, (c) 500 million dollars, or (d) 2 billion dollars?

Answer: d.

14. Are decongestants effective treatments for the common cold?

Topical decongestants are not recommended because prolonged use can result in rhinitis medicamentosa. Research in children less than 5 years old has been limited, but most studies have found little evidence that these medications are helpful. In fact, side effects of irritability and insomnolence may make young children feel worse. Studies in older children have been small and not always placebo-controlled. Some evidence suggests that a combination medication that includes a decongestant may improve nasal symptoms. Adult and adolescent studies have found subjective improvement in "sinus" symptoms after two doses of pseudoephedrine.

15. How do antihistamines affect cold symptoms?

First-generation antihistamines, such as clemastine fumarate, have been shown to reduce rhinorrhea. However, second-generation nonsedating antihistamines have not been shown to be effective. The first-generation antihistamines are thought to derive most of their efficacy from the anticholinergic effect. However, anticholinergic side effects, such as dry eyes, mouth, and nose, are sometimes subjectively worse than the symptoms that the drug is supposed to treat.

16. Are antitussives effective for the treatment of the cough associated with the common cold?

Research has been inconclusive; however, dextromethorphan and codeine are used frequently.

17. Should beta agonists be recommended to patients with cough and URI?

Three studies have shown improvement of cough when beta agonists are compared with antibiotics in the treatment of the common cold. One study, however, suggested that the benefit may be limited to patients with underlying reactive airway disease.

18. Is guaifenesin an effective treatment of congestion?

Results from adult studies have been variable. One older study reported significant subjective improvement in cough intensity and chest discomfort. Patients noted a thinning of sputum and increased sputum production with coughing.

19. What is the role of corticosteroids in the treatment of the common cold?

There is no proven benefit to the use of corticosteroids for treatment of cold viruses. Some evidence suggests that viral replication can be enhanced by the use of steroids.

20. A mother asks if she should give echinacea to her 8-year-old child, who has a cold. How should you respond?

Again, trials have shown variable results. No evidence supports the use of echinacea in children, but some evidence from adult studies supports its use in the treatment and prevention of acute URI. Randomized, controlled trials have shown a shorter duration of cold symptoms in adults taking echinacea to treat acute URI. Some evidence also suggests that echinacea may be helpful in the prevention of acute URI. However, study quality has been variable, and all trials have been small. Echinacea is also a variable product, with different preparations containing inconsistent doses of the herb or different parts of the plant. In addition, although small doses appear to be safe for short-term use, the safety of long-term use is uncertain.

21. What advice can you give patients about the use of vitamin C for the treatment of the common cold?

Three randomized control trials in adults reported that patients taking 1000 mg/day of vitamin C had symptoms for one-half day less than controls. Results have not been reproduced in children.

22. An adolescent patient tells you that she has been using zinc lozenges to treat cold symptoms. What can you tell her about zinc?

Two formulations of zinc are available: zinc gluconate and zinc acetate. A few small adult studies have shown a slight reduction in the length of URI symptoms in zinc users. However, statistical significance was variable among studies. It is unknown whether one formulation of zinc is better than the other. Significant adverse effects have been observed, including nausea, abdominal pain, headache, and dry mouth. Extended use of large doses also may result in neutropenia and immunosuppresion.

23. Do antibiotics have any role in the treatment of patients with symptoms of the common cold?

Studies have shown no improvement in symptoms of children with URI who are treated with systemic antibiotics. One study in adults suggests that 20% of cold sufferers also are colonized with *Haemophilus influenzae*, *Moraxella catarrhalis*, or *Streptococcus pneumoniae* and actually have a modest improvement in URI symptoms if treated with amoxicillin-clavulanate. However, it is difficult to assess which patients are truly colonized with bacteria, and antibiotics are not recommended.

24. Are any antiviral medications effective for treatment of the common cold?

There has been recent interest in the use of intranasal interferon for the treatment or prevention of the common cold. Although some studies have been optimistic that viral replication is decreased, many studies have found that the use of intranasal interferon results in nasal stuffiness, sneezing, and nasal discharge. Thus, even if the virus cannot replicate, the symptoms of the cold persist.

Preliminary research also has looked at other viral compounds. Dipyridamole and palmitate appear promising, but at this point little research has been done. Plecornaril is a compound currently under development with initially optimistic results. Further research is needed to investigate whether these compounds will be safe and cost-effective in the treatment or prevention of the common cold.

25. How long after a cold should a patient be considered infectious?

The infectious period is highly variable, but viral shedding can last for 2 weeks after symptoms resolve.

26. How many colds per year does the average person get?

Risk factors play a major role in the number of colds per year in children. Day care and schooling are risk factors in the spread of cold viruses. Most preschool children get 5–7 colds per year. Up to 10% of children get 12 colds per year. The frequency decreases over time toward the adult average of 2–3 colds per year.

27. Describe the mechanism of spread for rhinovirus.

There is actually no clear answer to this question. The most likely mechanism of spread is direct contact with infected nasal secretions. Studies suggest that people who have contact with contaminated secretions have a high rate of infection if they subsequently touch their own nose or eyes. Rhinovirus can live for hours on objects or on human skin. The ability to survive for an extended period outside the human body makes transmission from contact more likely. However, some researchers believe that the virus is also spread from respiratory droplets via an inhalation mechanism.

28. A day-care worker asks what she can do to reduce the spread of colds in her center. What can you tell her?

Because colds most likely are spread from infected secretions to hands and fomites, handwashing is essential. However, recent studies have shown that a strict handwashing policy in day-care centers reduced cold frequency only in children under 2 years of age.

29. Why has a vaccine not been developed to prevent the common cold?

Over 200 hundred different viruses cause the symptoms of the common cold. Most are rhinoviruses, but with over 100 different serotypes, a single vaccine to prevent the common cold appears almost impossible. Unless a common antigen or binding protein is found among all common cold viruses, vaccination development is unlikely.

BIBLIOGRAPHY

1. Glasziou P, Del Mar C: Upper respiratory tract infection. Clinical Evidence 6 Br J Med Clin Evid 6:1200–1207, 2001.
2. Goldman RA: Transmission of viral respiratory infections in the home. Pediatr Infect Dis J 19:S97–S102, 2000.
3. Jefferson TO, Tyrell D: Antivirals for the common cold. Cochrane Database of Systematic Reviews, issue 4, 2001.
4. Papadopoulos NG, Johnston SL: The rhinovirus—Not such an innocent? [editorial]. Q J Med 94:1–3, 2001.
5. Pitkäranta A, Virolainen A, Jero J, et al: Detection of rhinovirus, respiratory syncytial virus, and coronavirus infection in acute otitis media by reverse transcriptase polymerase chain reaction. Pediatrics 102:292–295, 1998.
6. Roberts L, Smith W, Jorn L, et al: Effect of infection control measures on the frequency of upper respiratory infection in child care: A randomized, controlled trial. Pediatrics 105:738–742, 2000.
7. Rotbart HA, Hayden FG: Picornavirus infections: A primer for the practitioner. Arch Fam Med 9:913–920, 2000.
8. Smith MBH, Feldman W: Over-the-counter cold medications: A critical review of clinical trials Between 1950 and 1991. JAMA 269:2258–2263, 1993.
9. Spencer SJ, Turner RB, Sorrentino JV, et al: Effectiveness of pseudoephedrine plus acetaminophen for the treatment of symptoms attributed to the paranasal sinuses associated with the common cold. Arch Fam Med 9:979–985, 2000.
10. Turner RB: The common cold. Pediatr Ann 27:700–795, 1998.

11. PERITONSILLAR, RETROPHARYNGEAL, AND PARAPHARYNGEAL SPACE INFECTIONS

Michael J. Muszynski, M.D.

1. How are deep neck space infections defined according to location?

Deep neck infections involve potential spaces of the neck, which are defined by fascial planes. The infectious process follows paths of least resistance within these planes but tends to be limited by local anatomy. Potential neck spaces with clinical significance are the masticator (masseteric, pterygoid, and temporal), buccal and parotid, submandibular and sublingual, lateral pharyngeal (parapharyngeal), retropharyngeal, pretracheal, and peritonsillar spaces. Peritonsillar, retropharyngeal, and parapharyngeal infections are the most important locations in children.

2. Compare the general incidence of neck space infections in childhood in relation to age.

Peritonsillar infections are the most common type of deep neck infection overall and tend to occur in older children; the average age is 10–11 years. Submandibular and submental infections, the second most common type, are otodontic in origin and are therefore limited to children with dentition.

Retropharyngeal abscesses are generally uncommon and occur in children less than 5 years old; 50% of cases present before the age of 2 years. Retropharyngeal abscess is distinctly unusual in older children and adolescents.

Parapharyngeal infections are rare in childhood and extremely rare in infants. They tend to occur from late childhood into adolescence.

3. Discuss the pathogenesis and source of peritonsillar abscesses.

Tonsillitis due to bacteria, respiratory viruses, and Epstein-Barr virus (infectious mononucleosis) may be severe enough to spread past the confines of the fibrous tonsil capsule. Bacterial contamination of the peritonsillar space results in local cellulitis with potential progression to abscess. Some authorities believe that infection of salivary and mucus glands (Weber's glands), which are located in the peritonsillar space and nest at the superior pole of the tonsil, is the initiating event. Supporting this theory is the fact that peritonsillar abscess occurs almost exclusively in the superior pole location.

4. Trace the pathologic processes leading to retropharyngeal abscess.

Bacterial infection of the paramedian lymph nodes in the retropharyngeal space leads to localized inflammation, edema, and ultimately suppuration. Purulence then ruptures into the potential space, as defined by the anatomy of the deep cervical fascia located between the posterior wall of the esophagus and the vertebral column. The infection is usually limited in extent by the anatomic fusion of the fascial layers at the level of the first thoracic vertebra. Occasionally penetrating trauma from sharp objects (e.g., pencils, swallowed safety pins, fish bones) can directly inoculate the retropharyngeal space with bacteria. Extension of vertebral osteomyelitis into the retropharyngeal space also has been described as a cause of retropharyngeal abscess.

5. Why is retropharyngeal abscess so unusual in adults?

Retropharyngeal abscesses form as a progression of infection within the paramedian chain of lymph nodes, which have atrophied by age 5 years.

6. What are the common presenting symptoms of peritonsillar abscess?

Patients present with an initial history of low-grade fever and sore throat. As the infection progresses toward abscess and anatomic displacement of tonsil tissue, symptoms of dysphagia, drooling, poor oral intake, and unilateral throat pain develop. Parents often note fetid breath. Subglottic and palate edema result in muffled speech commonly described as "hot potato voice" or "mouth full of pebbles." Trismus, a frequent and distressing symptom, results from spasm of the inflamed internal pterygoid muscle, which is located in intimate approximation to the lateral margin of the retropharyngeal space. Trismus often presents a challenge to routine examination of the mouth and throat.

7. Describe the clinical manifestations of retropharyngeal abscess.

As with peritonsillar abscess, fever and dysphagia are common. Drooling also may occur. However, as the abscess progresses, symptoms of stridor and respiratory distress become obvious. The patient may prefer a position of comfort such as sitting and leaning forward with the chin forward to maintain a maximal airway. Thus, it is important to consider retropharyngeal abscess in any child with fever, sore throat, and dysphagia followed by stridor. Lastly, stiff neck occurs because the inflammatory process is just anterior to the vertebral column.

8. Which symptoms best differentiate between peritonsillar and retropharyngeal abscess?

Unilateral throat pain, trismus, fetid breath, and muffled voice occur with peritonsillar but not retropharyngeal abscess. Findings of airway obstruction and stridor, respiratory distress, and stiff neck suggest retropharyngeal abscess. Chest pain is expected mainly with retropharyngeal abscess and is due to spread of infection beyond the inferior anatomic limit of the retropharyngeal space into the mediastinum.

9. Describe the presenting symptoms of parapharyngeal abscess.

The presentation varies according to the anatomic involvement of the parapharyngeal space, which may be conveniently divided into anterior and posterior compartments. Symptoms relate to inflammation or injury of the structures located in each compartment. The anterior compartment contains the internal pterygoid muscle and is contiguous with the retropharyngeal space. Not surprisingly, symptoms of parapharyngeal abscess in this location mimic those of peritonsillar abscess and include trismus and unilateral throat pain. The posterior compartment contains cranial nerves IX through XII, the sympathetic nerve chain, the carotid artery, and the jugular vein. Abscess in the posterior compartment results in facial nerve weakness, impaired gag reflex, vocal cord dysfunction or paralysis, trapezius muscle weakness, and unilateral impairment of tongue movement. Horner syndrome, hemorrhage from erosion of the carotid artery, and internal jugular vein thrombosis also have been described. Any patient with a clinical course suggestive of peritonsillar abscess followed by cranial nerve abnormalities should be suspected of having parapharyngeal abscess.

10. What are the expected physical examination findings in patients with peritonsillar abscess?

Often examination is difficult because of spasm and pain from trismus. On inspection of the oropharynx, the tonsil and soft palate on the affected side are displaced toward the midline. Inflammation of the pharynx is seen, usually with purulent material in tonsil crypts; pharyngeal inflammation may appear relatively mild, however, even in the face of significant abscess formation. The uvula is edematous with displacement away from its usual midline position in the direction away from the abscess. Fluctuation can be palpated at the superior pole of the tonsil. Examination of the neck shows ipsilateral, tender, enlarged anterior cervical lymph nodes. Unilateral spasm of neck muscles (torticollis) is common.

11. How does the clinical picture of peritonsillar cellulitis differ from that of peritonsillar abscess?

The distinction is one of degree relative to progression of the infectious process. If the unilateral inflammation and swelling of cellulitis occupy the same volume as a peritonsillar space abscess, the clinical distinction is quite difficult. Unilateral tender cervical lymphadentitis commonly occurs with both conditions. General differentiating findings are listed below, with the caveat that overlap is common.

FEATURE	PERITONSILLAR CELLULITIS	PERITONSILLAR ABSCESS
Age	Younger (mean = 10 yr)	Older (mean = 15 yr)
Symptoms	Trismus	Dysphagia, drooling
Voice	Relatively normal early	"Hot potato"
Appearance	Bilateral	Unilateral
Palpation	Firm	Soft, fluctuant

12. What are the expected physical findings of patients with retropharyngeal abscess?

The primary finding is anterior bulging of the posterior pharynx; however, it is often subtle or not readily apparent on inspection. Fullness and fluctuance are palpable, but digital examination of the posterior pharynx is generally not recommended because it may cause abscess rupture with subsequent aspiration. Nuchal rigidity may be a prominent finding and occasionally is confused with meningitis.

13. Why may the early physical findings of parapharyngeal abscess be difficult to distinguish from those of peritonsillar and retropharyngeal abscess?

1. Parapharyngeal abscess is so uncommon in childhood that the diagnosis may not even be considered.

2. Examination of the throat reveals a paucity of findings in both parapharyngeal and retropharyngeal abscesses.

3. Parapharyngeal abscess may cause unilateral swelling in the throat along with some degree of neck pain and trismus similar to the findings of peritonsillar abscess.

14. How does the tempo of clinical presentation vary for parapharyngeal, retropharyngeal, and peritonsillar abscesses?

Parapharyngeal abscess is somewhat insidious in presentation and is frequently overlooked until a complication leads the clinician to the diagnosis. Most peritonsillar and retropharyngeal abscesses are diagnosed before major complications develop. Symptoms of peritonsillar abscesses tend to be the most rapid in onset.

15. List conditions that occasionally may be confused with peritonsillar abscess.
- Epiglottitis and retropharyngeal and parapharyngeal abscesses. The "hot potato voice" of epiglottitis is indistinguishable from that of retropharyngeal abscess.
- Trismus may be similar to that seen in tetanus, hypocalcemic tetany, rabies, or the extrapyramidal and dystonic side effects of phenothiazines.
- Dental infections, parapharyngeal abscess, and lymphoid tumors of the tonsil may show similar unilateral displacement in the throat.
- Fever, toxicity, severe sore throat, drooling, and stiff neck can occur in cases of severe pharyngotonsillitis due to group A streptococci and/or infectious mononucleosis.

16. Which conditions should be considered in the differential diagnosis of retropharyngeal abscess?
- Epiglottitis also produces airway compromise and patient preference for a posture providing airway comfort (sitting, chin forward).
- Pressure on the airway from the anterior bulging of a retropharyngeal abscess can cause stridor similar to that associated with croup.
- Penetrating throat trauma and foreign bodies within the pharynx cause symptoms similar to those noted with retropharyngeal abscess.
- Cervical discitis and vertebral osteomyelitis, including tuberculosis, have similar presentations. Anterior extension of infection from vertebral osteomyelitis to the soft tissues also produces unilateral or generalized fullness of the retropharyngeal space.

17. Outline the general approach to the management of deep neck space infections.

When any deep neck space infection is suspected, the first step in management is to ensure an adequate airway. The next step is to assess the need for additional supportive measures, such as correcting dehydration and maintaining circulation and hydration. Hospitalization is required for all pediatric cases. The clinician then must define the condition and its extent by history, physical examination, and appropriate imaging studies. Definitive therapy involves specimen collection for culture, surgical approaches, and parenteral antimicrobial therapy. Otolaryngologic surgical consultation is strongly recommended.

18. Discuss the use of radiologic imaging studies to assess childhood neck infections.

The **lateral neck x-ray** is the time-honored study for upper airway infections. A normal lateral neck film effectively rules out retropharyngeal abscess. The presence of gas in the retropharyngeal space or any neck space points to infection with gas-forming bacteria or penetrating trauma. A lateral neck film is indicated in the initial evaluation of suspected pharyngeal foreign body. Care must be taken in the diagnosis of retropharyngeal abscess by lateral neck x-ray to minimize false-positive results. The film must be obtained with adequate extension of the neck. In such a view, the normal soft tissue of the posterior pharynx is less than 5 mm wide at the C3 vertebral level and has a width of less than 40% of the anteroposterior diameter of the vertebral body at the level of C4.

Computed tomography (CT) provides accurate definition of neck space infections and is readily available to most clinicians. It is especially helpful in the ill, uncooperative, or uncomfortable child in whom physical examination of the throat is difficult. Modern, rapid-sequence CT scanners avoid the need for sedation. CT findings effectively differentiate cellulitis from purulent collections and provide details about the extent of the process. The sensitivity of CT scan in the diagnosis of deep neck infections in children is said to be greater than 90%.

Ultrasound study of the neck structures distinguishes abscess from cellulitis or solid mass but provides less information and detail than CT images.

Magnetic resonance imaging (MRI) is emerging as the ultimate study for the definition of soft tissue anatomy of the neck but has the drawbacks of expense, poor availability at some locations, and need for significant sedation of young patients. Vascular complications secondary to deep neck infections, such as jugular vein thrombosis, are most often assessed by CT scan with administration of intravenous contrast material. Some experts believe that magnetic resonance angiography or venography is the most sensitive and accurate method to evaluate vascular complications.

19. Describe the microbiology of deep neck space infections.

Group A streptococcus (*Streptococcus pyogenes*) and *Staphylococcus aureus* are the classic causes. However, anaerobes are now recognized as equally or even more important pathogens. *Bacteroides*, *Fusobacterium*, and *Peptostreptococcus* species are the most prevalent isolates. Anaerobes may be the only isolates in a significant number of cases. Occasionally other aerobes, such as *Haemophilus* species, *Streptococcus pneumoniae*, and *Klebsiella pneumoniae*, are found. Most deep neck abscesses contain a mixture of organisms in virtually any combination of those noted above. Unusual organism, such as *Pseudomonas aeruginosa*, *Enterobacter* species, *Candida* species, and tuberculous or nontuberculous mycobacteria, may be found in immunocompromised hosts, including patients with acquired immunodeficiency syndrome (AIDS).

20. Discuss the options for antibiotic treatment of neck space infections.

Empirical antibiotic choice is directed toward the expected microbiology of the infection but is ideally guided by Gram stain and culture of aspirated abscess material. Appropriate specimen for culture is mandatory in the management of immunocompromised hosts with deep neck infections. Throat culture and swab cultures of drainage or pharyngeal surfaces are less reliable and may be misleading. Swab specimens often contain a mixture of oropharyngeal flora and, even if a possible pathogen is isolated from such specimens, the result does not necessarily correlate with the infection in the deep neck space. Initial antibiotic therapy should provide coverage for the most commonly described causes. Additional guidance is provided by Gram stain of the pus. Clindamycin or a beta-lactam/beta-lactamase inhibitor (e.g., ampicillin/sulbactam) is a reasonable choice. Methicillin-resistant *S. aureus* (MRSA) requiring intravenous vancomycin should be considered in recently hospitalized patients or patients not responding to empirical therapy. Other infrequently used regimens are a cephalosporin with anaerobic activity (e.g,. cefoxitin or cefotetan) or the combination of metronidazole with a second- or third-generation cephalosporin.

21. Identify the surgical approaches to peritonsillar abscess.
Tonsillectomy, incision and drainage, needle aspiration, and antibiotic therapy alone should be considered as options. The indication for abscess tonsillectomy is controversial. Older literature stresses the need for tonsillectomy or incision and drainage. Recent data suggest that children 1–6 years of age may respond to antibiotic therapy alone and that surgical intervention is required only if no improvement is seen within 48 hours of medical therapy. A common approach is to combine needle aspiration with antibiotic treatment and to consider abscess tonsillectomy if the abscess recurs or fails to respond. Bilateral tonsillectomy is usually performed because the risk of abscess formation around the contralateral tonsil is said to be 2–24%. There is general agreement that bilateral tonsillectomy is indicated for patients with a repeat episode of peritonsillar abscess. Algorithmic approaches for management have been proposed. These recommendations consider clinical efficacy and long-term outcome, operative risk, risk of disease recurrence, length of hospital stay, and cost of medical care. Below is an example of one such approach.

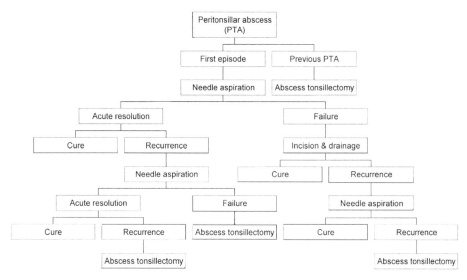

22. Summarize the advantages and disadvantages of the various surgical approaches to peritonsillar abscess.

PROCEDURE	ADVANTAGES	DISADVANTAGES

Needle aspiration	Simplest, least painful method
	Cost-effective
	Diagnostic and therapeutic
	Material for Gram stain and culture
	Avoids general anesthesia in older
	    patients
		May miss abscess space
		Repeat aspiration needed in 10–20%
		Requires patient cooperation
		General anesthesia needed in
		    young children
		Interval tonsillectomy more difficult
		    due to peritonsillar fibrosis

(Continued. on next page)

PROCEDURE	ADVANTAGES	DISADVANTAGES
Incision and drainage	Provides prompt symptomatic relief Useful in impending airway compromise Can be performed in an awake older patient	Less accurate culture results Painful and uncomfortable Requires calm, cooperative patient General anesthesia needed in young children
Tonsillectomy	Most effective method for patients with significant airway compromise Method with best surgical exposure; helpful in cases with severe trismus	Method with highest surgical risk General anesthesia required Expensive

23. Outline the management of retropharyngeal abscess.

As with all deep neck infections, attention is first directed to stabilization of the airway, then to supportive measures such as hydration. Immediate empirical antibiotic therapy by the intravenous route and otolaryngologic consultation are required. Incision and drainage are immediately indicated if any signs of airway obstruction are present or if the evolving abscess becomes fluctuant. The procedure is considered a surgical emergency and should be performed with protection of the airway by endotracheal intubation. The patient should be monitored for possible spontaneous rupture of the abscess and pulmonary aspiration.

24. List the most serious complications of peritonsillar, retropharyngeal, and parapharyngeal abscesses.

Peritonsillar abscess: extension into the retropharyngeal, pterygomaxillary, and/or mediastinum spaces; spontaneous rupture with aspiration pneumonia.

Retropharyngeal abscess: airway obstruction; spontaneous rupture with aspiration pneumonia; erosion through the fascia into the prevertebral space with inferior extension into the mediastinum or even past the diaphragm to the psoas musculature; extension into the parapharyngeal space with the complications associated with parapharyngeal abscess, the most feared of which are vascular.

Parapharyngeal abscess: extension into the retropharyngeal and mediastinum spaces; airway obstruction; cranial nerve damage; Horner syndrome; internal jugular vein thrombosis; cavernous sinus thrombosis; carotid artery erosion and rupture; arterial cerebral embolism.

25. How did George Washington die?

For two days the first president suffered with the symptoms of a cold and hoarse voice, which initially seemed a nuisance. Suddenly, between 2 and 3 AM on Saturday, December 14, 1799, he awakened Mrs. Washington and said that he felt ill, had pain on swallowing, difficulty with breathing, and pain on speaking. The first lady noted that over time his spoken words became more garbled and difficult to understand. Physicians summoned to his bedside later that morning noted redness of the president's throat. A diagnosis of "inflammatory quinsy" was announced. Quinsy is an outdated term for peritonsillar abscess derived from the Middle English *quinesie*, which in turn is a corruption of Latin for "sore throat." Washington's physicians were alarmed by his appearance and ordered various treatments, including extremity blisters, throat compresses, and multiple bleedings. As his condition deteriorated, the physicians concluded that Washington might well die from "cynache trachealis," an 18th century term describing upper airway inflammation that led to a cyanotic and critically ill patient. One of the physicians made the remarkable (for the time) suggestion of creating a hole in the president's trachea to relieve obstruction, but the more experienced and trusted physicians in attendance overruled him. They carried out more bleedings to an astounding estimated total volume of 5–9 pints. Just over 21 hours after alerting his wife in the middle of the night, Washington died. Medical historians have suggested peritonsillar abscess (quinsy), Ludwig's angina (another neck space infection), and diphtheria as possible diagnoses. Other historians believe that epiglottitis best describes Washington's symptoms, tempo of disease, and outcome. Whatever the primary diagnosis, all agree that airway obstruction due to infection of neck structures complicated by hypovolemia and anemia from massive blood letting ensured the tragic end.

BIBLIOGRAPHY

1. Blotter JW, Yin L, Glynn M, Wiet GJ: Otolaryngology consultation for peritonsillar abscess in the pediatric population. Laryngoscope 110:1698–1701, 2000.
2. Brook I: Peritonsillar, retropharyngeal, and parapharyngeal abscesses. In Long SS, Pickering LK, Prober CG (eds): Principles and Practice of Pediatric Infectious Diseases. New York, Churchhill Livingstone, 1997, pp 207–211.
3. Hammerschlag PE, Hammerschlag MR: Peritonsillar, retropharyngeal, and parapharyngeal abscesses. In Feigin RD, Cherry JD (eds): Textbook of Pediatric Infectious Diseases, 4th ed. Philadelphia, W.B. Saunders, 1998, pp 164–170.
4. Kirse DJ, Roberson DW: Surgical management of retropharyngeal space infections in children. Laryngoscope 111:1413–1422, 2001.
5. Lalakea M, Messner AH: Retropharyngeal abscess management in children: Current practices. Otolaryngol Head Neck Surg 121:398–405, 1999.
6. Parhiscar A, Har-El G: Deep neck abscess: A retrospective review of 210 cases. Ann Otol Rhinol Laryngol 110:1051–1054, 2001.
7. Scheidemandel HHE: Did George Washington die of quinsy? Arch Otolaryngol 102:519–521, 1976.
8. Schraff S, McGinn JD, Derkay CS: Peritonsillar abscess in children: A 10-year review of diagnosis and management. Int J Pediatr Otorhinolaryngol 57:213–218, 2001.
9. Scott PM, Loftus WK, Kew J, et al: Diagnosis of peritonsillar infections: A prospective study of ultrasound, computerized tomography and clinical diagnosis. J Laryngol Otol 113:229–232, 1999.
10. Sichel JY, Gomori JM, Saah D, Elidan J: Parapharyngeal abscess in children: The role of CT for diagnosis and treatment. Int J Pediatr Otorhinolaryngol 35:213–222, 1996.

12. INFECTIONS OF THE EYE AND ORBIT

Henry M. Feder, Jr., M.D.

1. How is viral conjunctivitis diagnosed? What are the causes?

Viral conjunctivitis is the most common cause of acute "red eye." The conjunctiva is injected (red) with follicles. The redness is usually greater peripherally. The discharge is watery and may cause the lids to stick together in the morning. Frequently both eyes are involved. There is more discomfort than pain. The principal viruses that cause conjunctivitis include adenovirus, enterovirus, and coxsackie virus.

2. A child presents with low-grade fever, bilateral conjunctivitis, and sore throat. The tonsils are enlarged and erythematous. What is the most likely diagnosis?

This is a classic description of pharyngoconjunctivitis, which is caused by adenovirus types 8 or 19 and is highly contagious.

3. What causes epidemic keratoconjunctivitis?

Adenovirus types 3 and 7. Epidemic keratoconjunctivitis is extremely contagious. It is spread most commonly by hand-to-eye contact, but it can even be spread in water (e.g., swimming pools). Also highly contagious are enterovirus 70 and coxsackie virus A24, which cause hemorrhagic conjunctivitis. These viral infections are severe and usually bilateral and may be associated with preauricular adenopathy and fever. Gram stain of the eye discharge shows lymphocytes without many bacteria. Treatments include eye compresses and perhaps artificial tears.

4. How is bacterial conjunctivitis diagnosed? What are the causes?

Bacterial conjunctivitis is associated with diffuse and marked conjunctival injection. Usually only one eye is involved. A purulent discharge is present, and the eye lids are stuck together in the morning and throughout the day. The eye is quite painful. The diagnosis is confirmed by Gram stain, which should show many neutrophils and gram-positive or gram-negative bacteria. The causes include *Haemophilus influenzae*, *Streptococcus pneumoniae*, *Moraxella catarrhalis*, *Staphylococcus aureus*, and *Neisseria gonorrhoeae*.

5. What are topical ophthalmic antibacterial agents? How do they differ with respect to clinical efficacy?

- Erythromycin ointment (AK-Mycin, Ilotycin)
- Sulfa agents: sulfacetamide (Sulamyd,Bleph-10, Sulf-10) drops and ointment; sulfisoxazole drops (Gantrisin)
- Quinolones: ciprofloxacin (Ciloxan), norfloxacin (Chibroxin, Noroxin), ofloxacin (Ocuflox)
- Bacitracin (AK Tracin) ointment
- Polymyxin B (always combined with another antibiotic): Neosporin (polymyxin B plus neomycin plus bacitracin), Polysporin (polymyxin B plus bacitracin)
- Aminoglycosides: gentamicin, tobramycin
- Tetracycline drops
- Trimethoprim combined with polymyxin B (Polytrim)

The bacterial spectrum for these agents is different; however, because of their high concentrations when applied locally, all of them can be used for bacterial conjunctivitis. Erythromycin ointment and sulfacetamide solution are inexpensive and well tolerated. Neosporin and Polysporin may cause contact allergic reactions and should be avoided.

6. For children with bacterial conjunctivitis and positive cultures for *H. influenzae* or *S. pneumoniae*, what were the cure rates at 3 and 9 days with polymyxin-bacitracin vs. placebo?

	POLYMYXIN-BACITRACIN	PLACEBO
Cure at 4 days	62%	28%
Cure at 9 days	91%	72%

For bacterial conjunctivitis, one topical antibiotic therapy, in general, has not been shown superior to another. Bacterial conjunctivitis is usually a self-limited infection but resolves more quickly with topical antibiotic therapy.

7. True or False: Treating presumed bacterial conjunctivitis with oral antibiotics prevents the development of acute otitis media.

False. In one study of bacterial conjunctivitis, 70% of patients had positive eye cultures, including *H. influenzae* (55%), *S. pneumoniae* (14%), and *M. catarrhalis* (17%). Patients were randomized to receive local polymyxin-bacitracin ointment or oral cefixime. The two therapies showed no difference in clinical efficacy for treating acute conjunctivitis, and about 10% of patients in each group developed acute otitis media. *H. influenzae* is the bacteria most frequently associated with otitis and conjunctivitis. Thus, oral antibiotic therapy for conjunctivitis does not prevent the development of otitis media.

8. What causes periorbital (preseptal) cellulitis?

Redness around the eye that involves the upper and lower eye lids is usually due to preseptal inflammation or infection. The causes of periorbital cellulitis are as follows:
- Reaction to bug bite (most common). Patients are afebrile, and the skin is not tender.
- Skin infection due to break in the skin and secondary group A beta-hemolytic streptococci or *S. aureus* infection.
- Underlying sinusitis, usually ethmoid. Patients are usually sick and need hospitalization for systemic antibiotics.
- Dental abscess. Patients are sick and have upper jaw tooth pain and/or tenderness. They require drainage and treatment with a penicillin or clindamycin.
- Conjunctivitis occasionally leads to periorbital cellulitis.

9. When should orbital cellulitis be suspected?

Children with either periorbital or orbital cellulitis present with red, swollen upper and lower eye lids. Clinically, orbital cellulitis is associated with reduced eye movement and proptosis. Postseptal cellulitis involves the area posterior to the septum in the eyelids and is much less common than preseptal cellulitis. Infection is usually due to orbital extension of underlying sinusitis.

10. A 10-year-old child with chronic seborrheic dermatitis develops recurrent red eyes that improve only slightly with over-the-counter Visine. The pediatrician notes red eye lids that are slightly swollen with scale at the eye lid margins. Blepharitis is suspected, and local erythromycin ointment is prescribed with little benefit. Why did the ointment fail?

The child has posterior blepharitis, which needs to be treated with systemic antibiotics. Posterior blepharitis is associated with seborrheic dermatitis and involves the meibomian sebaceous glands under the eye lid. Therapy involves aggressive treatment of the seborrhea dermatitis and systemic antibiotics such as cephalexin, doxycycline, or erythromycin. Local erythromycin also may be used

11. How is anterior blepharitis treated?

Anterior blepharitis is inflammation of eye lid margins, usually due to a local infection with *S. aureus*. Local erythromycin ointment is effective therapy. The infection takes weeks to resolve, and the erythromycin has to be used for 2–4 weeks after resolution to prevent relapse.

12. Which of the following infections require systemic antibiotics—sty, chalazion, or dacryocystitis?

A **sty**, or external hordeolum, is an inflammation of the superficial sebaceous glands at the anterior eye lid along the base of the eyelashes. Sties are common in patients with anterior blepharitis. They present as a tender red swelling at the lid margin. They usually resolve with warm soaks. Local antibiotics may also be used. Systemic antibiotics are not needed. If a sty persists, surgical drainage may be needed.

A **chalazion**, or internal hordeolum, is an inflammation of the meibomian glands. Chalazions are common in patients with posterior blepharitis. They present as a tender, red swelling anywhere on the eye lid. They are treated with twice-daily warm soaks, local antibiotics, and possibly systemic antibiotics (cephalexin, doxycycline, or erythromycin).

Dacryocystitis is an infection of the lacrimal sac caused by blockage of the nasolacrimal passage. It is a painful swelling below the medial lower eye lid. It is treated with warm soaks and systemic antibiotics (cephalexin, doxycycline, or erythromycin).

13. What is an Argyll Robertson pupil?

Argyll Robertson pupil is a small, irregular pupil that reacts to accommodation but not to light. It is a manifestation of neurosyphilis. Neurosyphilis can result from untreated congenital syphilis and may present after 2 years of age; it also can develop from 5 to more than 10 years after acquired syphilis. Neurosyphilis includes tabes dorsalis and paresis. Tabes dorsalis presents as wide-based gait with loss of reflexes and loss of position, pain, and temperature sensation in the legs.

14. What is paresis?

PARESIS is a mnemonic for the signs and symptoms of syphilis:

P = Personality (changed; irritable)
A = Affect (changed; flat)
R = Reflexes (increased)
E = Eye (Argyll Robertson pupil)
S = Sensorium (delusions)
I = Intellect (decreased)
S = Speech (changed; slowed)

15. A 5-year-old child presents with conjunctivitis of the left eye and a 2 × 2 cm tender left preauricular lymph node. The child has low grade fever. What pets should you ask about?

This is the classic presentation of Parinaud's oculoglandular fever and is due to *Bartonella henselae*, the agent of cat scratch disease. The child was exposed to multiple cats and kittens. Cats may have *B. henselae* in their blood (asymptomatic chronic infection), and when they scratch themselves, they can get the organism on their claws. Exactly how the organisms get from the cat's claws to the human's eye is not known. They can then infect humans by a scratch or occasionally by eye contamination. The diagnosis is confirmed serologically. In normal hosts, antibiotics, if begun early in the course of infection, may decrease the length of illness. Oral antibiotics with possible efficacy include rifampin, doxycycline, azithromycin, and trimethoprim-sulfamethoxazole.

16. What are the characteristics of the conjunctivitis of Kawasaki's syndrome?

The conjunctivitis of Kawasaki's is characterized by bilateral involvement of the bulbar conjunctiva. The injection is most intense in the periphery with sparing around the limbus. The eye has a clear discharge without exudate. Slit-lamp examination shows anterior uveitis.

17. A 15-year-old adolescent presents with fever and swelling above the medial right eye. This swelling is 4 cm in diameter and elevated by 1 cm. It is nontender and faintly red. Sinus x-rays show frontal sinusitis. What is the diagnosis?

The diagnosis is Pott's puffy tumor, which is a soft tissue swelling or abscess over the frontal sinus. The frontal bone is very thin over the anterior frontal sinus, and infection can break through and present as a painless mass. Pott was an English surgeon who first described this infection in 1760. Pott's puffy tumor requires surgical drainage because central nervous system complications are common.

18. What is uveitis?

The uveal tract consists of the iris, ciliary body, and choroid. Inflammation of the iris and ciliary body defines anterior uveitis (iritis), whereas inflammation of the choroid and retina defines posterior iritis. Multisystemic uveitis is associated with some pulmonary diseases, renal diseases, autoimmune diseases, and infections such as tuberculosis or syphilis. Anterior uveitis also occurs in Kawasaki's syndrome.

19. A 14-year-old girl presents with anterior uveitis. She has a history of severe aphthous stomatitis and genital ulcers. Both oral and genital ulcers sometimes leave scars. What is the likely diagnosis?

Behçet's disease, which is also associated with arthritis and meningitis.

20. A 4-year-old girl has had four episodes of high fever in the past 6 months, with each episode lasting 3–4 weeks. All laboratory studies are normal except the erythrocyte sedimentation rate, which is markedly elevated; she is also anemic. On the second day of fever, the patient develops anterior uveitis. What is the most likely diagnosis?

The likely diagnosis is systemic-onset juvenile rheumatoid arthritis (JRA). Patients with persistent high fevers and no other findings may have systemic-onset JRA. The development of arthritis and/or iritis make the diagnosis of JRA likely.

21. A 17-year-old girl was diagnosed by her gynecologist as having pubic crabs. Treatment with 1% lindane (Quell) cured the infestation. She comes to you because she removed a crab from an eyelash. What is the treatment?

The crab louse (*Phthirus pubis*) has wide-set pinchers that allow it to attach to hair spaced far apart (e.g., pubic hair, eyelashes). The head louse and body louse do not have pinchers and thus usually do not infest pubic hair or eyelashes. Sometimes examining the eyelashes may reveal nits. Treatment is local petrolatum jelly twice daily to smother the remaining lice. If this approach fails a lindane cream can be used on the eyelashes.

22. What are the incubation periods for neonatal conjunctivitis due to *Neisseria gonorrhoeae* or *Chlamydia trachomatis*?

The incubation period for *N. gonorrhoeae* is 1–14 days. Infection presents with a highly purulent conjunctivitis that on Gram stain shows gram-negative diplococci and neutrophils. The incubation period for *C. trachomatis* is 5–20 days. The discharge is usually mucopurulent, and Gram stain may reveal some polyneutrophils without bacteria. *N. gonorrhoeae* is proven by culture. *C. trachomatis* is best proven by tissue culture, which may not be available at all hospitals, or by polymerase chain reaction (PCR). Historically, *C. trachomatis* was diagnosed by Giemsa staining of conjunctival scrapings, which show blue-stained intracytoplasmic inclusions within epithelial cells. Hence the term inclusion conjunctivitis.

23. For newborn ophthalmic prophylaxis, erythromycin ointment and tetracycline ointment are more than 95% effective for preventing *N. gonorrhoeae*. How effective are they for preventing *C. trachomatis*?

In a large study comparing tetracycline ointment, erythromycin ointment, silver nitrate, and no prophylaxis, the incidence of chlamydial conjunctivitis was 1.3%, 1.5%, 1.6%, and 1.4%, respectively. Thus, erythromycin and tetracycline ointments were not effective for preventing *C. trachomatis* conjunctivitis.

24. How common is neonatal *C. trachomatis* conjunctivitis?

Eight to 20% of pregnant women have positive cervical cultures for *C. trachomatis*. The rate of transmission from mother to infant is 20–70%. Thus, more than 1% of infants develop chlamydial conjunctivitis. This rate is reduced by screening pregnant women for chlamydial infection and treating those who are positive.

25. What infections does *C. trachomatis* cause other than inclusion conjunctivitis of the newborn?

C. trachomatis serovars D through M cause pneumonitis of the newborn (in addition to newborn conjunctivitis), inclusion conjunctivitis in adults, nongonococcal urethritis, pelvic inflammatory disease, and proctitis. In addition, *C. trachomatis* serovars A, B, and C cause endemic trachoma of the eye— one of the most frequent causes of blindness in the world but rare in the United States. C. trachomatis serovars L1, L2, and L3 cause lymphogranuloma venereum. Two other important chlamydial species are *C. pneumoniae* (TWAR), which causes a mild respiratory flu-like illness in children and adults, and *C. psittaci*, which causes a potentially severe atypical pneumonia. *C. psittaci* is carried by more than 130 avian species (e.g., parrots, from the Greek word *psittakos*).

26. What is the probable serious diagnosis in a child who wears contact lenses and presents with a painful red eye?

Keratitis or corneal ulceration. These infections are more common with extended-wear lenses. The most common cause is *Pseudomonas aeruginosa*, but any gram-negative or gram-positive bacteria may be the culprit. Fungi or acanthamoeba (a free-living protozoan found in water) may also cause keratitis.

27. A 10-year-old child presents with multiple 2-mm, whitish papules on both eye lids. Examination with magnification reveals that some are umbilicated. What is the diagnosis? Describe the treatment.

The diagnosis is molluscum contagiosum (due to a poxvirus). Unfortunately, the only way to remove the papules from the eyelid is by curettage. They may also resolve spontaneously over time.

28. A 15-year-old adolescent has unilateral conjunctivitis characterized by pain, excessive tearing, injection, and photophobia. After 1 week of erythromycin ointment, it is getting worse. The pediatrician uses fluorescein, suspecting a foreign body. The fluorescein shows dendritic lesions. What is the diagnosis?

This is the classic presentation of herpes simplex keratitis. The pathogenesis of herpes keratitis is poorly understood. A primary herpes simplex infection may be asymptomatic or may cause a nonspecific bulbar and palpebral follicular conjunctivitis. If the skin of the eyelid is involved, typical herpes simplex vesicles are seen. After the primary infection, herpes simplex infection can recur, involving the corneal epithelium (keratitis) or corneal stroma. Herpes simplex keratitis is usually caused by herpes simplex type 1 and most commonly results in dendritic lesions. It is usually treated by an ophthalmologist with local antiviral drops (e.g., trifluridine).

29. A 6-year-old child presents with severe left eye pain, eye redness, and a cluster of blisters on the left side tip of the nose. What is the diagnosis?

This is a description of herpes zoster ophthalmicus (see figure on following page). Zoster involving the first division of the trigeminal nerve may begin with involvement of the forehead, the tip of the nose, or both. Zoster of the forehead is associated with ophthalmic zoster in 40% of patients, whereas zoster of the tip of the nose is associated with ophthalmic zoster in 80%. Manifestations of ophthalmic zoster include eye pain with cicatricial lid retraction, paralytic ptosis, conjunctivitis, keratitis, scleritis, iridocyclitis, retinitis, choroiditis, and optic neuritis. Corneal disease occurs in 66% of cases and includes epithelial ulceration, edema, or white-cell infiltration of the corneal stroma with loss of corneal sensation. Such cases need to be followed by an opthalmologist.

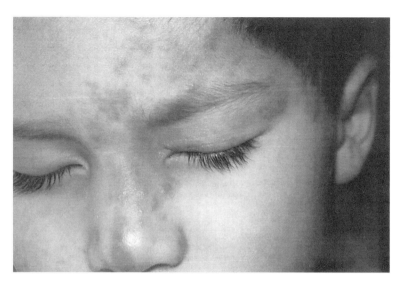

Herpes zoster ophthalmicus.

30. An adolescent boy with congenital toxoplasmosis has developmental delay but is otherwise healthy. He presents with blurry vision in one eye for 2 weeks. Could this be a sign of toxoplasmosis?

Congenital toxoplasmosis usually causes scarring of the retina. Occasionally congenital lesions can be reactivated and may present with blurry vision. The diagnosis can be confirmed by ophthalmologic examination, which shows acute inflammation.

31. A girl presents with fever and right sixth nerve palsy. She is unable to move her right eye laterally. She has had a chronic ear infection on the right and underwent a mastoidectomy 1 month before. An MRI shows petrous osteomyelitis. What is the diagnosis?

The diagnosis is Gradenigo's syndrome, which is sixth nerve (abducens) palsy due to petrous bone osteomyelitis. This is a rare complication of chronic ear infections.

BIBLIOGRAPHY

1. Baum J: Infections of the eye. Clin Infect Dis 21:479–488, 1995.
2. Bienfang PC, Kelly LD, Nicholson DH, Nussenblatt RB: Ophthalmology. N Engl J Med 323:956–963, 1990.
3. Chen J: Prophylaxis of ophthalmia neonatorum. Pediatr Infect Dis J 11:1026–1030, 1992.
4. Gigliotti G, Hendley JO, Morgan J, et al: Efficacy of topical antibiotic therapy in acute conjunctivitis in children. J Pediatr 104:623–628, 1984.
5. Melish ME: Kawasaki syndrome Pediatr Rev 17:153–162, 1996.
6. Trobe JD (ed): The Physician's Guide to Eye Care, 2nd ed. San Francisco, Foundation of the American Academy of Ophthalmology, 2001.
7. Wald ER, Greenberg D, Hoberman A: Short term oral cefixime therapy for treatment of bacterial conjunctivitis. Pediatr Infect Dis J 20:1039–1042, 2001.

III. Lower Respiratory Tract Infections

13. BRONCHIOLITIS, INFLUENZA, AND VIRAL PNEUMONIA

Edina H. Moylett, M.D., and Donough J. O'Donovan, M.D.

BRONCHIOLITIS

1. Define bronchiolitis.
Bronchiolitis is an acute inflammation of the airways, usually resulting from a viral infection, most notably respiratory syncytial virus (RSV), and is a common cause of wheezing in infants. Other terms used to describe bronchiolitis include "wheezy bronchitis" and "asthmatic bronchitis."

2. Name the viral pathogen responsible for most cases of bronchiolitis?
RSV is the leading pathogen isolated from infants with bronchiolitis, accounting for 60% of all cases.

3. List other infective agents causing bronchiolitis.

AGENT	PERCENT OF CASES
Respiratory syncytial virus	45–70
Parainfluenza viruses	
Type 1	8–15
Type 3	5–12
Rhinovirus	3–8
Adenovirus	3–10
Influenza virus	5–8
Mycoplasma pneumoniae	1–7
Enteroviruses	1–5

4. At what age is bronchiolitis most common?
Bronchiolitis is a common illness during the first two years of life, with a peak occurrence between 2 and 10 months of age. RSV infects approximately 50% of children during the first epidemic that they encounter and virtually all of the rest by the second epidemic.

5. Why is bronchiolitis more common during the winter months?
Bronchiolitis has a definite seasonal distribution in temperate climates, with an increase in the number of cases from winter to early spring, reflecting the epidemic nature of its prime agent, RSV.

6. List the epidemiologic risk factors associated with bronchiolitis.
- Passive smoke exposure
- Breast-fed for shorter periods
- Born during the months April through September
- Day-care attendance
- Living in crowded conditions
- More siblings

7. Is bronchiolitis a serious illness?

Although significant morbidity as a consequence of bronchiolitis is uncommon, approximately 2% of infants require hospitalization, and it is the leading cause of pediatric admissions for respiratory illness. Complications associated with bronchiolitis include otitis media (most common), secondary bacterial pneumonia (< 1% of hospitalized cases), apnea, respiratory failure, and bronchiolitis obliterans (very rare and usually associated with adenovirus-induced bronchiolitis/pneumonia).

8. Which infants are at increased risk for severe bronchiolitis?

• Premature infants (< 35 weeks' gestation)
• Infants with chronic lung disease
• Infants with congenital heart disease
• Infants with immunodeficiency disorders

9. List factors that increase of the risk of RSV infection in at-risk infants.

• Passive smoke exposure
• Birth within 6 months before the onset of the RSV season
• Day-care attendance
• School-aged siblings
• Two or more people sharing a bedroom
• Multiple births

10. How is bronchiolitis diagnosed?

Bronchiolitis is a clinical diagnosis. The diagnosis should be suspected in infants who present during the RSV season with the typical clinical features of bronchiolitis and supporting epidemiologic risk factors. The condition is commonly confused with asthma, particularly if it is the infant's first episode.

11. List the major clinical symptoms of bronchiolitis.

• Acute onset of wheezing
• Low-grade, short-lived fever
• Coryza and cough
• Apnea in younger infants
• Signs of lower tract involvement

Tachypnea	Apnea
Tachycardia	Hypoxemia
Irritability, lethargy, anorexia	Cyanosis (rare)

12. What are the major clinical findings in infants with bronchiolitis?

Infants with bronchiolitis demonstrate increased work of breathing, increased respiratory rate, retractions of the chest wall, flaring of the nasal alae, and grunting. Auscultatory findings, which may vary from hour to hour, include wheezing with or without crackles. Increasing dyspnea with decreasing lung sounds on auscultation and diminished movement of air may indicate progressive obstruction and impending respiratory failure.

13. Is apnea common in infants with bronchiolitis?

The incidence of apnea in infants with bronchiolitis is inversely proportional to the infant's age; the youngest infants and infants born prematurely are at greatest risk. Apnea is most often associated with RSV bronchiolitis but may occur in bronchiolitis due to other infective agents (parainfluenza viruses types 1 and 3, rhinovirus, adenovirus, influenza virus, and enterovirus). Severe recurrent apnea often requires mechanical ventilation until the apnea resolves, usually within a few days. The mechanisms leading to apnea in infants with bronchiolitis remain undetermined. Apnea may be the presenting finding in an infant with bronchiolitis.

14. What are the best predictors of the severity of bronchiolitis?

During the initial assessment the oxygen saturation in room air is a good predictor of the severity of bronchiolitis. Oxygen saturation (SaO_2) can be determined by pulse oximetry. SaO_2 < 95% correlates with more severe disease. Additional predictors of more severe illness include:
- Arterial blood gas with partial pressure of oxygen in arterial blood (PaO_2) < 65 mmHg or partial pressure of carbon dioxide in arterial blood ($PaCO_2$) > 40 mmHg
- At-risk infants (prematurity, bronchopulmonary dysplasia, congenital heart disease, or immunodeficiency disorders)
- Infant < 3 months old
- Lethargic and ill-appearing infants

15. Do laboratory tests help establish the diagnosis of bronchiolitis?

No. Routine laboratory tests offer little helpful information in the diagnosis of bronchiolitis. The total white cell count is usually within the normal range but may be elevated; polymorphonuclear predominance is noted in infants with more severe illness.

16. Are viral cultures of benefit in managing infants with bronchiolitis?

Yes. The diagnosis of bronchiolitis is usually established by the typical clinical presentation. However, the specific infective agent can be identified in a large proportion of infants by viral isolation from respiratory secretions, preferably, from a nasal wash. In most cases the viruses associated with bronchiolitis may be identified in tissue culture within 3–5 days. Rapid viral diagnostic tests, especially for RSV, are also available and can identify viral antigens in the respiratory secretions within hours.

17. Describe the typical changes in the chest radiograph of infants with bronchiolitis.

The hallmarks of the chest radiograph in acute bronchiolitis are hyperinflation, hyperlucency of the parenchyma, and decreased costophrenic angles. The bronchovascular markings are usually prominent, with linear densities radiating from the hila. Multiple areas of atelectasis are commonly present and difficult to distinguish from infiltrates of pneumonia. Bronchiolitis and pneumonia often coexist, especially with RSV infection.

18. Should hospitalized infants with bronchiolitis be treated with the antiviral agent ribavirin?

Ribavirin is a synthetic nucleotide that has in vitro antiviral activity against RSV, but ribavirin aerosol treatment for RSV infection is controversial. The high cost, aerosol route of administration, concern about potential toxic effects among exposed health care personnel, and conflicting results of efficacy trials contribute to this controversy. Decisions about ribavirin administration should be based on the particular clinical circumstances and physicians' experience.

Clinical circumstances in which ribavirin administration may be considered include risk for severe or complicated disease, congenital heart disease, cystic fibrosis, immunodeficiency, bronchopulmonary dysplasia, multiple congenital anomalies, and neurologic disease. It also may be considered in infants who are severely ill, as indicated by significant hypoxia, hypercapnia, or mechanical ventilation.

19. Should infants with bronchiolitis be treated with antibiotics?

No—unless there is a secondary bacterial infection.

20. Do bronchodilators have a role in the treatment of infants with bronchiolitis?

Although bronchodilators, mostly beta$_2$ agonists, are frequently used in the management of infants with bronchiolitis, no convincing data support their efficacy. In most young infants with bronchiolitis, the major cause of airway obstruction is inflammation caused by the viral infection rather than smooth muscle contraction. However, some infants with bronchiolitis have a positive response to bronchodilators; therefore, in infants with significant wheezing, a trial of albuterol may be indicated with continuation if a beneficial response is observed.

Kellner JD, et al: Bronchodilators for bronchiolitis. Oxford, Cochrane Library, Issue 4, 2001.

21. Does nebulized racemic epinephrine have a role in the treatment of infants with bronchiolitis?

Although only a small number of studies have addressed this issue, inhaled nebulized racemic epinephrine appears to be clinically effective in infants with acute bronchiolitis. Nebulized epinephrine has been shown to relieve symptoms and reduce hospital admissions in infants with mild-to-moderate bronchiolitis. Whereas epinephrine stimulates both alpha- and beta-adrenoreceptors, it is thought that the alpha-adrenergic properties are important in bronchiolitis, because vasoconstriction of the pulmonary vessels reduces mucosal edema and exudate, thereby reducing airway obstruction.

Menon K, et al: A randomized trial comparing the efficacy of epinephrine with salbutamol in the treatment of acute bronchiolitis. J Pediatr 126:1004-1007, 1995.

22. Discuss the role of corticosteroids in infants with bronchiolitis.

Systemic and inhaled corticosteroids are commonly used in infants with bronchiolitis, but most published studies do not support their efficacy. Some studies, however, have shown that corticosteroids, given orally or parenterally, improve clinical symptoms and reduce length of hospital stay, with the greatest benefit in patients with the most severe clinical course.

Garrison MM, et al: Systemic corticosteroids in infant bronchiolitis: A meta-analysis. Pediatrics 105:44, 2000.

Bulow SM, et al: Prednisolone treatment of respiratory syncytial virus infection: A randomized controlled trial of 147 infants. Pediatrics 104:77, 1999.

23. Should hospitalized infants with bronchiolitis be isolated and cared for with contact precautions?

Prevention is the primary method of defense. Hospitalized infants with bronchiolitis should be isolated. In addition to standard isolation precautions, contact precautions are also recommended for the duration of RSV-associated illness among infants and young children, including patients treated with ribavirin. The effectiveness of these precautions depends on compliance and necessitates scrupulous adherence to good hand-washing practices and use of gloves and gown when entering the patient's room. Patients with laboratory-documented RSV infection can be cared for in the same room.

24. Is there a vaccine to prevent RSV infection?

No.

25. What other immunoprophylaxis strategies are available for RSV infection?

Two forms of prophylactic therapy for RSV are available. RSV-IVIG (RespiGAM) is a high-titer purified immunoglobulin that results in a 41% reduction in hospitalizations due to RSV when given monthly throughout the RSV season; it also results in a significant decrease in the severity in symptoms in high-risk patients who acquire RSV. Palivizumab (Synagis) is a humanized monoclonal antibody formulation, directed against the RSV F protein, which exhibits neutralizing activity. When palivizumab is administered monthly by intramuscular injection, it has been shown to reduce RSV hospitalization by 55%. Both RSV-IVIG and palivizumab are indicated for prophylaxis against RSV disease in at-risk infants.

26. Can RSV-IVIG and palivizumab be used to treat infants with bronchiolitis?

No. However, RSV-IVIG may be considered for treatment of severe disease, especially in immunocompromised patients, in conjunction with ribavirin.

27. What is the association between RSV infection in infancy and recurrent wheezing episodes later in life?

An association between acute bronchiolitis in infancy and recurrent wheezing in later life has been recognized for some time and is supported by long-term follow-up studies. Almost 40% of infants with RSV bronchiolitis develop recurrent episodes of wheezing, particularly if there is a family history of wheezing, in the first year after the illness. Although some studies indicating respiratory RSV infection as a risk factor predisposing to asthma have been published, the relationship between RSV infection in early life and the development of asthma has not yet been fully defined.

INFLUENZA

28. What causes influenza?

Influenza is caused by infection with the influenza virus. The three serotypes of influenza virus, A, B, and C, are based on antigenic variation.

29. What are the differences among the different influenza serotypes?

FEATURE	SEROTYPE A	SEROTYPE B	SEROTYPE C
Host range	Humans, swine, equine, avian, marine mammals	Humans only	Humans and swine
Clinical manifestation	Can cause large pandemics with significant mortality among young people	Severe disease generally among the elderly and high risk, not associated with pandemics	Mild disease

30. When does the influenza virus circulate?

In temperate climates in either hemisphere, epidemics occur almost exclusively in the winter months (generally October to April in the Northern Hemisphere and May to September in the Southern Hemisphere), whereas influenza may be seen year-round in the tropics.

31. Who is most at risk for influenza?

Patients over 65 years old, very young patients, and patients with chronic cardiopulmonary disease. Other high-risk groups include patients with renal dysfunction, metabolic disorders, hemoglobinopathies, immunosuppression, and pregnant women.

32. How does someone become infected with influenza?

Influenza virus is acquired primarily by droplet spread of respiratory secretions (coughing, sneezing, or just talking). A single infected person can spread virus to a large number of susceptible persons. In addition, influenza virus may be spread by direct contact with an infected person or an object recently contaminated with influenza virus.

33. When is an infected patient contagious?

Patients are most infectious for the 24-hour period before clinical symptoms appear and during the most symptomatic period. The duration of the incubation period to the onset of illness and virus shedding ranges from 18 to 72 hours, depending in part on the inoculum size.

34. For how long is influenza virus shed after infection?

Influenza virus is usually shed in nasal secretions for up to 7 days after infection. The duration of viral shedding is longer in young children as well as immunocompromised patients.

35. Which of the following is the hallmark symptom of influenza: cough, sore throat, headache, or fever?

Fever is the hallmark symptom of influenza infection, distinguishing it from other viral respiratory syndromes. Clinical symptoms vary from asymptomatic infection to systemic involvement and death. Classically, 24–48 hours after inoculation, there is an abrupt onset of high-grade fever, myalgia, chills, headache, sore throat, dry cough, and malaise. In children, myalgias are particularly troublesome, and calf muscle myalgia may be a prominent symptom. In addition, cervical adenopathy is more common in children, and "croup" occurs exclusively in pediatric patients.

36. Are infants at risk for influenza infection?
Yes. Healthy children younger than 1 year of age are hospitalized for illness attributable to influenza at rates similar to those for adults at high risk for influenza. The rate of hospitalization decreases markedly with age. Clinical manifestations are nonspecific and include, fever, cough, lethargy, poor feeding, and respiratory distress.

37. What complications are associated with influenza infection?

Pulmonary	Nonpulmonary
Primary influenza pneumonia	Myositis with myoglobulinuria
Secondary bacterial pneumonia	Myocarditis
Tracheobronchitis	Pericarditis
Croup (laryngotracheobronchitis)	Toxic shock syndrome (secondary to
Exacerbation of chronic	*Staphylococcus aureus* infection)
obstructive pulmonary	Guillain Barré syndrome
disease and asthma	Transverse myelitis
	Encephalitis
	Reye's Syndrome

38. List the methods available for diagnosing influenza.
- Virus isolation by inoculation of appropriate cell lines (gold standard)
- Antigen detection on shell vial culture (using specific antibody)
- Detection of virus-specific RNA by reverse transcription DNA polymerase chain reaction (PCR)
- Rapid diagnosis by antigen detection, electroimmunoassay, radioimmunoassay, enzyme-linked immunosorbent assay, and immunofluorescence
- Documentation of a four-fold rise in antibody titer, acute and convalescent samples

39. Are antibiotics helpful in treating influenza?
Antibiotics are not indicated for the treatment of uncomplicated influenza infection. Primary influenza pneumonia is rare. Features of influenza pneumonia include bilateral nonconsolidative pulmonary infiltrates, absence of significant pathogens on sputum Gram stain, and worsening of symptoms soon after initial infection. Secondary bacterial pneumonia usually follows a recovery period of 4–14 days, is relatively common in the elderly population and responds to antibiotic therapy. *Streptococcus pneumoniae* and *Staphylococcus aureus* are the most common causes of secondary bacterial pneumonia.

40. Is it safe to administer steroids to a patient with influenza infection?
Yes. Steroid therapy for the exacerbation of reactive airways disease secondary to influenza infection should not be withheld. Steroids do not affect the course of natural influenza infection. Steroid therapy may be indicated for the rare occurrence of central nervous system complications associated with influenza infection.

41. List the available influenza antiviral therapies.
Amantadine (Symmetrel): active against all strains of influenza A; blocks the uncoating of influenza A virus through interaction with the M2 protein. Amantidine does not undergo metabolism and is excreted unchanged in the urine. No activity against influenza B virus.

Rimantadine (Flumadine): similar mode of action as amantidine. In contrast, rimantidine undergoes extensive metabolism; less than 15% is excreted unchanged in the urine.

Zanamivir (Relenza): a highly selective and potent inhibitor of neuraminidase of both influenza A and B viruses. The drug is not orally bioavailable and is therefore locally administered in nebulized form.

Oseltamivir (Tamiflu): a neuraminidase inhibitor active against influenza A and B; orally bioavailable.

42. What percentage of patients with influenza infection require hospital admission?

Estimated rates of influenza-associated hospitalizations have varied substantially by age group in studies conducted during different influenza epidemics. Among persons 65 years of age or older, hospitalization ranges from 200–1000 per 100,000 population. Among children aged 0–4 years rates have ranged from approximately 500 per 100,000 population for those with high-risk conditions to 100 per 100,000 population for those without high-risk conditions. For all other age groups the average hospitalization rate is 20–40 per 100,000 population for patients without comorbid conditions.

43. List the indications and dosage for influenza antiviral therapies.

Influenza Antiviral Agents

DRUG	INDICATION	DOSAGE
Amantadine	Prophylaxis: Dosing should be started in anticipation of an influenza A outbreak and before or after contact with people with influenza A virus respiratory tract illness. Amantadine should be continued daily for at least 10 days after a known exposure. Treatment: Dosing should be started as soon as possible, preferably within 24–48 hr after onset of signs and symptoms, and should be continued for 24–48 hr after the disappearance of signs and symptoms.	Adults: 200 mg/day (single or divided dose) Children (9–12 yr): 100 mg 2 times/day Children (1–9 yr): 4.4–8.8 mg/kg/day, not to exceed 150 mg (single or divided dose)
Rimantadine	Prophylaxis: as for amantadine. Treatment: as for amantadine. Not licensed for treatment of pediatric patients.	Children < 10 yr: 5 mg/kg/day; maximum = 150 mg Children > 10 yr and adults: 100 mg 2 times/day; reduce to 100 mg/day in elderly patients and patients with severe hepatic or renal impairment Adults: 100 mg 2 times/day; reduce to 100 mg/day in elderly patients and patients with severe hepatic or renal impairment ($Cl_{CR} < 10$ ml/min)
Oseltamivir	Prophylaxis: Oseltamivir is indicated for the prophylaxis of influenza in adult patients and adolescents 13 years and older. Treatment: Oseltamivir is indicated for the treatment of uncomplicated acute illness due to influenza infection in patients older than 4 years who have been symptomatic for no more than 2 days.	Adults and adolescents > 13 yr: 75 mg/day for at least 7 days Adults: 75 mg twice daily for 5 days Children > 1 yr: 15 kg, 30 mg 2 times/day > 15–23 kg, 45 mg 2 times/day > 23–40 kg, 60 mg 2 times/day > 40 kg, 75 mg 2 times/day
Zanamivir	Treatment: Zanamivir is indicated for treatment of uncomplicated acute illness due to influenza A and B virus in adults and pediatric patients 7 years and older who have been symptomatic for no more than 2 days.	Adults and children ≥ 7 yr: 2 inhalations (one 5 mg blister per inhalation for a total dose of 10 mg) twice daily (approximately 12 hr apart) for 5 days

44. What is the flu shot?

Influenza vaccine contains three strains (i.e., two type A and one type B), representing the influenza viruses likely to circulate in the United States in the upcoming winter. The process of selecting particular strains to be included in the vaccine is based on molecular and antigenic analysis of worldwide circulating strains, evaluation of antibody responses to previous vaccines, current epidemiologic trends, and growth characteristics in eggs of candidate strains.

45. What are the indications for influenza immunization?
- Persons 65 years of age or older
- Residents of nursing homes or chronic care facilities
- Adults and children with chronic pulmonary or cardiovascular disorders, including asthma
- Adults and children requiring regular medical follow-up for chronic medical conditions, such as metabolic disease, renal dysfunction, hemoglobinopathies, or immunosuppression.
- Children and adolescents taking long-term aspirin therapy (Reye's syndrome)
- Women who will be in their second or third trimester during the flu season

46. Who should not receive the flu shot?

Inactivated influenza vaccine should not be administered to patients with a history of anaphylaxis to egg protein or other components of the vaccine. In addition, vaccination should be deferred in patients with an acute febrile illness.

47. How is the influenza vaccine dosed?

The dose to be administered depends on age and prior receipt of the vaccine. Vaccine should be administered intramuscularly into the deltoid muscle of adults and the anterolateral aspect of the thigh in younger children and infants.

AGE	PRODUCT	DOSE	NUMBER OF DOSES
6–35 mo	Split virus only*	0.25 ml	1 or 2[†]
3–8 yr	Split virus only*	0.5 ml	1 or 2[†]
9–12 yr	Split virus only*	0.5 ml	1
> 12 yr	Whole or split virus*	0.5 ml	1

* Split-virus vaccines, including subvirion and purified surface-antigen vaccine, are associated with a lower rate of adverse effects in young children only.
[†] Two doses administered at least 1 month apart are recommended for children younger than 9 years who are receiving influenza vaccine for the first time.

48. When is the vaccine administered?

An annual influenza vaccine is given annually. The timing of administration depends on availability. If the vaccine is available, it should be administered in October or November. To avoid missed opportunities, vaccines may be offered as early as September.

49. How effective is the influenza vaccine?

The effectiveness of influenza vaccine depends primarily on the age and immuno-competence of the vaccine recipient and the degree of similarity between the viruses in the vaccine and the viruses in circulation. When the vaccine and circulating viruses are antigenically similar, influenza vaccine prevents influenza illness in approximately 70-90% of healthy persons younger than 65 years.

50. Can people get influenza from the vaccine?

Because the vaccine is inactivated, it does not have the ability to replicate and therefore cannot cause clinical disease.

51. List the two major adverse events associated with influenza immunization.

1. Hypersensitivity reactions, including anaphylaxis, to any component of the vaccine can occur. These reactions are rare.

2. A slight increase in the incidence of Guillain-Barré syndrome (GBS), an already rare disorder, is loosely associated with receipt of influenza vaccines (1 case of GBS per million persons immunized). The benefit of immunization against influenza outweighs the minimal increase in the incidence of GBS associated with influenza immunization.

VIRAL PNEUMONIA

52. Which of the following viruses is most frequently associated with viral pneumonia: parainfluenza virus, respiratory syncytial virus (RSV), adenovirus, or influenza A virus?

The answer is two-fold, depending on the patient population. For pediatric patients, the answer is RSV, which causes 50% of viral pneumonia cases in children younger than 2 years. Parainfluenza virus and influenza A virus are also isolated; adenovirus pneumonia is rare. In adult patients, influenza A virus is the clear answer; parainfluenza and RSV are uncommon pathogens. Adenovirus pneumonia is most commonly diagnosed in military recruits.

53. What clinical features differentiate viral from bacterial pneumonia?

FEATURE	VIRAL PNEUMONIA	BACTERIAL PNEUMONIA
Age	Peak age: 2–3 yr	Any age
Prodrome	Several days of upper respiratory symptoms	Similar clinical prodrome in young children and infants as viral pneumonia; older children may have a brief prodrome with acute onset of high fever and shaking chills
Fever	Present but lower than bacterial pneumonia	Acute onset of high fever
Cough	Present	Present
White cell count and differential	Normal or slightly elevated (< 20,000 cells/mm^3), lymphocytosis	Usually elevated (15,000–40,000 cells mm^3); preponderance of polymorphonuclear cells
ESR/CRP	Normal to slight elevation	Moderate elevation
Radiographic findings	Hyperinflation, diffuse infiltrates, transient lobar infiltrates	Lobar consolidation, often with pleural reaction and effusion/empyema

54. Which of the following radiologic findings is most typical of viral pneumonia: bronchopneumonia, diffuse bilateral reticulonodular pneumonia, lower lobe atelectasis, or normal radiograph?

The typical radiographic findings of viral pneumonia consist of a reticular or reticulonodular pattern that pathologically represents a hemorrhagic pulmonary edema, involving the bronchioles and interlobular septae. Influenza pneumonia can be localized or diffuse, unilateral or bilateral. Varicella pneumonia may present as patchy, bilateral air-space disease. Adenovirus and RSV may manifest as a lobar pneumonia not unlike a bacterial process.

55. Is specific antiviral therapy indicated in the treatment of viral pneumonia?

Yes. Specific therapy is available for the treatment of influenza A and B and RSV. Influenza therapies are reviewed in the section covering influenza virus. Ribavirin (a synthetic analog of guanosine) may be considered for the treatment of RSV in children who have serious underlying disorders; however, its efficacy has not been demonstrated conclusively. The Committee on Infectious Diseases of the American Academy of Pediatrics (AAP) currently recommends consideration of ribavirin for children at high risk for serious RSV disease.

56. Describe the role of steroids in the treatment of viral pneumonia.
There is no indication for steroids in the routine treatment of viral pneumonia. Steroids may aid in the treatment of secondary asthma exacerbation.

57. Are antibiotics of benefit for the treatment of viral pneumonia?
No. The lack of response to antibiotic therapy in the treatment of viral pneumonia is a diagnostic clue to the cause of the infection. Because of the overlap in clinical presentation of viral and bacterial pneumonia, antibiotics are usually initiated as part of therapy. Secondary bacterial pneumonia as a complication of viral pneumonia usually develops after a period of apparent improvement.

58. List the complications associated with viral pneumonia.
- Secondary bacterial pneumonia
- Bronchiolitis obliterans, bronchiectasis, and pulmonary fibrosis secondary to residual airway damage
- Airway plugging with debris, resulting in atelectasis, bronchospasm, and apnea and respiratory arrest
- Adult respiratory distress syndrome
- Chronic lung disease in adults secondary to recurrent viral pneumonia in childhood

59. Which patients are most at risk of developing viral pneumonia?
Viral pneumonia is typically a disease of childhood. In a prospective study of community-acquired pneumonia in adults, 10% were caused by viruses and 40% by bacteria; in 45% of cases, no etiologic agent was identified. Elderly patients, immunocompromised patients, and patients with chronic underlying cardiorespiratory disease are most at risk for developing pneumonia after influenza infection.

BIBLIOGRAPHY

1. American Academy of Pediatrics: Influenza. In Pickering LK (ed): 2000 Red Book: Report of the Committee on Infectious Diseases, 25th ed. Elk Grove Village, IL, American Academy of Pediatrics, 351–359, 2000.
2. American Academy of Pediatrics Committee on Infectious Diseases and Committee on Fetus and Newborn: Prevention of respiratory syncytial virus infections: Indications for the use of palivizumab and update on the use of RSV-IGIV. Pediatrics 102:1211–1216, 1998.
3. Bridges CB: Prevention and control of influenza: Recommendations of the Advisory Committee on Immunization Practices (ACIP). MMWR 50:1–44. 2001.
4. Hall CB: Bronchiolitis. In Mandell GL, Bennett JE, Dolin R (eds): Principles and Practice of Infectious Diseases, 5th ed. New York, Churchill Livingstone, 2000, pp 710–715.
5. Kneyber MCJ: Treatment and prevention of respiratory syncytial virus infection. Eur J Pediatr 159:399–411, 2000.
6. Kneyber MCJ: Long-term effects of respiratory syncytial virus (RSV) bronchiolitis in infants and young children: A quantitative review. Acta Paediatr 89:654–660, 2000.
7. Neuzil KM: The effect of influenza on hospitalizations, outpatient visits, and courses of antibiotics in children. N Engl J Med 342:225–231, 2000.
8. Orenstein DM: Bronchiolitis. In Behrman RE, Kliegman RM, Jenson HB (eds): Nelson Textbook of Pediatrics, 16th ed. Philadelphia, W.B. Saunders, 2000, pp 1285–1287.
9. Panitch HB: Bronchiolitis in infants. Curr Opin Pediatr 13:256–260, 2001.
10. Treanor JJ: Influenza virus. In Mandell GL, Bennett JE, Dolin R (eds): Principles and Practice of Infectious Diseases, 5th ed. New York, Churchill Livingstone, 2000, pp 1824–1849.

14. BACTERIAL PNEUMONIA IN CHILDREN

Aaron S. Chidekel, M.D.

1. What is the working definition of bacterial pneumonia?

Bacterial pneumonia can be considered an inflammation of the lung due to bacterial infection. This infection causes an inflammatory response with resultant consolidation of lung tissues. Possible associated features include involvement of the contiguous pleural space and development of a systemic response.

2. What are the most common causes of community-acquired bacterial pneumonia in children?

Respiratory viruses are the most common causes of lower respiratory tract infections in children, especially those less than 5-years of age, and respiratory syncytial virus is by far the dominant agent. In older children with pneumonia, however, bacterial causes, both typical and atypical, are more common, although most often no specific etiology for pneumonia is found.

The most common causes of pediatric community-acquired pneumonia (CAP) in developed countries have been studied extensively with reasonably consistent findings. *Streptococcus pneumoniae* is responsible for approximately 25–30% of CAP in children. Other commonly reported agents include *Mycoplasma pneumoniae* and the various *Chlamydia* species, most commonly, *C. pneumoniae*. The atypical agents are far more common in children older than 4–5 years, and in most recent studies, *S. aureus* and group A streptococci are infrequent causes of CAP in children. Similarly, *Legionella* species is far less common in children than in adults as a cause of pneumonia.

3. What are the most common causes of bacterial pneumonia among children who require hospitalization?

In the most recent studies of children with CAP who require hospitalization, the most common organism was *S. pneumoniae* (both above and below the age of 2 years). In children less than 2 years of age, *M. pneumoniae* was uncommon; the most common agent isolated in this age group was respiratory syncytial virus. In children older than 2 years, *M. pneumoniae* was more common, and overall viruses were less common. Even in these studies, *Staphyloccocus aureus*, group A streptococci, and *Legionella* species were notably uncommon.

4. What are some common causes of nosocomial bacterial pneumonia?

Few published data address the incidence and causes of nosocomial bacterial pneumonia in hospitalized children. Critical illness, trauma, and mechanical ventilation are important risk factors for nosocomial infection in general, and pneumonia is a common nosocomial infection in some studies. The organisms that are most commonly reported in these studies are *S. aureus*, *Haemophilus influenzae*, *Pseudomonas aeruginosa*, and gram-negative enteric bacteria.

Causes of Community-acquired Pneumonia in Children

Less than 2–3 years of age	
Streptococcus pneumoniae	*Moraxella catarrhalis*
Haemophilus influenzae (nontypable)	*Mycoplasma pneumoniae*
Greater than 3 years of age	
Streptococcus pneumoniae	*Haemophilus influenzae* (nontypable)
Mycoplasma pneumoniae	*Moraxella catarrhalis*
Chlamydia pneumoniae	

Continued. on next page

Causes of Community-acquired Pneumonia in Children (Continued)

Uncommon organisms that require high index of suspicion in patients of any age
Staphyloccocus aureus
Group A streptococci
Legionella pneumophilia

5. **When in the course of hospitalization are you most likely to encounter a nosocomial pneumonia with *Pseudomonas* species: (a) early, (b) late, or (c) never?**

(b) One study of pediatric trauma patients analyzed the causes according to the onset of pneumonia. In infections arising in the first week of hospitalization, the most common organism was *H. influenzae*, whereas infections arising after 1 week of hospitalization were more likely to be caused by *P. aeruginosa* and *Enterobacter* species. Notably, *S. aureus* was an important cause of pneumonia at any time during hospitalization. Not surprisingly, nosocomial pneumonia prolonged hospitalization significantly.

6. **What factors influence the mortality rate of bacterial pneumonia in children?**

In the developed world, the mortality of bacterial pneumonia has decreased dramatically, whereas in the developing world pneumonia remains a leading cause of death among children. Among the factors that have contributed to the decline in mortality include nutrition, hygiene, and access to health care. Other critical factors include the development of vaccines and use of antibiotics. Two of the most important risk factors for mortality in children include the severity of illness on presentation and the presence of a significant underlying medical condition.

7. **What are the major risk factors for acquiring and carrying antibiotic-resistant *S. pneumoniae*?**

Nasopharyngeal colonization with *S. pneumoniae* is common in children; colonization rates are as high as 25% in some cohorts. In fact, drug-resistant pneumococcal infections are far more common in young children than adults. Risk factors for acquiring drug-resistant *S. pneumoniae* include daycare attendance, which appears to most important, and recent or recurrent antibiotic use, especially use of beta-lactam antibiotics. Other factors include recurrent otitis media, young age, and season of the year. Antibiotic-resistant pneumonia is more common in winter than in summer.

8. **What is meant by the term antibiotic-resistant *S. pneumoniae*?**

In general, resistant pneumococci may be considered penicillin-resistant or multidrug-resistant. Organisms that demonstrate multidrug resistance are resistant to several classes of antibiotics. Penicillin resistance in pneumococci may be categorized as intermediate (minimal inhibitory concentration [MIC] ranges between 0.1 and 1 μg/ml) or high-grade (MIC ≥ 2 mg/ml). In general, high-grade resistance to penicillin among strains of pneumococci is more commonly associated with multidrug resistance.

9. **What is the mechanism of penicillin resistance in *S. pneumoniae*?**

Penicillin resistance is due to alterations in the penicillin-binding proteins. Changes in the binding affinities of these proteins causes resistance to the entire beta-lactam class of antimicrobial agents.

10. **Given the emergence of antibiotic-resistant *S. pneumoniae*, is the mortality rate of bacterial pneumonia likely to increase?**

Most studies that have evaluated the outcome of pneumonia caused by intermediately resistance *S. pneumoniae* have been encouraging. They found little or no difference in outcome among patients with sensitive or intermediately resistant pneumococci. The current data do not support the routine use of vancomycin for such patients, and the mortality rate has remained extremely low.

11. Is there any difference in the outcome of pneumonia caused by resistant versus susceptible S. *pneumoniae*?

The most recent data suggest little or no difference in outcome when patients are treated with standard antibiotic regimens. This finding has been dubbed the in vitro vs. in vivo paradox and is thought to be related to the excellent penetration of beta-lactam antibiotics into lung fluid, which overcomes the MICs of most organisms.

12. How should CAP in children be treated?

The management of CAP in children begins with a careful assessment of the severity of illness and underlying health status of the child. Attention to supportive measures such as hydration and fever control is also important. It is impossible to determine a specific cause for most cases of CAP, but good epidemiologic data provide guidance. *S. pneumoniae* is the most common cause of bacterial pneumonia in children, and, in general, atypical pathogens are rare in children under the age of 2 years. In addition, recent studies have shown good efficacy of standard antimicrobial therapy for patients with uncomplicated CAP. Therefore, beta-lactam antibiotics such as amoxicillin, high-dose amoxicillin, and amoxicillin/clavulanate remain the first-line agents along with macrolides such as erythromycin, azithromycin, or clarithromycin for children with beta-lactam sensitivity or older children in whom atypical pathogens such as *Mycoplasma* or *Chlamydia* species are more common.

13. How should hospitalized patients with bacterial pneumonia be treated?

Children with CAP who require hospitalization should be treated with aggressive supportive care and the appropriate antimicrobial therapy. First-line antibiotic choices include second- or third-generation cephalosporins, intravenous penicillin G, or high-dose ampicillin. In older patients, a macrolide may be added. The use of additional agents, such as linezolid or vancomycin, should be individualized; it is not the rule.

14. How should a patient with nosocomial pneumonia or severe underlying disease be treated?

Patients with nosocomial pneumonia need to be supported aggressively because patients with severe underlying illnesses or severe illness on presentation have the highest risk of poor outcome. A careful assessment of risk factors for nonbacterial infections such as fungi is indicated. The appropriate diagnostic studies such as blood and endotracheal tube cultures are important. Broad-spectrum antibiotic therapy with gram-negative coverage and coverage for methicillin-resistant *S. aureus* (MRSA) in certain patients is also important. An extended-spectrum penicillin in combination with an aminoglycoside, ceftazidime, or cefepime and agents such as imipenem and meropenem are reasonable choices. Vancomycin also should be considered to cover MRSA.

Note: The editors strongly suggest an infectious disease consultation for these patients.

Antibiotic Therapy for Pneumonia

Outpatients	
High-dose amoxicillin	Azithromycin
Amoxicillin/clavulanate	Clarithromycin
Erythromycin	
Inpatient community-acquired pneumonia	
Penicillin G	Cefuroxime
Ampicillin	Macrolides
Ceftriaxone	
Nosocomial pneumonia	
Combination antipseudomonal	Cefepime
beta-lactam and	Meropenem
aminoglycoside	Vancomycin (with risk of
Ceftazidime	methicillin-resistant *S. aureus*)

15. Is chest physical therapy helpful in bacterial pneumonia?

No evidence indicates that chest physical therapy is helpful in the management of bacterial pneumonia in an otherwise normal host. Important exceptions to this rule include patients with neuromuscular diseases and other conditions associated with impaired mucociliary clearance, such as cystic fibrosis.

16. Are bronchodilators helpful in bacterial pneumonia?

No evidence supports the routine use of bronchodilator medications in patients with bacterial pneumonia unless clinically indicated.

17. What factors affect the differential diagnosis of pediatric pneumonia?

Epidemiologic factors have an important influence on the differential diagnosis of pediatric pneumonia. Age is an extremely important consideration because neonates, infants, toddlers, and school-aged children represent unique populations in regard to etiologic organisms and host factors. Sociodemographic factors such as nutritional status, daycare attendance, travel, and other exposure risks may alter the differential diagnosis as well. Underlying medical conditions, which may cause or be associated with immunosuppression and other circumstances such as the possibility of hospital-acquired or even ventilator-associated pathogens, also need to be evaluated. Finally, a good working knowledge of community and hospital antibiotic resistance patterns is important.

18. What are some of the signs and symptoms of bacterial pneumonia?

Classic bacterial pneumonia—with high fever, toxicity, respiratory distress, and supporting laboratory data such as leukocytosis and lobar infiltrate—is easily recognized, but it is the exception rather than the rule. An additional scenario that is clinically recognized is the occurrence of viral prodrome, followed by more classic symptoms of acute bacterial pneumonia, which suggests bacterial (most commonly *S. pneumoniae*) superinfection after a viral respiratory infection.

19. What is the most common bacterial pneumonia after influenza?

S. pneumoniae. *S. aureus* also is associated with pneumonia after influenza

20. Many studies have evaluated the various diagnostic signs and symptoms for distinguishing the causes of pediatric pneumonia, both in the developed and developing world. What are the criteria of the World Health Organization (WHO)?

World Health Organization Definitions of Tachypnea and Pneumonia

RESPIRATORY RATE		AGE
> 60		0–2 months
> 50		2–11 months
> 40		1–4 years

CLINICAL SIGNS			DIAGNOSIS	ANTIBIOTIC
COUGH	TACHYPNEA	RETRACTIONS		
Present	Absent	Absent	Upper respiratory infection	No
Present	Present	Absent	Mild pneumonia	Yes
Present	Present	Present	Severe pneumonia	Yes

21. How specific is fever?

Fever is not specific to either bacterial or viral infections.

22. Is cough a reliable indicator of bacterial pneumonia in children?

No. In fact, cough may be absent in many cases.

23. Is wheezing commonly associated with bacterial pneumonia?

No. In general, wheezing is more commonly associated with viral or atypical lower respiratory tract infections than bacterial infections.

24. What about tachypnea?

WHO suggests that tachypnea is the most useful sign for identifying pneumonia in children. Tachypnea describes a pattern of rapid shallow breathing and is a hallmark of lower airway disease. Of importance, tachypnea is inversely correlated with oxygenation. Increasing tachypnea is associated with decreasing oxygenation. Several studies have found that tachypnea alone has the highest (but not perfect) sensitivity and specificity for pneumonia in pediatric patients. Sensitivity and specificity as high as 70% have been reported in some studies.

25. How does one count the respiratory rate in children?

The respiratory rate in a child can be extremely variable and is highly influenced by age, illness, and emotional factors. For example, the respiratory rate in a child can be increased by up to 5 breaths per minute per degree Celsius. Ideally, therefore, respiratory rate should be counted in a quiet, afebrile state for at least 1 minute, and age-specific normative values should be used.

26. Discuss the role of auscultation.

Auscultation in young children can be difficult for several reasons, including the generally uncooperative nature of ill children and the small tidal volumes and relatively low airflow rates, which may mask clinical findings. In a large Finnish study of hospitalized patients with pneumonia (bacterial or viral), rales were present in only 55% of 127 patients classified as having definite pneumonia. Fine rales (crepitations or crackles) were present in only 36% of patients. Crepitations were present in 44% of interstitial and 23% of alveolar pneumonias. Crepitations had a specificity of 78% and a sensitivity of only 36%.

Other signs, such as decreased breath sounds or egophony, are helpful, but their presence is far from the rule in cases of pediatric pneumonia.

27. What should I look for on physical examination?

The combination of fever, tachypnea, and crepitations in a child is highly suggestive of pneumonia. Many authorities believe that this combination of signs and symptoms alone is sufficient to warrant antibiotic therapy, without the need for radiographic or other studies.

28. What are the potential complications of bacterial pneumonia?

A detailed discussion of the complications of bacterial pneumonia is beyond the scope of this chapter. Relevant systemic complications of bacterial pneumonia include bacteremia and septicemia. Thoracic complications include pleural (parapneumonic) effusion and empyema. Pulmonary complications include abscess and/or pneumatocele formation. The management of these complications generally requires a team approach with multiple pediatric specialists, including infectious disease, pulmonology, pediatric surgery, and critical care medicine.

29. How should pneumonia complicated by parapneumonic effusion be managed?

Parapneumonic effusion is present in a significant minority of cases of bacterial pneumonia. It is thought to be present in 30–50% of adults with CAP. Thoracentesis may be indicated in bacterial pneumonia for either diagnostic or therapeutic reasons. The primary purpose of a diagnostic thoracentesis is to attempt to clarify an uncertain diagnosis. A large pleural fluid collection resulting in respiratory distress is an indication for a therapeutic drainage procedure. In patients with severe disease or risk factors for a poor outcome due to age or underlying conditions, parapneumonic effusion should be addressed early and aggressively both for diagnostic and therapeutic reasons.

Recommended Studies for Infectious Parapneumonic Fluid Analysis

White blood cell count and differential
Gram stain
Acid-fast bacillus (AFB) stain
Cultures for bacteria, AFB, and fungi
Total protein, pH, glucose, lactate dehydrogenase

30. Surgeons often perform thoracoscopy for parapneumonic effusions. Is this a reasonable approach?

Thoracoscopy has been shown in some studies to reduce length of hospitalization and speed recovery. Visualization and evacuation of empyemas via thoracoscopy may be useful in severe and complicated cases.

31. What kind of pleural effusion is seen in bacterial pneumonia?

By definition, parapneumonic effusions are due to pleural inflammation or infection (empyema) and are therefore exudative in nature.

32. What is the long-term outcome of bacterial pneumonia complicated by parapneumonic effusion?

In children with bacterial pneumonia complicated by parapneumonic effusion, the prognosis for complete resolution is excellent. Children with parapneumonic empyema have a more difficult time, with longer duration of fevers, toxicity, and hospital stay and require closer follow-up. The management of such patients varies and should be individualized and based on a collaborative approach. Certain children with empyema require chest tube or even video-assisted thoracoscopic drainage to facilitate recovery. However, even in this subgroup of children with severe pleural space disease, the long-term prognosis for complete pulmonary healing is excellent.

BIBLIOGRAPHY

1. Bartlett J, Mundy L: Community-acquired pneumonia. N Engl J Med 333:1618–1624, 1995.
2. Dowell S, Kupronis B, Zell E, Shay D: Mortality from pneumonia in children in the United States, 1939 through 1996. N Engl J Med 342:1399–1407, 2000.
3. Harwell J, Brown R: The drug-resistant pneumococcus: Clinical relevance, therapy and prevention. Chest 117:530–541, 2000.
4. Lerou P: Lower respiratory tract infections in children. Curr Opin Pediatr 13:200–206, 2001.
5. McCracken G: Etiology and treatment of pneumonia. Pediatr Infect Dis J 19:373–377, 2000.
6. McIntosh K: Community-acquired pneumonia in children. N Engl J Med 346:429–437, 2002.
7. Nelson J: Community-acquired pneumonia in children: Guidelines for treatment. Pediatr Infect Dis J 19:251–253, 2000.
8. Patel J, Mollitt D, Pieper P, Tepas JR: Nosocomial pneumonia in the pediatric trauma patient: A single center's experience. Crit Care Med 28:3530–3533, 2000.
9. Schaad U: Antibiotic therapy of childhood pneumonia. Pediatr Pulmonol 18(Suppl):146–149, 1999.
10. Korppi M: Physical signs in childhood pneumonia. Pediatr Infect Dis J 14:48–50, 1995.

15. ATYPICAL PNEUMONIA IN CHILDREN

Aaron S. Chidekel, M.D.

1. Define atypical pneumonia.

Atypical pneumonia can be many things; this nonspecific term refers to a respiratory process that does not have the classic features of bacterial pneumonia. The term implies a broad differential diagnosis, including infectious as well as noninfectious problems, and without further clinical clarification is of limited usefulness.

2. What are the common infectious causes of atypical pneumonia?

Common etiologic agents include atypical bacterial pathogens such as *Mycoplasma pneumoniae*, *Chlamydia pneumoniae*, and *Bordetella pertussis*. Other less common respiratory infections such as psittacosis and fungal infections due to histoplasmosis, blastomycosis or coccidioidomycosis can cause atypical pneumonia. Even tuberculosis can present with atypical pneumonia.

3. What are the noninfectious causes of atypical pneumonia?

No. Other causes of atypical pneumonias include various noninfectious causes of lung injury such as hypersensitivity pneumonitis, toxic pneumonitis, and inflammatory conditions such as sarcoidosis. Finally, although less relevant to pediatrics, the pneumoconioses are also causes of atypical pneumonia.

4. Summarize the differential diagnosis of atypical pneumonia.

Infectious causes	Noninfectious causes
Common	Hypersensitivity pneumonitis (e.g., allergic
M. pneumoniae	bronchopulmonary aspergillosis)
C. pneumoniae	Inflammatory processes (e.g., sarcoidosis)
Bordetella pertussis	Toxic pneumonitis
Respiratory viruses	Pneumoconioses
Less common	
Chlamydia psittaci	
Mycobacterium tuberculosis	
Histoplasma species	
Coccidioides species	

5. Describe the clinical presentation of atypical pneumonia.

In general, atypical pneumonia has a subacute presentation and a more indolent course than classic bacterial pneumonia. A syndrome of mixed upper and lower respiratory symptoms, malaise, fever, and prominent cough is most common. Most patients with atypical pneumonia do not require hospitalization, and it is rare for laboratory values, such as white blood cell count, to be markedly abnormal.

6. Is atypical pneumonia what my grandmother called "walking pneumonia"?

Yes.

7. Who gets atypical pneumonia?

Atypical pneumonia due to respiratory viruses is more common in younger children, whereas atypical pneumonia caused by Mycoplasma and Chlamydia species is most common in school-aged children. Infections with Mycoplasma and Chlamydia species are uncommon before the age of 2-years but become more common after the age of 5 years. Adolescents, college students, and military recruits are also commonly susceptible to atypical infectious pneumonias.

8. Describe the radiographic features of atypical pneumonia.

The radiographic features of atypical pneumonia are variable. Alveolar and/or interstitial infiltrates may be seen. Lobar consolidation and nodular densities are less common. Hilar adenopathy may occur, and pleural effusions are present in up to 30% of cases in some series.

9. What are *Mycoplasma* species?

Mycoplasma species, three of which cause disease in humans (*M. pneumoniae*, *M. hominis*, and *Ureaplasma urealyticum*), are the smallest free-living microorganisms that can survive extracellularly. To cause infection, however, the organism must adhere to and penetrate the respiratory epithelium.

10. Describe the pathogenesis of infection due to *M. pneumoniae*.

M. pneumoniae is spread by droplets from one person to another. It is highly infectious, although most often it causes mild disease. Like *B. pertussis*, *M. pneumoniae* is trophic for the respiratory epithelium, and infection causes damage to the airway epithelium and cilia. It primarily affects the small airways or bronchioles, although interstitial inflammation also may occur. This epithelial-based infection leads to a tracheobronchitis with a prominent and persistent cough.

11. Describe the clinical manifestations of infection with *M. pneumoniae*.

Infection with *M. pneumoniae* has a broad spectrum of manifestations, ranging from asymptomatic carriage or mild upper respiratory tract infections to severe pneumonia. Upper respiratory manifestations include pharyngitis and sinobronchitis. Pulmonary manifestations are also diverse. *M. pneumoniae* infection can cause lobar or interstitial pneumonia and pleural space disease and in rare cases leads to long-term pulmonary sequelae such as bronchiectasis and even bronchiolitis obliterans. *M. pneumoniae* infection also has been linked with extrapulmonary complications. In fact, *M. pneumoniae* has been associated with a broad range of extrapulmonary manifestations and epiphenomena, which remain well described but poorly understood.

Examples of Nonrespiratory Manifestations of M. pneumoniae *Infection*

Musculoskeletal	**Gastrointestinal**
Myalgia	Gastroenteritis
Arthralgia	Hepatitis (elevated liver enzymes)
Arthritis	Hepatosplenomegaly
Dermatologic	**Neurologic**
Erythematous rash	Meningitis/encephalitis
Erythema multiforme	Guillain-Barré syndrome
Stevens-Johnson syndrome	Transverse myelitis
Cardiovascular	Ataxia
Myocarditis	**Hematologic**
Pericarditis	Anemia
	Thrombocytopenia

12. Describe the clinical presentation of atypical pneumonia due to *M. pneumoniae*.

Although infection with *M. pneumoniae* may have an abrupt and acute onset that mirrors bacterial pneumonia, this presentation is by far the exception. In fact, it is thought that only up to 10% of mycoplasmal infections are accompanied by pneumonia. More commonly, *M. pneumoniae* infection begins as an upper respiratory infection that progresses in a subacute fashion to pneumonia. Pharyngitis, myringitis, and sinusitis tend to be the initial manifestations, followed by the development of lower respiratory symptoms. Lower respiratory symptoms include a prominent and troublesome cough, which is mostly nonproductive; wheezing; and chest pain and tightness. Fever and malaise may occur at any time and may be prolonged.

13. True or false: In atypical pneumonias, the clinical symptoms correlate poorly with objective findings on chest radiograph and clinical examination.

True. The radiographic and auscultatory findings are often disparate. The chest x-ray usually suggests a more severe pneumonia.

14. When can you expect to see cases of *M. pneumoniae* infection?

Infection with *M. pneumoniae* occurs throughout the year, although it is most common during the winter months. Hospitalization due to pneumonia caused by *M. pneumoniae* is uncommon, but mycoplasmal infections account for a significant minority of patients who require in-patient management. Mixed infections and *M. pneumoniae* infections in patients with underlying diseases such as sickle cell anemia or even asthma can be far more severe.

15. How is mycoplasmal infection diagnosed?

In general, because of the slow nature of its growth and difficulty in isolating it from respiratory tract secretions, cultures of *M. pneumoniae* are rarely performed in the clinical setting. The diagnosis of *M. pneumoniae* infection is most often serologic; more recently, polymerase chain reaction (PCR) has been used to detect mycoplasmal DNA. The most common serologic tests are enzyme-linked immunosorbent assays for IgM. These tests are useful for the diagnosis of acute mycoplasmal infection and have a reasonable sensitivity and specificity.

16. What about mycoplasmal cold agglutinins?

Cold hemagglutinins are IgM antibodies that agglutinate red blood cells at 4°C. This quick bedside test is performed by placing a small aliquot of blood in a "lavender top" tube containing sodium citrate and chilling it in ice. The tube is tilted and examined for agglutination. Only about 50% of patients with pneumonia due to *M. pneumoniae* develop cold agglutinins. The test is not specific for mycoplasmal infection, however; a variety of infections, including respiratory viruses and infectious mononucleosis, are associated with the presence of cold agglutinins.

17. How is mycoplasmal infection treated?

Because of the characteristics of the organism, beta-lactam antibiotics are ineffective in the treatment of mycoplasmal infections. Macrolide antibiotics are the treatment of choice, but tetracycline antibiotics are also options in older children. Treatment with antibiotics at best shortens the duration of symptoms and may reduce transmissibility. An additional possible advantage of treating community-acquired atypical pneumonia with macrolide antibiotics is that they cover a variety of pathogens, including *Chlamydia* species and even *B. pertussis*.

18. What about pneumonia caused by *Chlamydia* species?

Three species of *Chlamydia* cause infections in humans: *C. trachomatis*, which causes afebrile pneumonia in infants (see Chapter 12); *C. psittaci*, an avian pathogen that can also infect humans; and *C. pneumoniae*, the primary agent in this family that causes respiratory infections in children. *C. pneumoniae* is also called TWAR, although this term is used less commonly at present.

19. Is psittacosis the same as pigeon breeder's (bird-handler's) lung?

Bird-handler's lung is an example of hypersensitivity pneumonitis, whereas psittacosis is a true infectious pneumonia. A common term for psittacosis is "parrot fever," but any bird fancier can be exposed to psittacosis and become ill. In fact, the term parrot fever is misleading because over 130 bird species, including up to 30% of city pigeons, have evidence of *C. psittaci* infection. Diagnosis of *C. psittaci* infection is usually based on an epidemiologic association because its clinical manifestations are similar to those of other atypical pneumonias.

20. What are chlamydiae?

Chlamydiae are obligate intracellular pathogens that are classified as bacteria due to the presence of a cell wall as well as DNA, RNA, and ribosomes. However, they require a host cell to generate adenosine triphosphate (ATP). They exist extracellularly as infectious elementary bodies, which are phagocytosed after attaching to susceptible host cells.

21. Describe the clinical presentation of atypical pneumonia due to *C. pneumoniae*.

In general, pneumonia due to *C. pneumoniae* is even more indolent than that due to viruses or *M. pneumoniae*, but overall the presentations are similar. A subacute illness, beginning primarily with upper respiratory symptoms that progress to the lower respiratory tract, is most commonly reported presentation. A prominent and irritable cough may develop and have a prolonged duration. As with viral or mycoplasmal pneumonia, radiographic and laboratory findings correlate poorly with clinical findings on examination. Hospitalization is rarely needed. Extrapulmonary manifestations have been reported with *C. pneumoniae* infection, but they appear to be less common than with infection due to *M. pneumoniae*.

22. How is infection with *C. pneumoniae* diagnosed?

As with *M. pneumoniae*, infections with *C. pneumoniae* rely on serologic diagnosis because of the characteristics of the organism and the difficulty with culture techniques. IgM serology and PCR are the major diagnostic tests.

23. How is infection with *C. pneumoniae* treated?

Macrolide and tetracycline antibiotics are the treatments of choice. As with mycoplasmal infections, the response to antibiotics is slow and often incomplete. Beta-lactam antibiotics are not effective.

24. How can viral and atypical bacterial pneumonias be distinguished on clinical grounds?

It is nearly impossible to distinguish one cause of atypical pneumonia from another on clinical grounds alone. The table below summarizes the clinical characteristics of college students with atypical pneumonia syndromes due to a known pathogen.

CHARACTERISTIC	C. PNEUMONIAE (n = 14)	M. PNEUMONIAE (n = 17)	VIRAL (n = 17)
Fever	29%	47%	35%
Headache	57%	65%	53%
Cough	100%	94%	100%
Pharyngeal erythema	79%	82%	71%
Abnormal breath sounds	93%	94%	88%
WBC count > 10,000	15%	35%	19%
ESR > 15 mm/hr	85%	88%	56%

WBC = white blood cell, ESR = erythrocyte sedimentation rate.
Adapted from Luby J: Pneumonia caused by *Mycoplasma pneumoniae* infection. Clin Chest Med 12:237–244, 1991.

25. What antibiotics can be used to treat atypical pneumonia?

Macrolide antibiotics are first-line therapy: erythromycin, azithromycin, clarithromycin.
Tetracycline antibiotics are second-line therapy (older children): doxycycline, tetracycline.
Fluoroquinolone antibiotics (ofloxacin, levofloxacin) have activity against *C. pneumoniae* and *C. psittaci* but are not approved for use in children under age 18 years.

26. Is there an association between atypical pneumonia and asthma exacerbations?

Viral respiratory infections are the most important causes of asthma exacerbations in children. Rhinoviruses and respiratory syncytial virus (RSV) are the most important agents in this regard. Growing evidence supports a role for infection with both *M. pneumoniae* and *C. pneumoniae* in children with acute, difficult-to-control wheezing. In one study, antibiotic treatment was important in ameliorating the course of chronic wheezing in children with evidence of infection with *M. pneumoniae* and *C. pneumoniae*.

27. Discuss the role of atypical pathogens in the acute chest syndrome of sickle cell disease.
    Several studies have highlighted the importance of viral and other atypical respiratory infections in patients with acute chest syndrome. Both *M. pneumoniae* and *C. pneumoniae* have been well represented in these studies. It is now a part of standard management of patients with sickle cell disease and acute chest syndrome to add a macrolide antibiotic to cover these important pathogens. In the most recent and largest study of the etiology of acute chest syndrome, isolated infection with *M. pneumoniae*, *C. pneumoniae*, and viruses were found in 6.6%, 7.2%, and 6.4% of cases, respectively. Not surprisingly, RSV was the most commonly isolated virus.

BIBLIOGRAPHY

 1. Esposito S, Blasi F, Fioravanti L, et al: Importance of acute *Mycoplasma pneumoniae* and *Chlamydia pneumoniae* infections in children with wheezing. Eur Respir J 16:1142–1146, 2000.
 2. Esposito S, Blasi F, Bellini F, et al: *Mycoplasma pneumoniae* and *Chlamydia pneumoniae* infections in children with pneumonia. Mowgli Study Group. Eur Respir J 17:241–245, 2001.
 3. Ferwerda A, Moll H, de Groot R: Respiratory tract infections by *Mycoplasma pneumoniae* in children: A review of diagnostic and therapeutic measures. Eur Respir J 160:483–491, 2001.
 4. Gordon R: Community-acquired pneumonia in adolescents. Adolesc Med 11:681–695, 2000.
 5. Hindiyeh M, Carroll K: Laboratory diagnosis of atypical pneumonia. Semin Respir Infect 15:101–113, 2000.
 6. Luby J: Pneumonia caused by *Mycoplasma pneumoniae* infection. Clin Chest Med 12:237–244, 1991.
 7. Mak H: *Mycoplasma pneumoniae* infections. In Hilman B (ed): Pediatric Respiratory Disease: Diagnosis and Treatment. Philadelphia, W.B. Saunders, 1993, pp 282–285.
 8. Principi N, Esposito S, Blasi F, et al: Role of *Mycoplasma pneumoniae* and *Chlamydia pneumoniae* in children with community-acquired lower respiratory tract infections. Clin Infect Dis 32:1281–1289, 2001.
 9. Thom D, Grayston J: Infections with *Chlamydia pneumoniae* strain TWAR. Clin Chest Med 12:245–256, 1991.
10. Vichinski E, Neumayr L, Earles A, et al: Causes and outcomes of the acute chest syndrome in sickle cell disease. N Engl J Med 342:1855–1865, 2000.

16. NEONATAL PNEUMONIA AND PNEUMONIA IN EARLY INFANCY

Aaron S. Chidekel, M.D.

1. Define neonatal pneumonia.

The neonatal period is defined as the period between day 1 and day 28 of life. Pneumonia within this period may be described as neonatal pneumonia. A useful distinction that may guide the differential diagnosis of pneumonia in early life is early-onset newborn pneumonia vs. late-onset newborn pneumonia. In general, early-onset infections are either (1) vertically or transplacentally acquired or (2) nosocomial, whereas late-onset infections are acquired either (1) vertically or (2) in the community. Pneumonias also may be classified as congenital, perinatal, or postnatal, depending on time of acquisition.

2. How common is neonatal pneumonia?

It is estimated to occur in approximately 1% of full-term neonates and up to 10% of preterm neonates.

3. Is neonatal pneumonia a serious problem?

The mortality rate of neonatal pneumonia has remained fairly stable, despite great advances in neonatal intensive care. The mortality rate is highest in premature infants (as high as 50%). Even in full-term infants, the mortality rate may be as high as 20%. Neonatal pneumonia and treatment with oxygen and mechanical ventilation are also important contributors to the development of chronic lung disease in infants (bronchopulmonary dysplasia). In some studies, pulmonary infections such as *Ureaplasma urealyticum* have been linked to an increased risk of bronchopulmonary dysplasia, but other studies have found no similar association.

4. What are some of the noninfectious causes of neonatal respiratory distress?

Respiratory distress syndrome	Cardiac failure or defect
Transient tachypnea of the newborn	Pulmonary hypoplasia
Meconium aspiration syndrome	Diaphragmatic hernia
Pulmonary hemorrhage	Tracheoesophageal fistula
Pneumothorax	Central nervous system defect

5. What factors predispose an infant to neonatal pneumonia?

In general, all infants should be considered immunocompromised hosts, and pulmonary defenses are diminished in neonates as well. Preterm infants are at an even greater disadvantage. Immaturity of several important respiratory defenses, such as mucociliary clearance and cough, and decreased number and activity of pulmonary macrophages place infants at increased risk for severe respiratory infections. Systemic immune functions, including humoral and cell-mediated immunity, also are decreased in newborns; this factor also enhances susceptibility to lung infections.

6. Discuss important risk factors for neonatal pneumonia.

Maternal amnionitis is an important risk factor for early-onset neonatal pneumonia. In fact, early-onset neonatal pneumonia has been termed post-amnionitis pneumonia and most commonly is caused by group B streptococci (GBS) and gram-negative enteric organisms such as *Escherichia coli*. Maternal fever, prolonged rupture of fetal membranes (> 18–24 hours) with or without labor, preterm labor, invasive procedures during labor, and instrumentation of the fetus are also risk factors for neonatal infection. Maternal colonization with GBS is also significant.

All of these factors are important components of any complete neonatal history and should be reviewed in all cases. Other maternal factors, such as nutrition, socioeconomic status, and sexual activity history, are lesser risk factors. These historical features should lead to a high index of suspicion for early-onset pneumonia in an ill neonate.

7. What are the clinical signs of neonatal pneumonia?

One of the most important skills in the care of newborns is differentiating a well neonate from an ill neonate, because symptoms in the neonatal period are nonspecific. Decreased respiratory and systemic reserve in young infants warrants a rapid response to potential infection of any kind. Important respiratory features include signs of respiratory distress, such as dyspnea, tachypnea, grunting, flaring, or retractions. In some ill neonates with pneumonia, however, respiration may be suppressed, leading to apnea or respiratory irregularity. Cyanosis may be present. Nonspecific signs of illness in a newborn include listlessness, poor feeding, and hypo- or hyperthermia. Listen to the nurse who informs you that "the baby is not right or breathing funny."

8. What are the most common causes of neonatal bacterial pneumonia?

The most feared cause of neonatal pneumonia is GBS. Infection is usually severe and associated with a life-threatening sepsis syndrome. Approximately 50% of infants with GBS pneumonia have positive blood cultures, and 30–40% of infants with primary GBS sepsis also have pneumonia. Gram-negative enteric flora also can cause early-onset neonatal pneumonia but may be acquired nosocomially in hospitalized infants after the first week in the nursery. In select cases, *Listeria monocytogenes* can cause early-onset pneumonia in association with a sepsis syndrome.

9. How is neonatal pneumonia diagnosed?

The history and clinical examination remain the most important tools in making the diagnosing of any neonatal infection. Chest radiographic features such as bilateral airspace (alveolar) disease with air bronchograms are important but nonspecific indicators of pneumonia. Noninfectious causes of respiratory distress may be superimposed on or mimic infectious pneumonia in a newborn. A compete sepsis evaluation with cultures of blood, urine, cerebrospinal fluid, and tracheal aspirates is indicated, as are general hematologic, metabolic, and blood gas studies.

10. How is neonatal pneumonia treated?

Severe, early-onset pneumonia is a life-threatening emergency usually associated with a sepsis syndrome and respiratory failure. Major organ systems must be supported in a neonatal intensive care unit. Antibiotic choices for early-onset pneumonia are generally straightforward and include ampicillin and gentamicin. Cefotaxime may be added as well. In appropriate patients with risk factors for methicillin-resistant *Staphylococcus aureus*, vancomycin also should be considered. In some cases, coverage for nosocomial fungal pneumonia due to *Candida albicans* is necessary, especially in a preterm infant who has been in the special care nursery for a prolonged time.

11. Define congenital pneumonia.

Congenital pneumonia occurs when an infected mother transmits an organism to the fetus hematogenously across the placenta. Infants with congenital pneumonia usually have manifestations of a generalized congenital infection, such as microcephaly and hepatosplenomegaly; in fact, congenital pneumonia is generally a rare manifestation of congenital infections. In rare cases, it has been reported in association with cytomegalovirus and congenital rubella. Congenital tuberculosis is also uncommon, as is infection with *L. monocytogenes*. *Ureaplasma urealyticum* also has been associated with acute congenital pneumonia and, in some studies, with the development of bronchopulmonary dysplasia.

12. What is pneumonia alba?

Pneumonia associated with congenital syphilis.

13. What are the most common viral causes of perinatal pneumonia?

The most common cause of severe viral pneumonia is herpes simplex virus (HSV). The most common source of the virus is maternal cervical infection, which may be asymptomatic; the infant acquires the infection during birth. HSV pneumonitis occurs in approximately 40% of disseminated infections, and the fatality rate of severe infections is as high as 10–15%. Enteroviruses also can cause neonatal pneumonia, but infections are generally much less severe.

14. How common is community-acquired viral pneumonia in neonates?

Young infants are highly susceptible to respiratory tract infections with typical viral pathogens. Risk factors include the presence of siblings or another ill person in the home, exposure to environmental tobacco smoke, and season of hospital discharge or birth. Common causes include respiratory syncytial virus (RSV), rhinovirus, adenovirus, parainfluenza virus, and even enterovirus. Illnesses may range form mild to severe, and clinical manifestations may include respiratory as well as nonrespiratory signs. Tachypnea, cough, cyanosis, and signs of respiratory distress are the most common respiratory manifestations, but systemic features such as poor feeding, altered mental status, and even sepsis syndrome may occur. Apnea and bradycardia are also well-recognized manifestations of respiratory viral infection in young infants. RSV is classically associated with apnea and bradycardia, but many viruses may cause the same symptoms.

15. What are the characteristics of chlamydial infection in early infancy?

Infants actually acquire *Chlamydia trachomatis* vertically at the time of birth. The organism colonizes the respiratory tract and causes a distinctive pneumonia syndrome, which classically occurs between 2 and 12 weeks of age. Classic manifestations include chronic, afebrile respiratory illness that may be associated with conjunctivitis and otitis. Peripheral blood eosinophilia is also classically described. Pathophysiologically, *C. trachomatis* infection is an interstitial pneumonitis and may mimic bronchiolitis with a staccato cough and even wheezing.

16. Can *Bordetella pertussis* cause pneumonia in young infants?

Yes—although the most common manifestation of infection with *B. pertussis* is necrotizing tracheobronchitis. A young infant with *B. pertussis* infection may not have the ability to generate the respiratory force to whoop; therefore, classic whooping cough is not always present in neonates.

17. What are the most common bacterial causes of early-onset neonatal pneumonia?

GBS

Gram-negative enteric bacteria: *E. coli, Klebsiella pneumoniae*

L. monocytogenes

Nosocomial pathogens: *Pseudomonas aeruginosa, K. pneumoniae, Serratia marcescens, Enterobacter faecalis*, methicillin-resistant *S. aureus*, and *C. albicans*

18. What are the common causes of bacterial pneumonia in early infancy (1-4 months)?

C. trachomatis, S. pneumoniae, B. pertussis, and *S. aureus*.

19. Which antibiotics are appropriate treatments for neonatal bacterial and viral pneumonia?

Bacterial pneumonia	Viral pneumonia
Ampicillin	Acyclovir
Gentamicin	Ribavirin
Consider cefotaxime, vancomycin	

BIBLIOGRAPHY

1. Abzug M, Beam A, Gyorkos E, Levin M: Viral pneumonia in the first month of life. Pediatr Infect Dis J 9:881–885, 1990.
2. Beem M, Saxon E: Respiratory-tract colonization and a distinctive pneumonia syndrome in infants infected with *Chlamydia trachomatis*. N Engl J Med 296:306–310, 1977.

3. Bocchini J: The Chlamydiae. In Hilman B (ed): Pediatric Respiratory Disease: Diagnosis and Treatment. Philadelphia, W.B. Saunders, 1993, pp 266–271.
4. Campbell J: Neonatal pneumonia. Semin Respir Infect 11(3):155–162, 1996.
5. Da Silva O, Gregson D, Hammerberg O: Role of *Ureaplasma urealyticum* and *Chlamydia trachomatis* in development of bronchopulmonary dysplasia in very low birth weight infants. Pediatr Infect Dis J 16:364–369, 1997.
6. Jain S: Perinatally acquired *Chlamydia trachomatis* associated morbidity in young infants. J Matern Fetal Med 8(3):130–133, 1999.
7. Lyon A: Chronic lung disease of prematurity: The role of intra-uterine infection. Eur J Pediatr 159:798–802, 2000.
8. Thom D, Grayston J: Infections with *Chlamydia pneumoniae* strain TWAR. Clin Chest Med 12:245–256, 1991.
9. Tipple M, Beem M, Saxon E: Clinical characteristics of the afebrile pneumonia associated with *Chlamydia trachomatis* infection in infants less than 6 months of age. Pediatrics 63:192–197, 1979.
10. Whitsett J, Pryhuber G, Rice W, et al: Acute respiratory disorders. In Avery G, Fletcher M;, MacDonald M (eds): Neonatology: Pathophysiology and Management of the Newborn. Philadelphia, J.B. Lippincott, 1994, pp 429–452.

17. PULMONARY ASPIRATION SYNDROMES

Aaron S. Chidekel, M.D.

1. Define pulmonary aspiration.

Pulmonary aspiration involves the penetration of foreign material into the lower respiratory tract and tracheobronchial tree. A variety of airway defense mechanisms are in place to prevent pulmonary aspiration, beginning with a functional swallow and intact mucociliary escalator nd cough reflex. When these defenses are dysfunctional or overwhelmed, an aspiration syndrome may result.

2. Is aspiration a common event?

Aspiration is a common event in both normal and abnormal hosts. For example, normal adults commonly aspirate saliva and even food particles during sleep, and there is no reason to believe that children differ in this regard. This low-volume phenomenon rarely causes problems in otherwise normal hosts with intact pulmonary defenses. Aspiration or laryngeal penetration also may occur during eating or drinking, but the presence of an effective cough generally clears the offending agent without incident.

3. Give examples of pulmonary aspiration syndromes in pediatrics.

The best recognized example is the inhalation of a large foreign object into the main airway with resultant airway obstruction. Smaller particulate material also may be aspirated, either acutely or chronically, and produce tracheobronchitis, pneumonitis, and/or small airway disease, which may masquerade as or complicate asthma. Toxic substances may be inhaled, such as volatile liquids, and cause chemical pneumonitis; gastric acid also causes chemical pneumonitis. Oropharyngeal aspiration of infected secretions can lead to acute bacterial pneumonia or even lung abscess.

4. What is the triple threat of pulmonary aspiration?

Chemical pneumonitis, bacterial pneumonia, and airway obstruction.

5. Discuss the role of gastric acid in aspiration pneumonia.

Aspiration of gastric acid causes chemical pneumonitis, the severity of which is related to pH. The lower the pH, the more severe the injury. Gastric acid causes direct airway injury and induces an inflammatory response. This pneumonitis is clinically distinct from bacterial pneumonia. It has a more rapid onset than an infection; fever is generally absent; and lung injury is more diffuse and severe, resulting in worsened respiratory distress and hypoxia.

6. What other important features of the aspirate contribute to lung injury?

The frequency, quantity, and nature of the aspirate are important. The pH is critical. Other important features include volume, presence of foreign material or food, and high concentrations of bacteria.

7. What are the common risk factors for aspiration in infants and children?

Anatomic	Neuromuscular
Tracheoesophageal fistula	Swallowing immaturity and fatigue
Laryngeal cleft	Laryngeal/pharyngeal paralysis
Tracheostomy, endotracheal or nasogastric tube	Myopathies (congenital or acquired)
Craniofacial syndromes (e.g., Pierre-Robin syndrome, cleft lip or palate)	Cerebral palsy
	Altered consciousness/seizures
	Central nervous system abnormalities

Functional	**Pica**
Gastrointestinal dysmotility (gastroesophageal reflux/achalasia)	Foreign body aspiration
	Volatile liquid aspiration
Sinobronchitis	
Poor dentition	

8. Describe the symptoms of pediatric aspiration.

The symptoms of acute foreign body aspiration are self-evident. Choking and gagging, followed by severe coughing, are classically reported. The association of these symptoms is particularly important if the child was eating nuts, seeds, beans, or carrots or if the child was playing with a toy with small parts. A large object may lodge in the larynx or main trachea and cause significant, if not complete, airway obstruction. Airway obstruction may cause asphyxia and death. A smaller object passes more distally and causes symptoms such as focal wheezing and other less specific symptoms (e.g., stridor, hoarseness, congestion, cough). Fever may result from infection or reaction to the foreign body. The symptoms of chronic aspiration may be much more subtle and nonspecific. Examples range from apnea to chronic cough, congestion, and wheeze. An association with feedings is helpful but not always present. Chronic aspiration may be silent, because the laryngeal and pharyngeal receptors become insensitive to injury over time.

9. Discuss the role of gastroesophageal reflux.

Gastroesophageal reflux (GER) is an extremely important potential contributor to aspiration syndromes in pediatrics. GER is often a comorbidity in patients with chronic respiratory symptoms, and a high index of suspicion and aggressive evaluation and treatment are important. In addition to GER, dysphagia also may be an important contributor to lower respiratory symptoms.

10. List the possible respiratory consequences of GER.

- Chronic cough
- Wheezing
- Reactive airway disease/asthma
- Choking spells
- Stridor
- Apnea
- Aspiration pneumonia
- Lung abscess

11. What is the role of infection in aspiration syndromes?

Infection can play a significant role in the morbidity associated with aspiration. Many patients do not develop infection after aspiration. It is often difficult to determine the contribution of infection to the severity of disease related to the aspiration event. Hospitalized patients and patients with serious underlying illness, however, may develop oropharyngeal colonization with gram-negative hospital-acquired pathogens such as *Pseudomonas aeruginosa* and *Staphylococcus aureus* and develop a mixed aerobic-anaerobic infection.

12. List the infectious complications of aspiration.

- Tracheobronchitis (acute or chronic)
- Lobar pneumonia
- Multilobar pneumonia (Often in dependent segments)
- Necrotizing pneumonia
- Lung abscess

13. Which common bacteria are most commonly implicated in aspiration syndromes?

Anaerobes	**Aerobes**
Peptostreptococcus species	*Streptococcus pneumoniae*
Bacteroides melaninogenicus	*S. aureus*
Fusobacterium nucleatum	Gram-negative enteric organisms (usually hospital-acquired)

14. How is aspiration pneumonia treated?

Antibiotic choices for community-acquired aspiration pneumonia center on coverage for anaerobic bacteria and oropharyngeal flora. Penicillin, clindamycin, and ampicillin-sulbactam are potential options. In patients with underlying illnesses and risk factors for hospital-acquired infections, additional coverage for these organisms can be achieved with an extended-spectrum penicillin such as ticarcillin.

15. What antibiotics can be used to treat aspiration pneumonia with infection?

Treatment of infection in the setting of aspiration pneumonia is complicated and depends on the type of patient and potential risk factors.

16. Define choking.

Choking is the interruption of respiration by internal obstruction of the airway. This event leads to oxygen deprivation and death if not rapidly and effectively addressed. In young children, food and toys are the most common objects involved with accidental choking episodes. Objects that are small, round, and endowed with a pliable texture that allows them to conform to the shape of the airway or to adhere to the airway mucosa represent the greatest hazard. If the plug cannot be dislodged in a timely fashion because of lack of response by a supervising adult or the characteristics of the object, death will ultimately ensue from asphyxiation.

17. How common is choking?

In children aged 0–4 years, the death rate from unintentional suffocation, which includes aspiration or ingestion of foods, was approximately 2.96 per 100,000 between 1981 and 1998. This rate declined, by nearly a factor of 10, to 0.36 per 100,000 for children aged 5–9 years during the same period. Males have a higher risk of choking than females. Choking remains a major cause of preventable death and morbidity in the United States, although efforts by the federal government and public health community have made some progress in decreasing its occurrence.

18. Discuss risk factors for choking.

Choking results from a complex interaction among the victim, the environment, and the object involved. Young children with incompletely developed dentition and oral skills, smaller airways, immature swallowing mechanisms, and lack of experience and cognition are at highest risk of choking. Environmental factors such as distractions and lack of supervision are important, as are the circumstances surrounding meals and snacks. Meals and snacks should be a slow and steady process that is carefully supervised. Common choking hazards have been well studied and characterized. The following foods are present dangers to young, inexperienced children: hot dogs and sausages, chunks of meat, grapes, hard candy, popcorn, peanuts, raw carrots, and apples. Among toys, the most common choking hazards include balloons, small balls and marbles, toys with small parts, and small household items such as jewelry and watch batteries.

BIBLIOGRAPHY

1. Colombo J: Pulmonary aspiration. In Hilman B (ed): Pediatric Respiratory Disease: Diagnosis and Treatment. Philadelphia, W.B. Saunders, 1993.
2. DePaso W: Aspiration pneumonia. Clin Chest Med 12:269–284, 1991.
3. Herbst J, Hilman B: Gastroesophageal reflux and respiratory sequelae. In Hilman B (ed): Pediatric Respiratory Disease: Diagnosis and Treatment. Philadelphia, W.B. Saunders, 1993.
4. Kirsch C, Sanders A: Aspiration pneumonia: Medical management. Otolaryngol Clin North Am 21:677–689, 1988.
5. Reilly J, Cook S, Stool D, Rider G: Prevention and management of aerodigestive foreign body injuries in childhood. Pediatr Clin North Am 43:1403–1411, 1996.
6. Tarrago S: Prevention of choking, strangulation and suffocation in childhood. Wisc Med J 99(9):43–46, 2000.

18. TUBERCULOSIS

Aaron S. Chidekel, MD

1. How is tuberculosis spread?

Tuberculosis (TB) is transmitted from person to person by droplet nuclei. The tubercle bacillus is approximately 3–5 microns in size, which is ideal for airborne transmission and lung deposition. Young children (under the age of roughly 10–12 years) with primary pulmonary TB are rarely infectious; they contract the disease from adults around them.

2. How common is TB in children?

TB remains a major public health challenge worldwide. Particularly in the developing world, TB is extremely common; it is estimated that there are over 1 million new cases and approximately 450,000 deaths from TB each year among children less than age 15 years. In the United States, TB among children is much less common and occurs within specific at-risk groups. In 1994, for example, the case rate of TB in children was 2.85/100,000, but it is critical to note that 23% of these cases occurred in foreign-born children. In addition there is a higher case rate of TB among children with HIV and those less than 2 years of age.

3. Is it easy to catch TB?

Transmission of TB occurs when droplet nuclei are expectorated by one person and inhaled by another. Because of their small size, droplet nuclei may remain suspended in the air for hours. In addition to the physical factors of the environment (e.g., ventilation, proximity), the duration of exposure is important as well. In general, transmission requires between 4 and 8 hours of exposure; therefore, casual contact is not generally implicated.

4. How does this pattern of transmission affect hospital infection control procedures?

Not all children with TB, even pulmonary TB, require isolation, and institutional policies vary among children's hospitals. However, patients with TB who are isolated must be placed under airborne precautions until their infectious status is determined. A negative-pressure room is recommended, and the use of the appropriate mask or respirator is also necessary. Adult contacts also should wear masks in the hospital until the results of their skin tests and, if necessary, chest radiographs are available.

5. What is a Mantoux test?

The Mantoux test is the gold standard for both screening and diagnosing TB. Screening and diagnosis are major epidemiologic challenges, and the prior probability of infection should be considered in testing for TB. The Mantoux test involves the intradermal injection of a known quantity (5 tuberculin units) of antigen, and the technique of administration is extremely important, requiring practice. The tuberculin solution should result in an elevated wheal at the site of injection. TB is somewhat unique in that the same test (Mantoux) used for screening is used for diagnosis. Therefore, mass screening in populations at low risk for TB results in an increased number of false-positive results and a small number of true cases of TB.

6. Who should receive a skin test for TB?

The American Academy of Pediatrics does not recommend routine skin testing for all children. Only children at increased risk of acquiring TB should be tested. Indications for skin testing in children include the following:

Immediate skin testing
Symptomatic children
Contacts of known or suspected cases

Children with family members or contacts who have been incarcerated in the past 5 years

Children emigrating from or traveling to endemic regions and children with contacts from endemic regions

Annual skin testing

Children with HIV or living with HIV-infected people

Incarcerated adolescents

Children who should be tested every 2–3 years

Children exposed to high-risk contacts: HIV-infected people, homeless people, nursing home residents, institutionalized or incarcerated people, migrant farm workers

Children in whom skin testing should be considered at age 4–6 and 11–16 years

Children of immigrants or with either travel to endemic regions or exposure to people from endemic regions

Children residing in high-risk communities

7. Which children should have multipuncture (tine) TB tests?

Multipuncture tests are no longer recommended for any child.

8. What constitutes a positive purified protein derivative (PPD) test?

A PPD must be interpreted by a knowledgeable health care professional who can measure the induration in millimeters 48–72 hours after placement of the PPD. Skin test placement technique is critical because improper administration can result in false-negative results. The Mantoux skin test is the standard method and involves the intradermal injection of 5 tuberculin units in a volume 0.1 ml onto the volar aspect of the forearm. The induration needs to be measured at its widest point and recorded in millimeters (mm), not as "positive" or "negative." Many TB experts recommend using a ballpoint pen to aid in detecting and measuring induration.

9. How does the size of induration affect the interpretation of the test?

The skin test is interpreted as positive based on the clinical situation as described in the following guidelines:

Induration in mm

≥ 5 mm

Recent contacts

Immunocompromised host

≥ 10 mm

Children under 4 years of age

Children with risk factors (exposed to high-risk adults)

Foreign-born children from high prevalence country

Residents and employees in high-risk settings (includes health care workers)

IV drug users

Certain medical conditions (e.g., diabetes mellitus)

≥ 15 mm

Children with no known risk factors

Note: Positive tests also may result from atypical mycobacterial infection or previous vaccination with bacille Calmette-Guérin (BCG).

10. What factors may result in a false-negative PPD?

- Early TB infection
- Improper administration
- Improper interpretation
- Defective tuberculin
- Recent live virus vaccination with the measles vaccine
- Immunosuppression
- Age
- Severe stress or underlying illness

11. How is the PPD result interpreted in a person who has received BCG?

History of vaccination with BCG is not a contraindication for Mantoux skin testing for tuberculosis. BCG does not prevent TB infection, but it is most effective in preventing disseminated disease in very young children. Previous vaccination with BCG may result in false-positive results, but the BCG rarely causes an induration > 10 mm. The skin test should be interpreted based on the presence of risk factors, and any induration > 15 mm suggests that TB infection probably is present and requires further evaluation.

12. What if the child has a big red reaction?

Erythema must be differentiated from induration. Erythema does not constitute a positive reaction and should not be measured.

13. So what is an induration?

The pathophysiology of TB involves the activation of cell-mediated immunity. When a person who has been exposed to TB receives a Mantoux test, the antigen injected into the skin incites an immune response. This delayed-hypersensitivity reaction results in a positive response. Induration is identified as a hardened area in the skin due to the presence of white blood cells responding to antigen challenge.

14. Are "anergy panels" recommended in addition to a PPD, just to be sure?

No.

15. Why not simply have the family call me in 2-3 days if there is any change in the area of PPD placement?

Numerous studies have shown that parental reading of tuberculin skin tests is highly unreliable. The PPD must be evaluated by a trained health care professional.

16. What makes an adult or adolescent a member of a high-risk population?

Membership in the following categories increase the risk of contracting TB and should be included in the assessment of any child's risk for acquiring TB:

Household member with AIDS/HIV

Household member who uses intravenous or other illegal drugs

Household member who has worked in or been in prison in the past 5 years

Household member who has lived in a homeless shelter

Household member who has lived or worked in a long-term care facility

Household member who is foreign-born or has lived outside the United States

17. What are the three stages of TB?

Exposure, infection, and disease. This classification is useful because it guides both evaluation and therapy of a particular patient. For example, it is impossible to determine whether an exposed person will develop TB infection, but clinical monitoring and, in some cases, prophylaxis are recommended. A person who is infected with TB or has a positive skin test needs to be carefully evaluated for disease and treated accordingly. In a person with TB disease the appropriate therapeutic regimen must be arranged. In all cases, evaluation of possible contacts is required.

18. Which children should receive postexposure TB prophylaxis?

Infants and young children, children who are exposed to multiple drug-resistant TB, and immunosuppressed patients require postexposure prophylaxis, most often with isoniazid.

19. What is meant by tuberculosis infection?

When a person has a positive skin test for TB but no evidence of symptoms or laboratory or chest radiographic abnormality, infection is present. This scenario is also called latent tuberculosis infection. TB infection in childhood is treated with chemoprophylaxis, most often isoniazid, to prevent the progression to tuberculosis disease.

20. How is TB infection treated?

Isoniazid is the drug of choice for the treatment of patients with positive tuberculin skin tests. Daily therapy for 9 months is recommended. If isoniazid-resistant tuberculosis is suspected, rifampin is given daily for 6 months. If the patient has HIV, the period of treatment is extended up to 12 months.

21. What is meant by tuberculosis disease?

Tuberculosis disease is defined simply as the presence of symptoms and signs of TB. Examples include pulmonary or radiographic features and/or systemic manifestations.

22. Should every child with a positive PPD have a chest radiograph?

Yes. It is absolutely essential to evaluate every child with a positive tuberculin skin test for pulmonary disease. In some studies, up to 50% of children with primary pulmonary tuberculosis are asymptomatic despite the presence of extensive pulmonary involvement, which may not be evident on auscultation of the chest. It is particularly important to obtain both posterior-anterior and lateral views to evaluate fully for the presence of infiltrates and hilar adenopathy.

23. What should I expect to see on a chest radiograph in a child with primary TB?

Unlike adults, children with TB rarely develop cavitary disease. This is another reason that children are rarely infectious. Also unlike adults, children with TB may have disease in any lobe of the lung. The most common radiographic features include hilar or paratracheal lymphadenopathy, with or without an alveolar infiltrate. Miliary TB appears as a diffuse, micronodular pattern, which is evenly distributed throughout the lungs. Other findings may include atelectasis due to airway compression by an enlarged lymph node or even pleural effusion with or without a parenchymal infiltrate. The role of chest computed tomography (CT) in the evaluation of children with TB is evolving; CT may be considered in certain cases.

24. Describe the symptoms of primary TB disease in children.

Primary TB in children is often asymptomatic (50% of cases);therefore, a high index of suspicion may be required. Disseminated TB disease is uncommon, occurring in less than 5% of cases. Nonetheless, a thorough and careful multisystem evaluation is indicated. Infants are much more likely to have clinical symptoms of tuberculosis (80% of cases). In children, the most common presenting symptoms are fever and chronic cough. Children rarely have sputum production or hemoptysis. Constitutional symptoms, such as weight loss, decreased appetite, night sweats, and weakness, are possible. In infants, cough, fever, decreased appetite or weight loss, and focal findings on chest examination are the most common symptoms. TB meningitis is also possible in cases of disseminated disease and is fatal if not treated. TB meningitis presents with the typical symptoms of meningitis but is usually less acute than classic bacterial meningitis; it also may present with seizures and decreased consciousness.

25. What are the classic cerebrospinal fluid (CSF) characteristics of tuberculous meningitis?

The most commonly reported CSF findings in cases of TB meningitis include mild-to-moderate CSF pleocytosis, usually in the range of 10–500 WBC. Lymphocytes are the predominant cell type. Very high protein and low glucose levels are found. Acid-fast bacillus (AFB) smears and even cultures are usually negative because usually very few organisms are present in the CSF.

26. How can lymphadenitis due to tuberculosis be differentiated from other causes of lymph node infections?

Lymphadenitis is the second most common form of TB disease in children. Physical examination alone is insufficient to distinguish tuberculous lymphadenitis from bacterial or atypical mycobacterial infections. The lymph nodes are usually painless, firm, and discrete, but they may become fluctuant. Careful evaluation with attention to the clinical history, exposure risk, and complete differential diagnosis of lymphadenitis is therefore necessary. Even in cases of atypical mycobacterial infection, the tuberculin skin test may be reactive with 5–15 mm of induration. An induration > 15 mm is always attributed to *Mycobacterium tuberculosis*. When the cause of the lymphadenitis is unclear, excisional biopsy and culture may be necessary.

27. What is the preferred method for recovering *M. tuberculosis* from children?

Specimens are generally collected by gastric aspiration in children because they can rarely produce sputum, even with induction. Collecting gastric aspirates in the early morning allows the overnight accumulation of pulmonary secretions that are cleared via the mucociliary escalator, thereby increasing the yield.

28. When can children with TB infection return to school?

Children with primary TB are rarely infectious to others. A child who is a skin test converter needs to be evaluated for TB disease. If this evaluation is negative, the child may return to school immediately.

29. Why are children with TB rarely contagious to others?

Children rarely have cavitary disease or laryngeal TB, which can be highly contagious. Children with TB who are under the age of 10–12 years usually cannot expectorate AFB and, compared with adults with TB, harbor fewer organisms. These factors decrease the likelihood that any given child with TB is infectious and highlight the notion that children contract TB from adult contacts.

30. How do I know if an adolescent or adult with TB is infectious?

Hospitalized children under the age of 10–12 years rarely require isolation. Adult family members are more likely to be contagious. TB disease in adolescents, however, is more closely related to TB among adults; therefore, adolescents are much more likely to be infectious. Any person with a positive AFB smear of the sputum is contagious. Adults with cavitary disease or laryngeal TB are also assumed to be infectious. In general, a person with TB is considered infectious until the sputum becomes AFB-negative on three consecutive occasions or until they have received 2–4 weeks of antituberculous chemotherapy.

31. How is primary pulmonary TB treated?

One acceptable regimen is the daily administration of isoniazid, rifampin, and pyrazinamide for 2 months, followed by 4 months of isoniazid and rifampin. In areas where directly observed therapy (DOT) is available, twice weekly dosing is also possible. An alternative regimen is daily isoniazid and rifampin for 9 months, but this strategy should be used only in areas of low resistance to these medications.

32. Describe the treatment of complicated TB.

The management of disseminated (miliary) TB, bone and joint disease, and TB meningitis needs to be individualized and is based on clinical situation and epidemiologic factors. In general, such cases are treated with four drugs, including isoniazid, rifampin, pyrazinamide, and streptomycin or ethambutol, for at least 2 months. Specific changes in therapy can be based on microbiologic test results and clinical response. Antituberculous therapy is usually continued for at least 12 months, and in the absence of other factors can be simplified to daily isoniazid and rifampin after the initial 2 months of treatment. Do not try this approach at home without supervision by an infectious disease consultant.

33. What should be done for an infant born to a mother with TB?

Congenital TB (TB that has been spread to the fetus transplacentally) is extremely rare. Most often a young infant becomes infected with TB after birth from a contagious adult parent or caregiver. Management of the infant whose mother has TB depends on the clinical status of the mother and the potential presence of multidrug-resistant organisms. The mother who has TB infection but no disease poses no risk to the infant. A risk assessment should be done for the presence of other family members who may have TB disease, but no other specific interventions need to be taken at birth. Similarly, a mother who has extrapulmonary but not laryngeal TB is also noninfectious and poses no risk to her infant. Infants of mothers with miliary disease, however, should be evaluated thoroughly for congenital TB. An infant born to a mother with newly diagnosed pulmonary TB is considered at risk. In such cases, some experts recommend that the infant have a chest radiograph and skin test for tuberculosis (PPD 5TU). The infant should be treated with isoniazid for at least 3 months, at which time the PPD should be repeated. If the skin test and chest radiograph are negative and the infant is clinically well, isoniazid may be stopped. If compliance is poor, the infant should be treated for 9–12 months. If the skin test is positive, the infant requires a complete evaluation for TB and at least two-drug therapy for 12 months. Any infant taking isoniazid should receive pyridoxine supplementation. If the mother has active pulmonary TB, some experts recommend separating the mother and infant until she is no longer contagious. Others simply recommend treating the newborn with isoniazid and returning the infant to the mother immediately. Breast-feeding is permitted if the mother has TB, but small amounts of medication will pass into breast milk. Breast-feeding mothers also should receive pyridoxine supplementation.

34. Discuss the general features of TB medications.

Isoniazid (INH), rifampin, and pyrazinamide (PZA)are the most commonly used medications in the treatment of TB. Of these, isoniazid is the most often prescribed. All patients treated for TB should have baseline laboratory studies that include at least a complete blood count with differential and platelet count and liver function studies. Patients should be monitored regularly during therapy for the occurrence of side effects and to improve compliance if DOT is unavailable. Dosing is once daily for all medications, unless DOT is used, and medication is most often given as crushed tablets.

35. What particular considerations apply to INH?

INH is bactericidal, well absorbed, well tolerated, and easy to administer. It penetrates all body tissues well. In children it is generally administered as crushed tablets, which are given with food. Side effects of INH are rare but may include pyridoxine (vitamin B_6) deficiency, and hepatotoxicity. Pyridoxine deficiency causes peripheral neuropathy, but this side effect is rare in children and supplementation is not usually indicated. Hepatotoxicity is more common; in some series, up to 10% of children have minor elevations of liver function studies. These abnormalities are rarely severe and generally asymptomatic. Some experts recommend clinical follow-up only, whereas others obtain liver function studies at intervals during treatment with INH. INH is administered at doses of 10–15 mg/kg/day with a maximal dose of 300 mg.

36. Discuss the most relevant clinical features of rifampin.

Rifampin is bactericidal and also well tolerated and safe. It penetrates well into most bodily tissues but penetrates the meninges only in the presence of inflammation. The most common side effects are gastrointestinal (GI) upset, but hepatotoxicity also may occur. Rifampin causes a reddish-orange discoloration of the urine, tears, and other bodily fluids and may permanently stain soft contact lenses. Because rifampin is metabolized in the liver, it has several important drug interactions, including accelerated clearance of oral contraceptives, which renders them ineffective. Rifampin is contraindicated in patients with HIV who are taking protease inhibitors. The dose of rifampin is 10–20 mg/kg/day, with a maximal dose of 600 mg. As with INH, most experts recommend clinical monitoring and defer laboratory testing unless the patient is symptomatic.

37. What are the distinguishing features of PZA?

PZA is bactericidal and is active against *M. tuberculosis* within macrophages. PZA is well absorbed from the GI tract, and the most common side effect is GI upset. Other factors unique to PZA include that it may cause hyperuricemia, but only rarely does it lead to gout in children. PZA should be avoided in the first trimester of pregnancy and may worsen glucose control in diabetes. The usual dose is 15-20 mg/kg/day with a maximal dose of 2 gm. PZA typically is used during the first 2 months of treatment.

38. How is ethambutol used for the treatment of TB in children?

Ethambutol is used with care and only in the treatment of complicated childhood TB because of the possibility of optic neuritis and red-green color blindness. Although this complication is reversible on discontinuation of the medication, ethambutol is often avoided in children because of the difficulty in monitoring ocular function.

39. Summarize the most commonly used TB medications.

AGENT	ACTIVITY	DOSE (mg/kg/day)	SIDE-EFFECTS	OTHER POINTS
Isoniazid	Bactericidal	10–20	Elevated liver function tests Hepatitis Peripheral neuropathy Mild CNS effects	Age related B_6 deficiency
Rifampin	Bactericidal	10–20	Rash Hepatitis Fever Thrombocytopenia (rare)	Orange secretions Drug interactions
Pyrazinamide	Bactericidal	20	Gastrointestinal upset Hepatitis Rash Hyperuricemia (rare)	
Streptomycin	Bactericidal	20	Ototoxicity Vertigo	Intramuscular use only
Ethambutol	Bactericidal Bacteriostatic	25 15	Optic neuritis	

40. What about the use of corticosteroids in childhood TB?

The evidence is incomplete, but corticosteroids may be used in the treatment of TB meningitis as an attempt to decrease the inflammatory destruction of central nervous system structures and to ameliorate severe neurologic sequelae. Other potential uses include in cases of pleural, pericardial, or severe miliary TB. A tapering course of 4–8 weeks' duration is most often recommended.

41. How does drug resistance affect the treatment of TB?

Multidrug-resistant (MDR) TB is a major worldwide public health concern. Although the occurrence of MDR-TB has been declining in the United States, the general rate of resistance to a single drug has held steady at roughly 10%. TB resistance varies widely depending on the community and place of origin of the index case. It is widely agreed that if MDR-TB exposure or infection is suspected, a physician with expertise in this area should be consulted as because it dramatically alters treatment strategies and options for individual patients.

BIBLIOGRAPHY

1. American Thoracic Society: Treatment of tuberculosis and tuberculosis infection in adults and children. Am J Respir Crit Care Med 149:1359–1374, 1994.
2. American Thoracic Society: Targeted tuberculin testing and treatment of latent tuberculosis infection. Am J Respir Crit Care Med 161(4 Pt 2):S221–S247, 2000.
3. American Thoracic Society: Diagnostic standards and classification of tuberculosis in adults and children. Am J Respir Crit Care Med 161(4 Pt 1):1376–1395, 2000.
4. Correa A: Unique aspects of tuberculosis in the pediatric population. Clin Chest Med 18:89–98, 1997.
5. Froehlich H, Ackerson L, Morozumi P, for the Pediatric Tuberculosis Study Group of Kaiser Permanente NC: Targeted testing of children for tuberculosis: Validation of a risk assessment questionnaire. Pediatrics 107(4):54, 2001.
6. Inselman L: Tuberculosis in children: An update. Pediatr Pulmonol 21:101–120, 1996.
7. Mazade M, Evans E, Starke J, Correa A: Congenital tuberculosis presenting as sepsis syndrome: A case report and review of the literature. Pediatr Infect Dis J 20:439–442, 2001.
8. Pomputius W III, Rost J, Dennehy P, Carter E: Standardization of gastric aspirate technique improves yield in the diagnosis of tuberculosis in children. Pediatr Infect Dis J 16:222–226, 1997.
9. Smith K: Tuberculosis in children. Curr Probl Pediatr 31:1–30, 2001.
10. Starke J: Tuberculosis in children. Prim Care 23:861–881, 1996.
11. Starke J: Tuberculosis: An old disease but a new threat to mother, fetus, and neonate. Clin Perinatol 24:107–127, 1997.
12. Vallejo J, Starke J: Intrathoracic tuberculosis in children. Semin Respir Infect 11(3):184–195, 1996.

IV. Lymphatic System

19. LYMPHADENOPATHY AND LYMPHADENITIS

Dwight A. Powell, M.D.

1. What lymph node size should raise concern?

Generally, lymph nodes in normal children are ≤ 1.0 cm in diameter. Given difficulties with precise measurements, lymph nodes that exceed 1.5 cm in diameter should be considered abnormally enlarged. The exceptions are inguinal lymph nodes, which are normal up to 1.5 cm; epitrochlear nodes, which should not exceed 0.5 cm; and supraclavicular nodes ,which should not exceed 0.2 cm in diameter.

2. At what age are lymph nodes the largest relative to body size?

Lymph nodes tend to enlarge through age 8–12 years, then undergo atrophy beginning in adolescence.

3. Define lymphadenopathy and lymphadenitis.

Lymphadenopathy refers to any disease of the lymph nodes. The size of the node usually increases because of proliferation of T or B lymphocytes within the nodes, infiltration of cells into the node (inflammatory or metastatic tumor cells), development of tumor cells within the nodes, local cytokine release that leads to granulomatous changes, or tissue necrosis that results in caseation or suppuration. **Lymphadenitis** refers specifically to inflammation of lymph nodes.

4. In evaluating a child with a possible infectious cause of lymphadenopathy, what type of epidemiologic information is important?

Information that should be routinely sought includes travel history, exposure to pets or insects, trauma, recent infections, past history of frequent infections or recurrent lymphadenopathy, underlying illnesses, and rate of the lymph node enlargement. The rate of enlargement helps to classify the lymphadenopathy as acute (< 1 week) or subacute (1–3 weeks).

5. What should be included in the examination of all children with lymphadenopathy?

Determine whether the involved node(s) are focal or part of generalized lymphadenopathy and whether involvement is bilateral or unilateral. The area of the body draining to the nodes should be carefully examined. Nodes should then be examined for size, texture (hard, rubbery, soft), pain, warmth, redness, movement vs fixation to overlying skin, and whether the node is fluctuant. Malignancies and chronically infected nodes tend to be firm and painless without surrounding redness or cellulitis and to increase steadily in size. Acute lymphadenitis of bacterial origin usually enlarges rapidly, is very tender, has overlying redness or surrounding cellulitis, and frequently is fluctuant.

6. Although infections are the most common cause of generalized and focal lymphadenopathy of childhood, what other causes may be seen?

Malignancies: primary lymphomas and metastatic neoplasms, non-Hodgkin lymphoproliferative disorders, childhood histiocytic disorders.

Autoimmune disorders: rheumatoid arthritis, lupus erythematosus.

Lipid storage disorders: Gaucher disease, Niemann-Pick disease.

Drug reactions: phenytoin, serum sickness.

Inherited immunodeficiency disorders: chronic granulomatous diseases, Wiskott-Aldrich syndrome, Chediak-Higashi syndrome,

Others: sarcoidosis, hyperparathyroidism, Gianotti-Crosti syndrome, Kawasaki disease.

7. You find ulcers and vesicles in the mouth of a 2-year-old child with fever and bilateral 2-cm enlargement of the submandibular and upper anterior cervical lymph nodes. What are the two most likely causes? How can they be differentiated?

Both herpes simplex virus (HSV) gingivostomatitis and enteroviral herpangina infection can cause this illness. HSV lesions can appear anywhere in the mouth or pharynx, whereas enteroviral lesions are limited to the tonsils, pharynx, and soft palate structures. This distinction is important because early treatment of HSV gingivostomatitis with oral acyclovir may reduce the severity and duration of infection, whereas enteroviral infections do not require therapy.

8. In a 5-year-old child who presents with fever and sore throat, you find bilateral 2-cm enlargement of the jugulodigastric (tonsillar) lymph nodes and reddened, swollen tonsils without exudate. What are the most likely infectious agents? What criteria are used to decide whether a throat swab for rapid streptococcal assay or culture is indicated?

Many causes of pharyngitis are associated with bilateral cervical lymphadenitis. Non-exudative tonsillitis may be caused by numerous respiratory viruses, *Mycoplasma pneumoniae*, and several bacterial pathogens. For practical purposes, it is most important to identify and properly treat only *Streptococcus pyogenes* (GAS), which may present with exudative or nonexudative pharyngitis. Viral and mycoplasmal pharyngitis are usually associated with coryza and cough, both of which are rare in GAS infections. Thus, in presence of coryza and cough streptococcal studies are unnecessary; in their absence, throat swab for rapid antigen assay, DNA probe, or culture is the only immediate way to determine the presence of GAS.

9. When a 3-year-old child presents with rapidly enlarging, painful, unilateral cervical lymphadenitis, what are the two most likely bacterial agents?

Staphylococcus aureus and *S. pyogenes* account for 40–80% of acute unilateral cervical lymphadenitis in young children. Children with this infection are usually 1–4 years of age, and the lymphadenitis may or may not be associated with pharyngitis, impetigo, or other obvious infections of the face, ears, mouth, or throat.

10. Describe a reasonable initial diagnostic and therapeutic approach to the same child.

If the child is not toxic and does not have extensive surrounding cellulitis or major infection proximal to the involved lymph node and if the lymph node is not fluctuant, diagnostic studies are probably unnecessary. Such a child may reasonably be started on an oral beta-lactam antibiotic (e.g., cephalexin, cefadroxil, or amoxicillin-clavulanate) and observed closely. For penicillin-allergic children, oral clindamycin is a reasonable initial antibiotic. Toxic children or those with extensive cellulitis or serious proximal infections should be hospitalized, and parenteral antibiotics should be initiated. If the node is fluctuant, it probably requires incision and drainage; consult a surgeon along with beginning parenteral antibiotic therapy.

11. What if the same child is given oral antibiotics and returns to your office in 48 hours with no improvement?

Although the temptation is simply to try a different antibiotic, this strategy is probably not the most appropriate. Ideally, one should be more aggressive at determining the cause of the infection. Safe techniques include a needle aspiration of the node to be sent for Gram stain and culture. Use an 18-gauge needle and 3-ml syringe; if no return is seen, remove the empty 3-ml syringe and replace it with a syringe containing 0.5 ml of nonbacteriostatic saline. Inject the saline, and withdraw the bloody fluid to be sent for Gram stain and culture. Culture is becoming increasingly important because cases of community-acquired methicillin-resistant *S. aureus* are becoming more prevalent and sensitivities are required to guide therapy.

12. What concerns should you have if the same child returns in 48 hours with further enlargement of the node, spiking fevers, and worsening pain despite good compliance with an antibiotic to which the organism is susceptible (Fig. 1)?

Lymph nodes infected with *S. aureus* and *S. pyogenes* may develop into large abscesses in up to 30% of cases despite appropriate antibiotic therapy. They are not always fluctuant. Either ultrasonography or computed tomography (CT) scan of the node will determine the presence and size of an abscess and help to determine whether surgical drainage in necessary (Fig. 2).

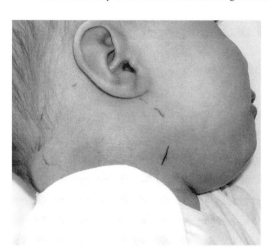 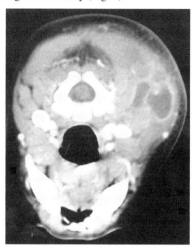

FIGURE 1 *(left).*   Three-year-old child with further enlargement of lymph node, spiking fevers, and worsening pain.

FIGURE 2 *(right).*   CT scan of involved node.

13. A 4-year-old child presents with a subacute unilateral anterior cervical lymph node measuring 2 × 3 cm. The node has developed slowly over the past 2 weeks, has not been associated with fever or systemic illness, and on exam is firm, moveable, nontender, nonerythematous, and nonfluctuant (Fig. 3). What is the most likely infectious agent?

Nontuberculous mycobacterial lymphadenitis due to *Mycobacterium avium-intracellulare* is the most likely cause. Other infections that present as subacute unilateral cervical lymphadenitis include chronic bacterial adenitis, cat-scratch disease, toxoplasmosis, histoplasmosis, and tuberculous lymphadenitis.

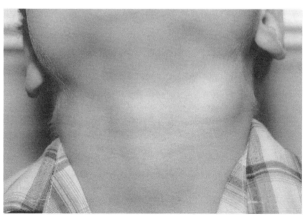

FIGURE   3.   Four-year-old child with a subacute unilateral anterior cervical lymph node measuring 2 × 3 cm.

14. What is the simplest diagnostic test to detect the presence of nontuberculous mycobacterial lymphadenitis?

Most children with nontuberculous mycobacterial lymphadenitis respond with at least 5 mm of induration to an intermediate-strength purified protein derivative (PPD) intradermal skin test.

15. Distinguish between tuberculous and nontuberculous cervical lymphadenitis.

FEATURE	TUBERCULOUS	NONTUBERCULOUS
Age	Any, but most > 5 years	1–6 years
Sex	Females predominate	No difference
Race	Foreign born (Asian, black, Hispanic)	Non–foreign-born Caucasian
Exposure	Exposure to tuberculous adult common	Tuberculous exposure rare
Node involvement	Posterior cervical, bilateral	Anterior cervical, unilateral
Chest radiograph	Abnormal (20–70%)	Normal (97%)
PPD skin test	Usually > 15 mm induration	Usually 5–15 mm induration

16. What is the usual outcome of nontuberculous lymphadenitis if left untreated?

Although some nodes may spontaneously resolve, most eventually caseate, resulting in tenderness, erythema, and central fluctuance. If still untreated, these nodes rupture and develop constant drainage of foul-smelling caseous material identical to the scrofulous tuberculous nodes of antiquity (Fig. 4).

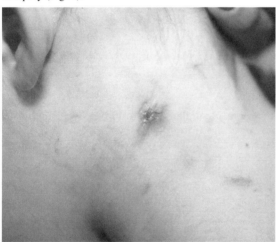

FIGURE 4. Lesion of untreated nontuberculous lymphadenitis.

17. If the interpretation of the PPD skin test is questionable, how else can nontuberculous mycobacterial lymphadenitis be diagnosed?

It is safe to perform a needle aspiration of the node for culture and smear. Unfortunately, acid-fast staining is often negative, culture requires 4–8 weeks, and cultures are positive in < 50% of cases. Biopsy provides the benefit of histology to identify caseating granulomas, maximal opportunity to identify acid-fast bacilli, and a large amount of tissue for culture. Surgeons should always remove the entire lymph node when performing a biopsy for nontuberculous mycobacteria. Partially biopsied nodes are very likely to develop chronically draining sinus tracts.

18. What is the therapy of choice for nontuberculous mycobacterial lymphadenitis?

Complete removal of the infected lymph node and all surrounding nodes that appear to be infected is optimal therapy. *M. avium-intracellulare* is resistant to most antituberculous antibiotics.

19. How should a child with nontuberculous lymphadenopathy be managed when caseation and a chronically draining sinus tract have developed?

Surgical removal at this stage becomes much more difficult with potential damage to surrounding structures such as the seventh cranial nerve. Limited data support a trial of clarithromycin or azithromycin with rifabutin. Management of such patients requires input from an infectious diseases expert.

20. What is the optimal therapy for a child with tuberculous lymphadenitis?

Surgical excision of tuberculous lymph nodes is not required. The diagnosis is confirmed by a strongly positive PPD skin test, tuberculous exposure history, and chest x-ray evidence of tuberculosis. If an adult contact has been identified (mycobacteria in sputum), the sensitivities of the adult's organism can reliably guide therapy. Otherwise a fine-needle biopsy of the infected node can be performed to obtain material for mycobacterial polymerase chain reaction (PCR) or mycobacterial culture and drug susceptibility testing. Tuberculous lymph nodes respond well to the same 6-month antituberculous regimens used to treat pulmonary tuberculosis.

21. In an adolescent who presents with subacute enlarging unilateral posterior lymphadenitis with no tuberculous exposure, a negative chest x-ray, and a negative PPD skin test, what other diagnoses should be considered?

The most likely infections include Epstein-Barr virus, toxoplasmosis, cytomegalovirus, or anicteric hepatitis A or B. These infections usually are associated with a mononucleosis syndrome of pharyngitis, fatigue, and possibly hepatosplenomegaly. In adolescents who are sexually active or involved in intravenous drug abuse, human immunodeficiency virus infection is a concern. Generalized lymphadenopathy is common, and after the acute mononucleosis symptoms resolve, persistent generalized lymphadenopathy persists for $\geq$ 3 months. If an infection is not readily apparent, malignancies, particularly lymphomas, must be excluded with a lymph node biopsy.

22. Boggy, painful scalp lesions in association with bilateral painfully enlarged occipital lymph nodes are most suggestive of what infection?

Tinea capitis, usually due to *Trichophyton tonsurans*. The boggy swelling is a heightened immune response to the infection called kerion. The scalp lesion occasionally becomes secondarily infected with bacterial pathogens, particularly *S. aureus*. However, suppurative lymphadenitis is rare, and even though a course of antibiotics may be beneficial, the infection will not clear without prolonged antifungal therapy. Griseofulvin is still the initial therapy of choice. Corticosteroids may be beneficial for the treatment of kerions.

23. Pruritus of the scalp and occipital lymphadenopathy should bring to mind what conditions?

Tinea capitis (early infections manifest as dandruff and "black-dot" alopecia), seborrhea, and head lice.

24. What viral infections are most likely associated with a rash and postauricular lymphadenopathy?

Rubella, rubeola, and roseola.

25. What is Parinaud's oculoglandular syndrome?

The oculoglandular syndrome of Parinaud refers to the complex of unilateral conjunctivitis and ipsilateral preauricular lymphadenitis. The most common cause is *Bartonella henselae*, the bacterial agent of cat-scratch disease. Other infections presenting with this syndrome include oculoglandular tularemia, sporotrichosis, tuberculosis, syphilis, and coccidioidomycosis. Epidemic adenoviral conjunctivitis frequently results in preauricular lymph node swelling, whereas endemic adenoviral pharyngeal-conjunctival fever rarely does so.

26. Do anaerobic bacteria play a role in cervical lymphadenitis?

Depending on the study cited, anaerobic bacteria have been isolated in up to 40% of cases of submandibular or anterior cervical lymphadenitis. However, it is not clear that these organisms are pathogenic or require specific therapy in most cases of cervical lymphadenitis. Patients with dental caries or dental gum disease are at highest risk of having true anaerobic bacterial lymphadenitis. Such infections should be treated with antibiotics effective against beta-lactamase–producing bacteria (amoxicillin-clavulanate or ampicillin-sulbactam).

27. Which enlarged lymph nodes in the head and neck should always raise suspicion of a noninfectious cause?

The supraclavicular lymph nodes are rarely enlarged in infections; palpable supraclavicular nodes with no other explanation raise should raise concern for malignancy, particularly Hodgkin or non-Hodgkin lymphoma. Biopsy is warranted, particularly in the presence of fever or weight loss.

28. Normal newborn infants rarely have generalized lymphadenopathy. What infections should be considered in such cases?

Generalized lymph node enlargement in a newborn usually represents a congenital infection. Toxoplasmosis, rubella, and congenital syphilis are the most likely infections to present with generalized lymphadenopathy. Abnormalities of the eyes, brain, skin, liver, spleen, heart, and bone marrow may be present as well.

29. Congenital syphilis is the leading candidate to cause a congenital infection if which lymph nodes are found to be enlarged?

The epitrochlear nodes, which are rarely enlarged in other congenital infections.

30. What causes the "cellulitis-adenitis" syndrome of infancy?

In very young infants (usually 3–7 weeks of age), cervical lymphadenitis with surrounding cellulitis may be caused by *S. aureus* or *S. pyogenes*, as in older children. However, the most likely cause is group B streptococci. Infants with this infection are febrile and toxic-appearing and have associated bacteremia. Hospitalization and parenteral antibiotics are indicated.

31. In infants from 2 months to 2 years of age, what are the main infections to consider in the evaluation of generalized lymphadenopathy and hepatosplenomegaly?

Although becoming rare with maternal prenatal testing and antiviral therapy, perinatal HIV infection should still lead the differential diagnostic list in such children. Miliary tuberculosis or fungal infection (particularly histoplasmosis) also may present in this manner. Extensive pulmonary involvement and failure to thrive are components of all three infections.

32. How does one diagnose HIV, miliary tuberculosis, or histoplasmosis in a very ill infant?

In infants, HIV should be confirmed with two positive HIV virologic tests performed on two separate blood samples (HIV DNA or RNA detection, HIV p24 antigen, or HIV viral isolation). Infants with miliary tuberculosis have a high probability of skin test anergy; in addition to PPD skin testing, therefore, an aggressive search for adult contacts with active tuberculosis is essential. Three successive morning gastric washings for mycobacterial culture should be positive > 50% of the time. Biopsy of lymph nodes or liver for histology and culture may be helpful. Histoplasmosis is considered when exposure risk is high (e.g., bats in the attic, exposure to a barn or old shed). Histoplasma antigens can be detected in urine, and serologic assays (complement fixation and immunodiffusion) are usually positive.

33. A child recently returned from a trip to Arkansas with her family. The mother reports that a tick was removed from the child's scalp 10 days ago. Now the child has a scabbed sore at the site of the tick bite and ipsilateral swollen postauricular lymphadenitis. What is the most likely infection?

Ulceroglandular tularemia caused by *Francisella tularensis*. This form of tularemia accounts for approximately 70% of all tularemia cases. If you knew the answer, skip the rest of the chapter.

34. True or false: Tularemia is caused primarily by handling dead animals, particularly rabbits.

False. Handling dead animals is now a rare cause of tularemia. Most cases are associated with tick bites, particularly in the south central and western states. Ticks capable of transmitting disease include *Dermacentor andersoni* (wood tick), *Dermacentor variabilis* (dog tick), and *Amblyomma americanum* (lone star tick). Fever, chills, headache, myalgias, and arthralgias usually develop 2–12 days after the bite of an infected tick. A nonhealing ulcer with a red rim develops at the site of the bite, followed by large, tender regional lymph nodes. In the head and neck, lymphadenopathy in multiple sites along the cervical drainage pathway is common.

35. How quickly can you confirm the diagnosis of tularemia? Can initiation of therapy be delayed for test results?

Lymph node aspirates can be obtained for culture, but the laboratory must be notified so that level 2 biosafety precautions can be enacted. In most cases, the diagnoses is made with serology. A single agglutination titer of 1:160 is highly suggestive, but usually a fourfold rise in antibody titer over 2–3 weeks is required for confirmation. Therefore, therapy should be started based on a clinical diagnosis before serologic confirmation.

36. Which antibiotics are appropriate for suspected tularemia?

A 7- to 10-day course of intravenous gentamicin is generally recommended. Oral doxycycline is effective, but relapses have been described. Oral ciprofloxacin (not licensed for children < 18 years old) has been effective in a limited number of adults and children.

37. What clinical features should raise suspicion of cat-scratch disease in a child?

The most common presentation is a scratch from a kitten that is followed in 1–2 weeks by one or more papular lesions over the scratch area (Fig. 5) that may be ulcerated. These lesions are followed in 1–3 weeks by a slowly evolving lymphadenitis proximal to the scratch site (Fig. 6). Initially the node is painless, nonerythematous, firm, and associated only with low-grade fever. Affected nodes appear most commonly on the extremities, but often cervical lymph nodes are involved. Because the scratch and papular lesions are not always present, consider cat-scratch disease in any child with a subacute lymphadenopathy and feline contact.

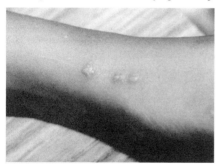

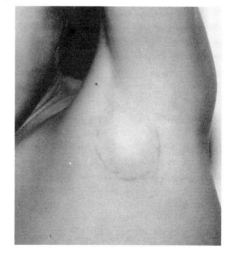

FIGURE 5 *(above).* Papular lesions of cat-scratch disease.

FIGURE 6 *(right).* Enlarged lymph node associated with cat-scratch disease.

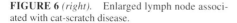

38. Is it essential to confirm the diagnosis of cat scratch disease? If so, what are the diagnostic options?

Because few other conditions mimic the classic presentation of cat scratch disease, a clinical diagnosis is satisfactory. *Bartonella henselae*, the causative organism of cat-scratch disease, cannot be cultured in most laboratories; if diagnosis is required, one must rely on serology (indirect fluorescent antibody or enzyme immunoassay) or PCR from infected tissue. IgM and IgG serologic assays are available, and both are usually positive at the onset of clinical symptoms. A positive IgM or a rising IgG antibody level is diagnostic.

39. Describe the natural course of untreated cat-scratch lymphadenitis.

In many children, the lymphadenitis resolves without any complications. About 25% of nodes eventually suppurate. Such nodes usually can be aspirated with an 18-gauge needle; occasionally repeated aspirations are required. Drainage by surgical incision is rarely required.

40. What about the possibility of medical therapy for cat scratch disease?

Data are limited, but one prospective controlled study demonstrated that azithromycin in a dose of 10 mg/kg/day, followed by 5 mg/kg/day for 4 additional days, resulted in an 80% decrease in the size of treated lymph nodes in 7 of 14 treated patients compared with 1 of 15 patients receiving placebo. Data about treatment of complications are limited. One report of children with hepatosplenic granulomatous cat-scratch disease described probable benefit from rifampin used alone or in conjunction with other antibiotics.

41. Is cat-scratch disease limited to lymphadenopathy, or can complications develop?

There are a growing number of complications, which occur in approximately 15% of immunocompetent patients with cat-scratch disease. Most often complications occur in patients with lymphadenopathy, but occasionally complications present without lymphadenopathy.

Complications of Cat-scratch Disease in Immunocompetent Patients

MOST COMMON	LEAST COMMON
Parinaud's oculoglandular fever	Neuroretinitis
Osteolytic bone lesions	Pneumonia
Encephalitis	Peripheral neuropathy
Granulomatous hepatitis/splenitis	Arthritis
Henoch-Schönlein purpura	Mesenteric lymphadenitis
	Epidural or paraspinal abscess
	Pleural effusion

42. You order a chest x-ray of a 3-year-old child with suspected pneumonia. The radiologist confirms your suspicion of a left upper lobe infiltrate but also observes that the child has left-sided hilar lymphadenopathy. What should be the next diagnostic study?

Tuberculosis is the most concerning infection that causes hilar lymphadenopathy in association with a pulmonary infiltrate. Therefore, an intermediate-strength PPD skin test should be applied. It is unusual to see hilar lymphadenopathy in association with the common bacterial or viral causes of pediatric pneumonia.

43. What if the PPD is negative in the above case? What other infections can cause hilar lymphadenopathy?

First, consider whether the child may be anergic to the PPD skin test (highest risk in young infants, infants with rapidly progressive disease, malnourished infants, or infants with immunodeficiencies such as HIV infection). If anergy is unlikely, nontuberculous mycobacteria (rare causes of pulmonary disease), *Mycoplasma pneumoniae* (20% of cases), histoplasmosis, coccidioidomycosis, blastomycosis, and cryptococcosis are the most likely infections. Sarcoidosis presents with pulmonary parenchymal disease and bilateral hilar lymph node enlargement in > 95% of children. If there is no obvious infectious cause of mediastinal lymphadenopathy, one must be concerned for malignancy. A chest CT scan and consultation with a thoracic surgeon for a mediastinal biopsy are indicated.

44. In a sexually active adolescent, what are the agents of concern in the presence of inguinal lymphadenitis?

In the Unites States the most common infections are genital herpes simplex virus (HSV), syphilis, and chancroid.

45. Does lymphadenitis occur in both primary and recurrent genital herpes simplex viral infections?

Bilateral, tender, nonsuppurative inguinal lymphadenitis lasting up to 2–3 weeks occurs in approximately 80% of patients with primary genital HSV infections. With recurrent genital HSV, lymphadenitis occurs in only approximately 20% of males and 30% of females. It is much less intense and shorter in duration than with primary infection.

46. Does inguinal lymphadenitis accompany syphilis and gonorrhea?

Bilateral painless inguinal lymphadenopathy develops in 50–70% of patients with primary syphilis approximately 7 days after development of the painless chancre. Inguinal lymphadenopathy also may be seen with secondary syphilis, but lymphadenitis is not present in gonorrhea.

47. While examining a sexually active adolescent boy with inguinal lymphadenopathy, you note a genital ulcer. What clinical features distinguish syphilis from chancroid?

Syphilis (*Treponema pallidum*) causes painless genital ulcers and relatively painless inguinal lymphadenopathy. Chancroid (*Haemophilus ducreyi*) presents with painful genital ulcerations and inflamed inguinal lymph nodes that often suppurate and rupture. Syphilis is diagnosed by identification of spirochetes on a dark-field examination of material scrapped from the base of the ulcer and by a positive fluorescent treponemal antibody titer. Chancroid is diagnosed by finding gram-negative coccobacilli on a smear from the ulcer base and by culture of *H. ducreyi* from the lesions.

BIBLIOGRAPHY

1. Arisoy ES, Armando GC, Wagner ML, Kaplan SL: Hepatosplenic cat-scratch disease in children: selected clinical features and treatment. Clin Infect Dis 28:778–784, 1999.
2. Bass JW, Freitas BC, Freitas AD, et al: Prospective randomized double blind placebo-controlled evaluation of azithromycin for treatment of cat-scratch disease. Pediatr Infect Dis J 17:447–452, 1998.
3. Bryant KA: Tularemia: Lymphadenitis with a twist. Pediatr Ann 31:187–190, 2002.
4. Chesney PJ: Cervical lymphadenitis and neck infections. In Long SS, Pickering LK, Prober CG (eds): Principles and Practice of Pediatric Infectious Diseases. New York, Churchill Livingstone, 1997, pp 186–197.
5. Darville T, Jacobs RF: Lymphadenopathy, lymphadenitis, and lymphangitis. In Jensen HB, Baltimore RS (eds): Pediatric Infectious Diseases: Principles and Practice. Philadelphia, W.B. Saunders, 2002, pp 610629.
6. Powell DA: Tuberculous lymphadenitis. In Schlossberg D (ed): Tuberculosis and Nontuberculous Mycobacterial Infections, 4th ed. Philadelphia, W.B. Saunders, 1999, pp 186–194.
7. Powell DA: Atypical mycobacteria. In Behrman RE, Kliegman RM, Jenson HB (eds). Nelson Textbook of Pediatrics, 16th ed. Philadelphia, W.B. Saunders, 2000, pp 900–903.
8. Starke JR: Management of nontuberculous mycobacterial cervical adenitis. Pediatr Infect Dis J 19:674–675, 2000.
9. Young G, Toretsky JA, Campbell AB, Eskenazi AE: Recognition of common childhood malignancies. Am Fam Physician 61:2144–2154, 2000.

V. Cardiac Infections

20. ACUTE RHEUMATIC FEVER

Anne Marie C. Brescia, M.D.

1. Who first described acute rheumatic fever (ARF)? When?
Thomas Sydenham in 1848.

2. What are the Jones criteria for diagnosis of ARF?

Major criteria	Minor criteria
1. Arthritis	1. Fever
2. Carditis	2. Arthralgia
3. Chorea	3. High C-reactive protein (CRP) or
4. Erythema marginatum	erythrocyte sedimentation rate (ESR)
5. Subcutaneous nodules	4. Prolonged PR interval

3. What are the guidelines for diagnosing ARF with the Jones criteria?
A patient must have two major criteria or one major plus two minor criteria, with supporting evidence of antecedent group A streptococcal (GAS) infection.

4. What is the most common symptom of ARF?
Painful, migratory arthritis of short duration is present in 80% of patients. The pain responds to salicylates. Larger joints are typically affected, especially knees, ankles, wrists, and elbows. Affected joints are swollen, erythematous, and warm as well as painful. Arthritis usually does not last more than 1 week in each joint.

5. What is the most serious feature of ARF?
Carditis, which is estimated to affect 41–83% of patients. Cardiac involvement is detected by tachycardia, murmur, cardiomegaly, rhythm disturbance, prolonged PR interval, pericardial friction rub, or cardiac failure. Valvulitis is most likely to lead to mitral or aortic regurgitation. The myocardium and endocardium are usually involved. Involvement of the pericardium indicates pancarditis, the most life-threatening complication of ARF.

6. Define Sydenham's chorea.
Sydenham's chorea is characterized by fast, clonic, involuntary movements, muscular hypotonus, and emotional lability. It is estimated to affect 15% of patients and is attributed to inflammation of basal ganglia and caudate nucleus. This symptom usually appears later than the others (approximately 2–4 months after the initial infection, sometimes as late as 12 months). Of interest, symptoms disappear during sleep.

7. Is chorea pathognomonic for ARF?
Yes. A presumptive diagnosis of ARF can be made when isolated chorea is present.

8. Is erythema marginatum just another red rash?
No. Erythema marginatum, which is evanescent and nonpruritic, affects about 5% of patients with ARF. It usually is seen on the trunk and limbs but not the face. The outer edge is serpiginous

(snakelike) and sharp, whereas the inner edge is diffuse. Central skin gradually returns to normal. Individual lesions may last for hours. They may become more prominent after a hot shower.

9. Where are subcutaneous nodules found?

Nodules are found on extensor surfaces of joints, bony prominences, dorsum of feet, occipital region, and cervical spinous processes. They last a few days and are firm and painless. Elbows are most frequently involved. ARF nodules are typically located on the olecranon, whereas rheumatoid nodules are 3–4 cm distal to the olecranon.

10. Do all patients with ACF have fever?

No. Fever is a minor criterion. When present, it ranges from 38.4°–40°C and lasts approximately 1 week.

11. Which laboratory tests are useful?

Although nonspecific, CRP and ESR may be helpful. The electrocardiogram may show a prolonged PR interval.

12. What are the most common laboratory abnormalities in ARF?

Anemia, leukocytosis, thrombocytosis, and the presence of antistreptococcal antibodies.

13. What evidence supports a preceding streptococcal infection?

Increased antistreptolysin O (ASO) or other streptococcal antibodies, positive throat culture for GAS, or recent scarlet fever.

14. Which antibody tests are useful?

Throat cultures may be negative by the time rheumatic fever is apparent, making antibody titers more useful. ASO is the most widely used antibody test. Other available tests are anti-DNase B, antihyaluronidase, and antistreptokinase. The streptozyme test measures antibodies to multiple antigens. An elevated ASO or anti-DNase B may be expected in 85% of patients. To demonstrate a rising antibody titer, most authors recommend checking titers 2 weeks after the initial titer.

15. Describe the pathologic process of ARF.

The pathologic process is a diffuse vasculitis mediated by an immune reaction to streptococcal infection. It is typically a small-vessel vasculitis that affects joints, heart, brain, and peripheral vascular system.

16. What is the precipitating cause?

Tonsillopharyngitis with group A beta-hemolytic streptococci (GABHS).

17. Why does the vasculitis occur?

The theory of molecular mimicry is based on shared epitopes (common antigenic sequences) between GAS and heart valve and brain. In the confusing presence of shared epitopes, the immune system has difficulty distinguishing between self and nonself. Partial tolerance develops, and an inflammatory reaction is directed at self antigens that share common epitopes with GAS.

18. What is the most important antigenic structure of GAS?

The M protein, located in the external layer of the cell wall, is responsible for type-specific immunity and has antiphagocytic action. It is thought to be a marker of streptococcal rheumatogenic potential.

19. What are Aschoff bodies?

Aschoff bodies are pathognomonic for rheumatic carditis. They consist of a perivascular infiltrate of large cells with polymorphous nuclei and basophilic cytoplasm arranged in a rosette around an avascular center of fibrinoid.

20. Is GAS the most common cause of acquired heart disease in children?

No. It has been replaced by Kawasaki disease in this dubious place of honor.

21. How much time passes between infection with GAS and development of ARF?

The asymptomatic latency period is 2–3 weeks.

22. What is the peak age of incidence of ARF?

The typical age at onset is 5–18 years. Not surprisingly, this is the age range in which GAS pharyngitis is most prevalent. Sydenham's chorea has a higher incidence in females after puberty.

23. When are recurrences of ARF most common?

Within the first 2 years after the initial attack—but they can occur any time.

24. When does rheumatic heart disease manifest?

About 10–20 years after the original attack. The mitral valve is involved most frequently, followed by the aortic valve.

25. Describe the recommended treatment.

First, eradicate the GAS. One method is a single intramuscular dose of benzathine penicillin G. The arthritis may be treated with salicylates and nonsteroidal anti-inflammatory drugs and usually responds within 3 days. Mild-to-moderate carditis may be treated with aspirin. Severe rheumatic carditis requires steroid therapy for 10–15 days, followed by a taper. However, neither aspirin nor steroids have been shown to influence evolution of valvular disease. Chorea may be difficult to treat; haloperidol and valproate have been used.

26. Is antibiotic prophylaxis warranted?

Yes. The usual choice is oral or intramuscular penicillin.

27. How long should prophylaxis be given?

This issue is hotly debated. Most authors agree that prophylaxis should be continued at least until young adulthood. Some authors recommend that patients with carditis receive prophylaxis for life, whereas in patients without cardiac involvement prophylaxis should be given for at least 5 years and until 21 years of age.

28. What is the animal model of ARF?

Trick question. There is no animal model; humans are the only species known to be susceptible to ARF.

29. What is the other nonsuppurative complication of streptococcal pharyngitis?

Poststreptococcal glomerulonephritis.

30. What are PANDAS?

In this context, they are not furry bears that love to climb trees and eat bamboo. PANDAS is an acronym for **p**ediatric **a**utoimmune **n**europsychiatric **d**isorders **a**ssociated with **s**treptococcal infections. The term refers to a group of disorders, particularly obsessive-compulsive disease and tic disorders (e.g., Tourette's syndrome), for which a possible relationship to GABHS infection has been suggested.

31. What is the suggested treatments for PANDAS: (a) daily bamboo, (b) penicillin prophylaxis, (c) IVIG, or (d) none of the above?

None of the above. Because the clinical entity of PANDAS is poorly defined and few data about appropriate management are available, the editors suggest neuropsychiatric intervention. Establishing a causal relationship in this case is difficult because the two common entities often occur together.

BIBLIOGRAPHY

1. Ayoub EM: Acute rheumatic fever. In Textbook of Pediatric Rheumatology, 4th ed. Philadelphia, W.B. Saunders, 2001, pp 690–701.
2. DaSilva NA, de Faria-Pereira BA: Acute rheumatic fever: Still a challenge. Rheum Dis Clin North Am 23:545–568, 1997.
3. Gibofsky A, Kerwar S, Zabriskie JB: Rheumatic fever: The relationships between host, microbe, and genetics. Rheum Dis Clin North Am 24:237–259, 1998.

21. KAWASAKI DISEASE

Anne Marie C. Brescia, M.D.

1. When was Kawasaki syndrome first described?

Kawasaki syndrome (KS) was first described in 1967 by Kawasaki as mucocutaneous lymph node syndrome. It was originally identified in postmortem examination and called infantile periarteritis nodosa, which is now thought to be indistinguishable from fatal KS.

2. What are the diagnostic criteria for KS?

Fever for at least 5 days *and* four of the five following criteria:

1. Bilateral nonpurulent conjunctival injection (usually bulbar)
2. Mucosal changes such as erythematous, dry, fissured lips or pharyngeal erythema or strawberry tongue
3. Peripheral extremity changes, such as swelling and erythema of hands and feet during the acute phase or periungual desquamation during the subacute phase
4. Rash, which may be maculopapular, erythema multiforme, or scarlatiniform
5. Cervical lymphadenopathy

In addition, the clinician must exclude all other diseases that could explain the patient's symptoms.

3. What other diseases can mimic KS?

Measles	Adenovirus
Staphylococcal toxin-mediated diseases	Leptospirosis
Streptococcal toxin-mediated diseases	Acrodynia
Scarlet fever	Other rheumatologic disorders

4. What is the least common feature of KS?

Ironically, for a disease originally called mucocutaneous lymph node syndrome, cervical lymphadenopathy is the least common feature and is seen in 50–75% of patients.

5. How high is the fever? How long does it last?

Fevers that may exceed 39°C typically last 1–2 weeks if not treated and usually resolve within 1–2 days after therapy with intravenous gamma globulin (IVIG).

6. On day 5 of fever, does the patient suddenly have KS?

In the presence of fever and all other diagnostic criteria for KS, experienced physicians may make the diagnosis before the fifth day of fever and choose to give IVIG accordingly.

7. What other associated features did not quite make the cut for diagnostic criteria?

Believe it or not, cardiac disease is not one of the diagnostic criteria. Other features may include irritability, aseptic meningitis, arthralgias, arthritis, hepatic involvement, hydrops of the gallbladder, diarrhea, otitis media, bacille Calmette-Guérin induration, and pneumonitis.

8. Describe the three clinical phases of KS.

1. **Acute febrile phase** (1–2 weeks): fever, conjunctival injection, oral mucosa erythema, erythema of hands and feet, rash, cervical adenopathy, aseptic meningitis, diarrhea, hepatic involvement.
2. **Subacute phase:** desquamation, irritability, anorexia, conjunctival injection, thrombocytosis.
3. **Convalescent phase:** clinical signs have disappeared; this phase continues until the sedimentation rate is normal (usually 6–8 weeks after onset).

9. What are the most common cardiac abnormalities?

Dilatation (ectasia) and aneurysm formation. The study by Kato et al. found that 1–3 months after the onset of KS, 15% of patients had angiographic evidence of aneurysms. Fifty percent of aneurysms resolved by 18 months later. One-half of the unresolved aneurysms were smaller, one-third eventually resolved but were associated with stenosis, and the remainder were associated with irregularities of the vessel wall without stenosis.

10. During which stage do coronary artery aneurysms usually develop?

During the second (subacute) stage. The risk for sudden death is highest during this stage. In the acute phase, patients may have myocarditis and pericardial effusion.

11. Are patients with atypical KS at risk for coronary artery aneurysms?

Yes. Atypical KS, which is most common in young infants, is associated with fever and fewer than four of the other criteria.

12. How big is a giant aneurysm?

To be considered a giant aneurysm, internal luminal diameter must be ≥ 8 mm. Kato et al. showed that 4.4% of patients develop giant aneurysms, which are more likely to thrombose, rupture, and become stenotic.

13. Are coronary aneurysms the only cardiac complication of KS?

Of course not. Patients are also at risk for myocarditis (50% of patients with acute KS), valvulitis (1% of patients; usually mitral), pericardial effusion (25% of patients with acute KS), systemic arterial aneurysms, myocardial infarction, and hemopericardium secondary to ruptured coronary artery aneurysm.

14. What are the typical laboratory findings in KS?

White blood cell (WBC) count ranges from normal to elevated; sedimentation rate is elevated. Normocytic anemia may be present and becomes more severe in coronary disease and with a prolonged febrile stage. Thrombocytosis appears in the second-to-third week. Sterile pyuria is present in one-third of patients. IgG may be low in the acute phase and Ig elevated in the subacute phase. Hypoalbuminemia and mild elevations in liver transaminases are often found in patients with KS.

15. What is the cerebrospinal fluid (CSF) profile in KS?

When patients are irritable enough to undergo lumbar puncture, the typical CSF profile includes 25–100 WBC/μl, lymphocyte predominance, normal glucose, and normal or elevated protein.

16. What are Beau's lines?

Transverse grooves that develop across the nails 1–2 months after KS.

17. How is KS distinguished from toxic shock?

Typical patients with KS are not hypotensive and do not usually have renal involvement or elevations of creatine kinase, as may be seen in toxic shock.

18. Describe the pathophysiology of KS.

KS is a medium-sized arterial vasculitis. Also affected are small arterioles, larger arteries, capillaries, and veins. In the coronary arteries, the entire vascular wall is involved. The coronary artery media develops inflammation with edema and necrosis of smooth muscle cells. Eventually, the arterial wall loses structural integrity.

19. What causes KS?

The cause is unknown. The prevalent theory, of course, is to blame an infectious agent. It is thought that symptoms are manifest in genetically susceptible people. No causative agent has been identified.

20. Who gets KS? When?

Eighty percent of cases occur in children less than 4 years old. Asians are at the highest risk. The seasonal predilection is from winter to early spring.

21. What is the risk of coronary artery disease?

About 20–25% of untreated patients develop coronary abnormalities. Dilitation is first detected at 10 days, with peak frequency within 4 weeks of onset.

22. What features are associated with a poorer prognosis?

Fever for more than 16 days, fever recurring after 48 hours, arrhythmias other than first-degree heart block, male gender, age less than 1 year, cardiomegaly, and low platelet count, low hematocrit, and low albumin at presentation.

23. What is the major cause of mortality in KS?

Mortality results from myocardial infarction due to thrombosis of a coronary aneurysm or rupture of a large aneurysm. Death is most likely to occur within 2–12 weeks after onset of illness.

24. Describe the recommended treatment.

In the first 10 days, treatment with a single dose of IVIG (2 gm/kg) and aspirin (80–100 mg/kg/day) has been shown to decrease coronary artery abnormalities from 20–25% to 2–4%. IVIG also leads to more rapid defervesence, correction of acute-phase reactants, and improved myocardial function.

25. What about patients who have persistent fever 48 hours after receiving IVIG?

10% of patients still have fever 48 hours after receiving IVIG. Many patients receive a second dose of IVIG because prolonged fever is a risk factor for more severe coronary disease.

26. Has IVIG been proven to work?

Newburger et al. showed that, after 2 weeks of therapy, 8% of patients who received IVIG for 4 days, in addition to aspirin, had coronary artery abnormalities compared with 23% of patients treated with aspirin alone. Seven weeks after therapy, 4% of patients treated with IVIG plus aspirin had cardiac abnormalities compared with 18% of the group treated with aspirin alone.

27. How long should low-dose aspirin therapy continue?

This issue is hotly debated. According to one recommendation, if at 8 weeks the sedimentation rate has normalized and the echocardiogram has always been normal, aspirin may be discontinued. It is highly unlikely that patients with normal coronary arteries at 2 months after onset of illness will develop abnormalities. Because it has been shown that the vessel wall remains abnormal even after resolution of dilatation or aneurysms, patients with such abnormalities receive aspirin indefinitely even after the echocardiogram appears normal.

28. Why do patients not develop aspirin toxicity?

Acute KS is associated with decreased absorption and increased clearance of aspirin.

29. How often are echocardiograms recommended?

A baseline echocardiogram should be taken at initial presentation; echocardiograms should be repeated at 2–3 weeks and 6–8 weeks after presentation. Complete blood count and sedimentation rates are followed in a similar pattern.

30. Should a patient with KS be vaccinated?

Because specific antiviral antibodies in IVIG may interfere with immune response, administration of live virus vaccines (measles-mumps-rubella and varicella) should be delayed for 6–11 months after IVIG has been given.

BIBLIOGRAPHY

1. Kato H, Ichinose E, et al: Fate of coronary aneurysms in Kawasaki disease: Serial coronary angiography and long-term follow-up study. Am J Cardiology 49:1758–1766, 1982.
2. Kato H, Sugimura T, et al: Long-term consequences of Kawasaki disease. Circulation 94:1279–1285, 1996.
3. Newburger JW, Takahashi M, et al: The treatment of Kawasaki syndrome with intravenous gamma globulin. N Engl J Med 315:341–347, 1986.
4. Rowley AH, Shulman ST: Kawasaki syndrome. Pediatr Clin North Am 46:313–329, 1999.

22. OTHER CARDIAC INFECTIONS

Jeffrey M. Bergelson, M.D.

1. Who gets endocarditis?

- In the United States, most cases of endocarditis occur in children with congenital heart disease, many of whom have undergone surgical repair.
- Hospitalized patients with central venous catheters are at increased risk, as are children with bacteremia caused by *Staphylococcus aureus*.
- In developing countries, rheumatic heart disease is still the major predisposing factor.
- Patients with prosthetic valves, calcified valves, or arteriovenous dialysis shunts; burn patients; and intravenous drug users are also at risk.

2. What are the typical symptoms and signs of endocarditis?

The classic picture of the patient with longstanding subacute endocarditis includes fever, a changing murmur, vascular or embolic phenomena, splenomegaly, and immune-mediated arthritis and glomerulonephritis. However, many patients present with less specific findings, such as fever, fatigue, myalgia, or arthralgia. Endocarditis should be considered whenever children at risk—particularly those with congenital heart disease—have persistent, unexplained fever or malaise.

3. Describe the evaluation of patients with possible endocarditis.

The evaluation should emphasize predisposing conditions, diagnostic signs, and evidence of complications.

History
- Known cardiac lesions
- Fever
- Symptoms of congestive failure
- Neurologic symptoms
- Allergies

Physical exam
- Cardiac exam: underlying lesion (including mitral valve prolapse/regurgitation), new valvular insufficiency
- Pulses: emboli
- Neurologic exam: emboli, vasculitis, aseptic meningitis, intracranial hemorrhage
- Peripheral signs: conjunctival petechiae, splinter hemorrhages, skin lesions
- Joints: arthritis

Laboratory tests
- Multiple blood cultures: evidence of sustained bacteremia; organism and sensitivities
- Electrocardiogram: conduction defects
- Chest x-ray: congestive failure, septic emboli
- Urinalysis: hematuria, glomerulonephritis
- Baseline complete blood count (CBC)
- Baseline renal function
- Echocardiogram: underlying cardiac lesion, cardiac function, vegetations, cardiac abscess, dehiscence of prosthetic valve

4. How is the diagnosis made?

The diagnosis is most strongly supported by persistent bacteremia with an organism likely to cause endocarditis, echocardiographic evidence of vegetations or intracardiac abscess, and new valvular incompetence. Other suggestive evidence includes:

- Vascular phenomena, such as emboli
- Pulmonary infarction

- Conjunctival hemorrhages
- Purpuric skin lesions (Janeway lesions)
- Immunologic phenomena, such as glomerulonephritis
- Retinal lesions (Roth spots)
- Painful nodules on the fingers (Osler's nodes)

Many patients also have fever, a predisposing cardiac lesion, and an increased erythryocyte sedimentation rate (ESR), and some have splinter hemorrhages, positive rheumatoid factor, false-positive Venereal Disease Research Laboratory (VDRL) test for syphilis, splenomegaly, anemia, or arthralgias.

5. A famous university defined a set of major and minor diagnostic criteria that combine clinical, microbiologic, pathologic, and echocardiographic information. These criteria have been found to be sensitive and specific in both adult and pediatric populations. Name the university.

Duke University.

6. Endocarditis results in sustained bacteremia and is often caused by relatively nonvirulent organisms that may sometimes be dismissed as culture contaminants. How many blood cultures should I draw?

Isolation of the same organism from repeated cultures provides valuable supportive evidence for the diagnosis; taking multiple samples for culture also increases the likelihood of identifying the pathogen. In clinically stable patients, at least three blood cultures should be drawn over a period of 24 hours. If the patient has recently received antibiotics, antibiotics should be withheld, and if the initial cultures are negative, an additional series should be drawn in 48–72 hours. In acutely ill patients, cultures should be drawn from independent sites before antibiotics are given.

7. Discuss the role of echocardiography.

Echocardiographic evidence of endocarditis greatly improves diagnostic accuracy and is invaluable in detecting complications. An echocardiogram should be performed whenever endocarditis is suspected, and it should be repeated if there is a clinical change during therapy. However, not all "lumps" seen on echocardiography are vegetations, and not all vegetations can be visualized. When endocarditis is believed likely but the echocardiogram is negative, a repeat study in 7–10 days may be useful.

Transesophageal echocardiography (TEE) has greater sensitivity than transthoracic echocardiography in detecting small vegetations, prosthetic valve endocarditis, and complications such as perivalvular abscess. TEE is recommended for adults in whom endocarditis is strongly suspected. However, the indications for TEE in children have not been defined.

Vegetations typically decrease in size within 2 weeks of antibiotic therapy, but in most patient vegetations are still visible at the end of an adequate course of therapy.

8. Which organisms cause endocarditis?

- Infection of native valves is most often caused by viridans streptococci, enterococci, and *S. aureus;* coagulase-negative staphylococci (such as *S. epidermidis*) are much less common.
- Viridans streptococci most often cause relatively indolent infections.
- *S. aureus* may cause acute endocarditis, with overwhelming sepsis, metastatic infection, and rapid destruction of the affected valve. Unlike viridans streptococci, *S. aureus* attacks valves that were previously normal. The propensity of these organisms to infect native valves reflects their capacity to adhere to the endocardium.
- In animal models, other organisms, such as *Escherichia coli,* are very inefficient in establishing infection, even of damaged valves.
- Prosthetic valve endocarditis is commonly caused by *S. epidermidis* as well as by the organisms that infect native valves. In the first months after surgery, prosthetic valves can be infected by nosocomial pathogens, including *Pseudomonas* spp. and fungi.

• Various other organisms—including gram-negative bacilli, fungi, diphtheroids, *Coxiella burnetii* (Q fever), and rickettsiae—also may cause endocarditis.

9. Which antibiotics are used for the initial treatment of endocarditis?

For **native valve** endocarditis the combination of ampicillin, oxacillin (or nafcillin), and gentamicin provides bactericidal activity against viridans streptococci, enterococci and *S. aureus*. Vancomycin plus gentamicin can be used for patients allergic to penicillin. The empirical regimen for **prosthetic valve** endocarditis includes vancomycin, gentamicin, and rifampin.

In patients who are not acutely ill, it is preferable to wait until the diagnosis is confirmed and the organism is identified before antibiotic treatment is begun. In patients who require immediate treatment (e.g., patients who are toxic,or have evidence of congestive failure or new valvular insufficiency), antibiotics should be directed against the common pathogens.

10. What causes culture-negative endocarditis?

Fungi, *Bartonella* spp., *Brucella* spp., rickettsiae (Q fever), mycobacteria, and *Chlamydia* spp. have been identified as causes of endocarditis with negative cultures. These organisms can be identified by serologic tests or polymerase chain reaction (PCR).

11. What are the reasons for failure to isolate culturable organisms?
   • Administration of antibiotics before blood cultures were obtained
   • Small culture volumes (the density of organisms in blood samples is often very low)
   • Inadequate culture technique
   • Infection by fastidious bacteria (nutritionally deficient streptococci or HACEK organisms)

12. What are HACEK organisms?

Oral gram-negative bacilli cause 5–10% of native valve endocarditis. These organisms are summarized by the acronym **HACEK**: *H*aemophilus species (*H. parainfluenzae, H. aphrophilus,* and *H. paraphrophilus*), *A*ctinobacillus actinomycetemcomitans, *C*ardiobacterium hominis, *E*ikenella corrodens, and *K*ingella species.

13. Why should we care about the HACEK organisms?

They have specific nutritional requirements, grow slowly in routine culture medium, and may be responsible for cases of endocarditis with negative cultures. When endocarditis is a consideration, the microbiology laboratory should be notified so that blood cultures can be retained for at least two weeks. Some HACEK organisms produce beta-lactamases; they are best treated with a third-generation cephalosporin such as cefotaxime.

14. Is all endocarditis due to infection?

No. Valvular lesions can occur in noninfectious conditions (e.g., Libman-Sacks endocarditis associated with systemic lupus). In marantic endocarditis (nonbacterial thrombotic endocarditis), large sterile vegetations may become evident only when embolic phenomena occur. Marantic endocarditis is often associated with cancers and is rarely observed in children.

15. Does antibiotic prophylaxis prevent endocarditis?

No randomized clinical trials have been performed to support the use of antibiotic prophylaxis. However, based on information about the incidence of endocarditis with particular cardiac lesions, the incidence of bacteremia after specific procedures, the organisms that cause endocarditis, and the results of animal studies, most experts believe that prophylaxis is indicated. Recommendations for prophylaxis are published periodically by the American Heart Association.

16. Who should receive prophylactic antibiotics before dental procedures?
   • Patients at highest risk are those with prosthetic valves, previous episodes of bacterial endocarditis, complex cyanotic congenital heart disease, and systemic-pulmonary shunts or conduits.

- Patients with many other congenital cardiac defects, hypertrophic cardiomyopathy, or valves damaged by rheumatic fever are also at risk.
- Certain conditions do not put patients at increased risk and do not necessitate prophylaxis. Examples include innocent murmurs, isolated secundum atrial septal defect, mitral valve prolapse without regurgitation, and atrial or ventricular septal defects corrected more than 6 months in the past.
- Prophylactic antibiotics are recommended for at-risk patients undergoing dental extractions, initial placement of orthodontic bands, periodontal procedures, and prophylactic cleaning of teeth that is expected to cause bleeding. No prophylaxis is recommended for routine fillings, taking of x-rays, injection of local anesthetics, or adjustment of orthodontic appliances.

17. Which antibiotics are appropriate for endocarditis prophylaxis?

Antibiotics are aimed at viridans streptococci. Oral amoxicillin (50 mg/kg, up to 2 gm in adults) should be given 1 hour before the procedure. Patients allergic to penicillin can receive clindamycin (20 mg/kg, up to 600 mg) or clarithromycin (15 mg/kg, up to 500 mg).

18. In a patient with bacteremia, when should I be concerned about endocarditis?

Consider the underlying anatomy, organism, and nature of the bacteremia. Endocarditis is more likely in a patient with a predisposing cardiac lesion who has sustained bacteremia with no obvious focus of infection and whose bacteremia is caused by an organism likely to be involved in endocarditis. For example, a patient with no evidence of cardiac disease who has an *E. coli* urinary tract infection and a single positive blood culture is unlikely to have endocarditis. On the other hand, a patient with a bicuspid aortic valve who has had multiple cultures positive for viridans streptococci or *S. aureus*, is very likely to have an endocardial focus of infection and should be evaluated thoroughly.

A common source of confusion is the presence of a central venous catheter. Because the catheter may traumatize a valve or the endovascular surface, patients with catheters are at increased risk even if they have normal anatomy. When *S. aureus* bacteremia occurs, many clinicians consider it prudent to perform an echocardiogram even when the catheter is believed to be the site of infection. However, bacteremia that resolves quickly when the catheter is removed is unlikely to reflect endovascular infection.

19. What are the symptoms of myocarditis?

Children with myocarditis may present with symptoms of congestive heart failure or low cardiac output (fatigue, dyspnea, hypotension); with chest pain due to ischemia or pericardial inflammation; or with cardiac arrhythmias. The onset may be fulminant or insidious. The patient may be febrile or may recently have had a flu-like illness.

20. What causes myocarditis?

Most cases of myocarditis in the U.S. are believed to be caused by viruses. Although viruses are rarely cultured, viral nucleic acid can be detected in many biopsy specimens. Enteroviruses, adenoviruses, cytomegalovirus, and HIV have been implicated. Bacteria, fungi, and parasites also may be involved. Approximately 5% of patients with Lyme disease have myocardial involvement, typically some degree of atrioventricular block. In South America, Chagas disease (*Trypanosoma cruzi*) commonly affects the heart.

Rheumatologic diseases, such as juvenile rheumatic arthritis, also may cause cardiac inflammation. Metabolic and genetic disorders can cause myocardial dysfunction without associated inflammation.

21. Describe the evaluation of a child with suspected myocarditis.

The physical exam should focus on evidence of congestive failure and low cardiac output as well as evaluation of heart sounds and rhythm. The chest x-ray may show pulmonary edema or cardiac enlargement. An electrocardiogram may show voltage abnormalities, ischemic changes, or abnormal rhythm. The echocardiogram is probably the most useful test and is performed to evaluate cardiac size, cardiac function, and presence of a pericardial effusion; it is also important for excluding unsuspected cardiac malformations. The definitive diagnosis is established by a myocardial biopsy showing both inflammation and myocyte necrosis. Viral cultures of the nasopharynx and stool, and PCR testing of biopsy specimens may suggest a specific viral etiology.

22. Is there a definitive treatment for viral myocarditis?

No specific antiviral therapy has been shown to be effective. Pleconaril, an anti-enteroviral drug, has been tried in some patients, but no data are available to show its usefulness. Several immunosuppressive therapies have been tried. Corticosteroids have not been shown to be effective. Based on its efficacy in reducing cardiac sequelae of Kawasaki disease,and on a clinical trial with historical controls, high-dose IV immunoglobulin has been used in a number of centers. A randomized trial in adults did not show efficacy for IVIG, but some pediatric cardiologists believe that it is effective in children.

23. What are the clinical findings in a child with pericarditis?

The characteristic symptoms are chest pain and fever, but children may not complain of pain. Tachycardia and tachypnea are common, and a paradoxical pulse (decreased blood pressure during inspiration) or dyspnea may suggest cardiac tamponade. Heart sounds may be muffled. A biphasic or triphasic friction rub may be present and is often heard best when the patient is leaning forward. *Editor's note:* Good luck at hearing a friction rub.

24. What causes pericarditis?

- Purulent pericarditis in children typically results from bacteremia and is most often caused by *S. aureus, Streptococcus pneumoniae, H. influenzae,* or *Neisseria meningitidis.*
- Tuberculosis should be considered in all patients with pericarditis.
- Viruses (such as enteroviruses) may cause pericardial effusions and pericarditis.
- Noninfectious causes include collagen-vascular disease, rheumatic fever, hypersensitivity reactions, uremia, and post-pericardiotomy syndrome.

25. What diagnostic tests should be performed?

The echocardiogram is the best way of demonstrating a pericardial effusion. A chest x-ray may show pneumonia, suggesting a bacterial pathogen. A blood culture should be performed, and a purified protein derivative test for tuberculosis should be done. If a significant effusion or tamponade is present or if bacterial infection is suspected, the effusion should be drained, examined, and cultured. Patients should be monitored carefully because of the possibility of tamponade.

26. What therapy is appropriate for pericarditis?

Viral pericarditis is treated with nonsteroidal anti-inflammatory agents. **Bacterial** pericarditis is treated with drainage and prolonged (3–4 week) courses of antibiotics.

BIBLIOGRAPHY

1. Dajani AS, et al: AHA Scientific Statement: Prevention of bacterial endocarditis. JAMA 277:1794–1801, 1997.
2. Beyer AS, et al: AHA Scientific Statement: Diagnosis and management of infectious endocarditis and its complications. Circulation 98:2936–2948, 1998.
3. Wilson WR, et al: AHA Scientific Statement: Antibiotic treatment of adults with infective endocarditis due to streptococci, enterococci, staphylococci, and HACEK organisms. JAMA 274:1709–1713, 1995.
4. P. Ferrieri, et al: Unique features of infective endocarditis in childhood. Pediatrics 109:931–941, 2002.
5. Feldman AM, McNamara DM: Myocarditis. N Engl J Med 343: 1388–1398, 2000.

VI. Gastrointestinal Infections

23. GASTROENTERITIS

Mark R. Magnusson, M.D., Ph.D.

1. When is antibiotic treatment for *Salmonella* gastroenteritis indicated?
Antibiotic therapy is indicated for patients at high risk for invasive disease (bacteremia):
• Infants younger than 3 months
• Patients with malignancies
• Patients with hemoglobinopathies
• Patients with HIV, AIDS, or other immunodeficiency
• Patients with chronic gastrointestinal disease or severe colitis

2. What is the single most effective control measure to decrease transmission rates of bacterial gastroenteritis in developed countries: (a) hand-washing, (b) vegetarianism, (c) living alone, or (d) Saran wrap?
(a). Hand-washing decreases the transmission via the fecal-oral route.

3. What measure is the most effective in developing countries?
A water supply free from contamination by sewage.

4. What causes of gastroenteritis are associated with travel?

MICROORGANISM	AVERAGE FREQUENCY (%)	RANGE (%)
Toxigenic *Escherichia coli*	40–60	0–72
Invasive *E. coli*	< 5	0–5
Shigella species	10	0–30
Salmonella species	< 5	0–15
Campylobacter jejune	< 5	0–15
Vibrio parahaemolyticus	< 5	0–30
Aeromonas species	< 5	0–30
Giardia lamblia	< 5	0–6
Entamoeba histolytica	< 5	0–6
Rotavirus	5	0–36
No pathogen identified	40	20–85

From Gorbach SL, et al: Infectious diarrhea and bacterial food poisoning. In Sleisinger MH, Fordtran JS (eds): Gastrointestinal Disease, 5th ed. Philadelphia, W.B. Saunders, 1993, p 1153, with permission.

5. What common causes of vomiting should be considered in the differential diagnosis of infectious gastroenteritis?
Newborn (birth to 2 weeks)
• Normal variations ("spitting up")
• Gastroesophageal reflux

- Gastrointestinal (GI) obstruction–congenital anomalies
- Necrotizing enterocolitis (premature birth)
- Infection: meningitis, sepsis

Older infant (2 weeks to 12 months)
- Normal variations
- Gastroesophageal reflux
- GI obstruction, especially pyloric stenosis, intussusception, or incarcerated hernia
- Gastroenteritis
- Infection: sepsis, meningitis, urinary tract infection, otitis media, pertussis
- Drug overdose: aspirin, iron, lead, acetaminophen

Older child (over 12 months)
- GI obstruction: incarcerated hernia, intussusception
- Other GI causes: gastroenteritis, gastroesophageal reflux, appendicitis
- Infection: meningitis, urinary tract infection, upper respiratory infection
- Metabolic disorder: diabetic ketoacidosis
- Toxins/drugs: aspirin, iron, lead, alcohol, acetaminophen
- Pregnancy

Henretig FM:Vomiting. In Fleishek GR, Ludwig S (eds): Textbook of Pediatric Emergency Medicine, 3rd ed. Baltimore, Williams & Wilkins, 1993, p 508.

6. **What less common but severe, life-threatening causes of vomiting should be considered in the differential diagnosis of infectious gastroenteritis?**

Newborn (birth to 2 weeks)
- Anatomic anomalies: esophageal stenosis/atresia, intestinal obstructions, especially malrotation and volvulus, Hirschsprung's disease
- Other GI causes
- Necrotizing enterocolitis
- Peritonitis
- Neurologic disorders: kernicterus, mass lesions, hydrocephalus
- Renal disorders: obstructive anomalies, uremia
- Infection: sepsis, meningitis
- Metabolic disorders: inborn errors, especially congenital adrenal hyperplasia

Older infant (2 weeks to 12 months)
- Gastroesophageal reflux (severe)
- Esophageal disorders
- Rumination
- Intestinal obstruction, especially pyloric stenosis, intussusception, or incarcerated hernia
- Other GI causes, especially gastroenteritis (with dehydration)
- Neurologic disorders: mass lesions, hydrocephalus
- Renal disorders: obstruction, uremia
- Infection: sepsis, meningitis, pertussis
- Metabolic disorders: inborn errors
- Drugs: aspirin, digoxin

Older child (over 12 months)
- GI obstruction, especially intussusception
- Other GI causes, especially appendicitis or peptic ulcer disease
- Neurologic disorders: mass lesion
- Renal disorders: uremia
- Infection: meningitis
- Metabolic disorders: diabetic ketoacidosis, adrenal insufficiency
- Toxins/drugs: aspirin, ipecac, digoxin, iron, lead

Henretig FM:Vomiting. In Fleishek GR, Ludwig S (eds): Textbook of Pediatric Emergency Medicine, 3rd ed. Baltimore, Williams & Wilkins, 1993, p 508.

7. What infectious causes of diarrhea should be considered in the differential diagnosis of gastroenteritis?

Viruses: rotavirus, Norwalk virus, enteroviruses, astroviruses

Bacteria: *Salmonella, Shigella, Yersinia,* and *Campylobacter* spp.; pathogenic *Escherichia coli, Aeromonas hydrophila, Vibrio* spp.; *Clostridium difficile*; tuberculosis

Parasites: *Giardia lamblia, Entamoeba histolytica, Cryptosporidium parvum*

8. List the indications and potential benefits of antimicrobial therapy in bacterial gastroenteritis according to pathogen.

ENTEROPATHOGEN	INDICATION OR EFFECT
Shigella species	Shortens duration of diarrhea
	Eliminates organisms from feces
Campylobacter jejuni	Shortens duration
	Prevents relapse
Salmonella species	Indicated for infants < 12 mo
	Bacteremia
	Disseminated foci (e.g., osteomyelitis)
	Enteric fever
Escherichia coli	
Enteropathogenic	Use primarily in infants
	Intravenous use for invasive disease
Enterotoxigenic	Most illnesses brief and self-limited
Enteroinvasive	Information incomplete
Yersinia enterocolitica	None for gastroenteritis alone
	Indicated if septicemia or other
	localized infection is suspected
Clostridium difficile	10–20% relapse rate
Aeromonas hydrophila	Efficacy not clearly established

9. Match the infection with the pertinent history.

a. Recent antibiotic use
b. Immunosuppression
c. Illnesses in other family members or close contacts
d. Travel outside the United States
e. Consumption of untreated water, raw shellfish
f. Recent intake of chitterlings
g. Presence of family pets

1. *Entamoeba histolytica*
2. *Clostridium difficile*
3. Rotavirus or Norwalk agent
4. *Cryptosporidium parvum*
5. *Vibrio* spp.
6. *Campylobacter* spp.
7. *Yersinia enterocolitica*

Answers: a, 2; b, 4; c, 3; d, 1; e, 5; f, 7; g, 6.

10. Describe the natural history of viral gastroenteritis.

Normally the intestinal epithelium is replaced every 3–5 days. After a self-limited episode of viral gastroenteritis, the intestinal epithelium recovers in 7–10 days with functional recovery within 2 weeks. Occasionally, especially in infants < 12 months of age, postviral enteritis may be prolonged, probably as a result of transient disaccharidase deficiency.

11. What is pseudoappendicitis?

Pseudoappendicitis is a clinical syndrome that includes fever, abdominal pain, right lower quadrant tenderness, and leukocytosis. It occurs primarily in older children and adults.

12. What enteric bacterial pathogens are associated with pseudoappendicitis?

Intestinal lymphoid hyperplasia, particularly in the appendix and cecum, associated with *Yersinia* and *Salmonella* enteric infection is the presumed etiology.

13. How does the pathobiology of the various causative agents of acute infectious gastroenteritis relate to their clinical presentation?

PATHOBIOLOGY/AGENT	INCUBATION PERIOD	VOMITING	ABDOMINAL PAIN	FEVER	DIARRHEA
Toxin producers					
Preformed toxin					
Bacillus cereus	1–8 hr	3–4+	1–2+	0–1+	3–4+, watery
Staphylococcus aureus,					
Clostridium perfringens	8–24 hr				
Enterotoxin					
Vibrio cholerae, entero-	8–72 hr	2–4+	1–2+	0–1+	3–4+, watery
toxigenic *E. coli,*					
Klebsiella pneumoniae,					
Aeromonas species					
Enteroadherent					
Enteropathogenic and	1–8 days	0–1+	1–3+	1–2+	1–2+, watery
enteroadherent *E. coli,*					
Giardia organisms,					
cryptosporidosis					
Cytotoxin producers					
Clostridium difficile	1–3 days	0–1+	3–4+	1–2+	1–3+, usually watery, occasionally bloody
Hemorrhagic *E. coli*	12–72 hr	0–1+	3–4+	1–2+	1–3+, initially watery, then quickly bloody
Invasive organisms					
Minimal inflammation					
Rotavirus and Norwalk agent	1–3 days	1–2+	2–3+	3–4+	1–3+, watery
Variable inflammation					
Salmonella, Campylobacter, Aeromonas species, *Vibrio parahaemolyticus, Yersinia* species	12 hr–11 days	0–3+	2–4+	3–4+	1–4+, watery or bloody
Severe inflammation					
Shigella species, enteroinvasive *E. coli, Entamoeba histolytica*	12 hr–8 days	0–1+	3–4+	3–4+	1–2+, bloody

From Ahlquist DA, Camilleri M: Diarrhea and constipation. In Braunwald et al (eds): Harrison's Principles of Internal Medicine. New York, McGraw-Hill, 2000, p 243, with permission.

14. What are the key features of the viral pathogens seen in acute gastroenteritis?

VIRUS	MAJOR RISK GROUP	SEASONALITY	DIAGNOSTIC TEST	TREATMENT
Rotavirus (group A)	Children < 3 yr	Winter	ELISA	Oral rehydration, ? vaccination
Adenovirus (types 40, 41)	Children < 3 yr	Year-round	ELISA	Oral rehydration

Table continued on following page

VIRUS	MAJOR RISK GROUP	SEASONALITY	DIAGNOSTIC TEST	TREATMENT
Caliciviruses (genogroup III, SLVs)	Young children	Unknown	Experimental and EM	Oral rehydration
Astrovirus	Young children, immunocompromised hosts	Winter	Experimental and EM	Oral rehydration
Norwalk-like virus	Children and adults, epidemics	Winter	Experimental and EM	Oral rehydration

ELISA = enzyme-linked immunosorbent assay, EM = electron microscopy.

15. Describe the enteric virus that shares a name with a major league baseball team.

Astroviruses, which are 27–32 nm in diameter, have a characteristic icosahedral ultrastructure and contain a unique plus-sense, single-stranded RNA. This virus is a fairly common cause of mild to moderate gastroenteritis in children accounting for about one-quarter to one-half as much illness as rotavirus.

16. Many children with gastroenteritis become dehydrated. How can the severity of dehydration in children with gastroenteritis be estimated?

NO DEHYDRATION	MILD-TO-MODERATE DEHYDRATION*	SEVERE DEHYDRATION*
< 3% weight los	3–8% weight loss	> 9% weight loss
No signs	Dry mucous membranes	Signs from mild-to-moderate group
	Sunken eyes (and minimal or no tears)	*plus*
	Diminished skin turgor (pinch test > 1 sec)	Decreased peripheral perfusion (cool, mottled, pale; capillary refill time > 2 sec)
	Altered neurologic status (drowsiness, irritability	Circulatory collapse
	Deep (acidotic) breathing	

* Signs are listed in each column in order of increasing severity.
Note: If in doubt clinicians should err by overestimating the % dehydration.
From Armon K, Elliott EJ: Acute gastroenteritis. In Moyer VA, et al (eds): Evidence-based Pediatrics and Child Health. London, BMJ Books, 2000, p 277, with permission.

17. Which signs, symptoms, and laboratory data are most useful in caring for children with dehydration from gastroenteritis?

SIGN, SYMPTOM, TEST	SENSITIVITY (%)	SPECIFICITY (%)	LR+	LR
Skin turgor	65	56	1.4	0.6
Peripheral perfusion	35	86	2.5	0.8
Sunken eyes	81	27	1.1	0.7
Pulse > 130/min	56	49	1.1	0.9
Restless/lethargic	91	10	1.1	0.9
No urine for many hours	41	48	0.8	1.2
Sunken fontanel	54	25	0.7	2.6
Systolic BP < 100 mmHg	45	62	1.2	0.8
Absent tears	43	66	1.3	0.9
Deep breathing (acidotic)	50	74	1.9	0.7
Respiratory rate <30/min	51	69	1.7	0.7

Table continued on following page

SIGN, SYMPTOM, TEST	SENSITIVITY (%)	SPECIFICITY (%)	LR+	LR
Dry mouth	85	29	1.2	0.5
Increased thirst	66	49	1.3	0.7
Serum urea >6.5 mmol/liter	71	71	2.5	0.4
Capillary pH < 7.35	43	80	2.2	0.7
Base deficit >7	67	52	1.4	0.6

LR+ = positive likelihood ratio, LR = negative likelihood ratio.
Editors note: Careful review of the above chart will qualify you to edit the statistical secrets book yet to be published.
From Armon K, Elliott EJ: Acute gastroenteritis. In Moyer VA, et al (eds): Evidende-based Pediatrics and amd Child Health. London, BMJ Books, 2000, p 276, with permission.

18. What are the effects of antimotility agents for diarrhea in children with gastroenteritis?
Loperamide has been shown to shorten the duration of diarrhea in both randomized controlled trials and uncontrolled studies. However, the side-effect profile includes drowsiness, necrotizing enterocolitis, delirium, respiratory suppression, constipation, coma, and death. These risks may be excessive for a typically self-limited illnesses such as viral gastoenteritis. No studies have examined the use of other opiates or anticholinergics in children.

19. Why is *Lactobacillus* species (a probiotic) important in the biology of gastroenteritis?
Lactobacillus species are a component of the normal bowel flora responsible for homeostasis in the uninfected state.Several trials, both controlled and uncontrolled, demonstrate reductions in length of hospitalization and duration of diarrhea with the addition of *Lactobacillus* spp. to the oral rehydration solution on children with viral gastroenteritis.

20. Which therapies for infectious gastroenteritis are helpful? Which are harmful?
Likely to be beneficial
• Amino acid oral rehydration solution (vs. standard oral rehydration solution)
• Rice-based oral rehydration solution
Trade-offs between benefits and harms
• Empirical antibiotic treatment of travellers' diarrhea
• Empirical antibiotic treatment of community-acquired diarrhea
Unlikely to be beneficial
• Bicarbonate-free oral rehydration solution (vs. standard oral rehydration solution)
Likely to be ineffective or harmful
• Reduced-osmolarity oral rehydration solution (vs. standard oral rehydration solution)

21. What are some infrequent complications of *Shigella* infection?
Reiter syndrome after infection with *S. flexneri*, hemolytic-uremic syndrome from *S. dysenteriae* type 1, colonic perforation, and convulsions.

22. What is ekiri syndrome?
A potentially lethal fulminant toxic encephalopathy associated with *Shigella* infection.

23. One of the risks of *Salmonella* gastroenteritis is bacteremia. How many patients with Salmonella gastroenteritis develop recognizable focal infection?
Focal complications can occur in as many as 10% of patients.

24. Bacteremia is uncommon in *Campylobacter* infection, but what other several complications may occur during convalescence?
Immunoreactive complications include Guillain-Barré syndrome, Reiter syndrome, and erythema nodosum.

25. How is *Escherichia coli*-associated diarrhea classified?

TYPE OF *E. COLI*	EPIDEMIOLOGY	TYPE OF DIARRHEA	MECHANISM OF ACTION
Enteropathogenic	Acute and chronic endemic and epidemic diarrhea in infants	Watery	Adherence, effacement
Enterotoxigenic	Infantile diarrhea in developing countries and travelers' diarrhea	Watery	Adherence, enterotoxin production
Enteroinvasive	Diarrhea with fever in all ages	Bloody or nonbloody	Adherence, invasion of mucosa
Enterohemorrhagic	Hemorrhagic colitis and hemo-lytiuremic syndrome in all ages and thrombotic and throm-bocytopenic purpura in adults	Bloody or nonbloody	Cytotoxin production, adherence, effacement
Enteroaggregative	Incompletely defined	Watery	Adherence

26. A 3-month old infant with diarrhea tests positive for *Clostridium difficile*. Which of the following statements is not true?

(a) Up to 25–50% of infants less than 1 year of age are asymptomatic carriers of *C. difficile*.
(b) Patients with *C. difficile* in the stool pose a nosocomial risk if hospitalized.
(c) The treatment of choice is metronidazole.
(d) In addition to colitis, *C. difficile* is associated with some forms of tetanus.
Answer: (d). You must be thinking of *Clostridium tetani*.

27. Name a bacterial agent found in salt water that is associated with gastroenteritis and severe sepsis with distinctive skin manifestations.

Vibrio vulnificus. The infection occurs in patients who suffer traumatic injuries in a marine environment

28. A child in day care is reported to have *E. coli* 0157:H7 in the stool. Should the child be treated with antibiotics?

No. Antibiotic treatment may be associated with an increased risk of developing hemolytic uremic syndrome.

BIBLIOGRAPHY

1. American Academy of Pediatrics: Practice parameter: The management of acute gastroenteritis in young children. Pediatrics 97:424–432, 1996.
2. American Academy of Pediatrics, Committee on Infectious Diseases: 2000 Red Book. American Academy of Pediatrics, 2000.
3. Guerrant RL, Gilder TV, et al: Practice guidelines for the management of infectious diarrhea. Clin Infect Dis 32:331–350, 2001.
4. Henretig FM: Vomiting. In Fleishnek GR, Ludwig S (eds): Textbook of Pediatric Emergency Medicine, 3rd ed. Baltimore, Williams & Wilkins, p 508.
5. Moyer VA, et al (eds): Evidence-Based Pediatrics and Child Health. London, BMJ Books, 2000.
6. Murphy MS. Guidelines for managing acute gastroenteritis based on a systematic review of published research. Arch Dis Childhood 79:279–284, 1998.

24. INFECTIOUS HEPATITIS

Lisa B. Zaoutis, M.D.

1. What agents are responsible for infectious hepatitis?

Viral agents are the most common causes of hepatitis, whether the liver is the primary site of infection or affected as part of a more generalized viral process. Hepatitis viruses A, B, C, D, E, and G are the most common causes of hepatitis and are considered primarily hepatotropic. Other viral agents that cause hepatitis as part of a more generalized infection include the following:

- Epstein-Barr virus
- Cytomegalovirus
- Varicella zoster
- Herpes simplex
- Yellow fever
- Measles
- Mumps
- Rubeola
- Rubella
- Enterovirus
- Adenovirus
- Human immunodeficiency virus

Bacterial, parasitic, and fungal causes of hepatitis are less common; in such cases, the liver is often involved as part of a systemic or extrahepatic illness.

2. Describe the key features of hepatitis A.

The hepatitis A virus (HAV) causes a self-limited illness with abrupt onset of fever and diarrhea initially, followed by nausea, anorexia, malaise, dark urine, and jaundice. The incubation period is 2–5 weeks, the prodrome lasts for 1–7 days, and the icteric phase usually lasts less than 2 weeks. Hepatitis A can range from an asymptomatic infection to hepatomegaly with or without splenomegaly. Evidence of hepatocellular injury predominates with elevations in serum levels of alanine aminotransferases (ALT) and aspartate aminotransferase (AST); elevated serum levels of conjugated bilirubin and gamma glutamyl transpeptidase (GGT) reflect a cholestatic picture as well. Most children under 2 years of age with HAV infection are asymptomatic, but the trend reverses after the age of 5 years with only 20% of infected children remaining asymptomatic. Liver enzymes may remain elevated for several weeks. HAV does not cause chronic infection and rarely causes fulminant hepatitis.

3. Describe the typical illness caused by hepatitis B virus (HBV).

The typical illness is divided into the prodromal, icteric (or symptomatic), and convalescent phases, but the disease can range from a completely asymptomatic illness to fulminant lethal hepatitis. The prolonged incubation period ranges from 1 to 6 months and is followed by the insidious onset of nonspecific constitutional symptoms such as fatigue, nausea, and malaise. Often extrahepatic symptoms, including arthritis or rash, precede or accompany clinical hepatitis. This icteric phase typically lasts more than 2 weeks, and the convalescent or recovery phase may extend for weeks to months. Asymptomatic or nonicteric forms of the illness can occur and are more common in children less than 5 years of age. The pattern of liver enzyme elevations is similar to that seen hepatitis A.

Chronic HBV infection is more common in younger patients, who may remain asymptomatic throughout the course (carrier state). Alternatively, evidence of chronic or progressive liver disease may be detectable. The vast majority of neonates infected at birth (up to 90%) become chronic carriers of hepatitis B antigen, whereas only 20% of children and less than 10% of adults develop carrier states.

4. What are the key features of hepatitis C?

Perinatally acquired infection may present with no clear clinical signs or symptoms. Older children, who mainly acquire infection through transfusion of blood products, may report only nonspecific complaints of fatigue or abdominal pain, which are difficult to differentiate from the underlying illness. Extrahepatic manifestations, such as vasculitis or serum sickness-like illness, are very uncommon, as is jaundice. Liver enzymes may be normal or only mildly elevated and may vary widely throughout the course of the infection. During childhood, hepatitis C infection is usually a benign illness, but chronic infection often leads to cirrhosis and cancer after many years.

5. What is unique about infection with hepatitis D virus (HDV)?

HDV infection is associated only with HBV infection. It can take two forms: coinfection or superinfection. Coinfection refers to acquisition of HBV and HDV infection at the same time. Superinfection occurs when a person with chronic HBV infection subsequently develops infection with HDV. The features of the clinical manifestations are those of the underlying HBV infection, although the HDV infection usually causes a more severe illness.

6. Where is infection with hepatitis E virus (HEV) most commonly found?

HEV is the cause of endemic non-A, non-B hepatitis in the Indian subcontinent, Asia, and Africa. It is very rare in developed countries. The clinical manifestations closely resemble HAV infection, but the illness has a higher fatality rate, especially in pregnant women.

7. What is the plural form of the word *hepatitis*?

The plural of hepatitis is hepatitides (pronounced hep-e-*tit*-e-*dez*). Before you say the plural in public, practice several times out loud in private so that it rolls off your tongue in a nonchalant manner.

8. How is hepatitis A diagnosed?

The immunoassay for anti-HAV IgM is the standard for diagnosis. This antibody is detectable at the onset of the illness and remains detectable for months. The presence of anti-HAV IgG follows and denotes protection from reinfection. The available immunoassays cannot distinguish between natural infection and vaccine-induced antibodies. A specific assay, not commercially available, can identify antibody to the P2 antigen found only in patients with natural infection and not in patients with vaccine-induced immunity (try to get your lab to do this test).

9. How is hepatitis B diagnosed?
- Hepatitis B surface antigen (HBsAg) is present in acute and chronic HBV infection.
- Hepatitis B core IgM antibody (anti-HBc IgM) is evidence of acute hepatitis B infection.
- Hepatitis B core IgG antibody (anti-HBc IgG) is found in resolving or chronic hepatitis B infection but not in patients with immunity from the hepatitis B vaccine.
- Hepatitis B e antigen (HBeAg) is present with active viral replication and is associated with high infectivity.
- Hepatitis B envelope antibody (anti-HBe) heralds the end of viral replication.
- Hepatitis B surface antibody (anti-HBs) indicates lasting immunity after infection or hepatitis B vaccination.

Note: See Chapter 50 (Fast Facts) for the test on interpretation of these secrets.

10. How are hepatitis C nd hepatitis D diagnosed?

The diagnosis of **hepatitis C** is suggested by the detection of anti-hepatitis C IgG (IgG anti-HCV) on enzyme-linked immunosorbent assay (ELISA) but must be confirmed by recombinant immunoblot assay or HCV RNA polymerase chain reaction (PCR).

Because **hepatitis D** occurs only with acute or chronic hepatitis B, the IgM antibody to HDV (IgM anti-HDV) is sought only if HBsAg is present.

11. What initial panel of serologic tests should be performed if hepatitis B and C are suspected?

Newborn: HbsAg, anti-HbsAg, anti-IgM Hbc, HCV PCR (if the mother is seropositive for hepatitis C).

All others: IgM anti-HAV, HbsAg, HbsAb, IgM anti-HBc, anti-HCV Ab.

12. What is the mode of transmission of HAV?

Person-to-person transmission via the fecal-oral route is the most common mode of transmission. Foodborne outbreaks occur, but waterborne outbreaks are rare.

13. How is HBV transmitted?

- Transmission occurs via blood or body fluids from a person with acute or chronic HBV infection (i.e., positive for HBsAg).
- Transmission by infected blood products is rare in the U.S. because of routine screening.
- Needle sharing
- Sexual activity (homosexual or heterosexual)
- Interpersonal household contacts over an extended period: child-to-child and mother-to-child are the most common patterns. Young children remain at highest risk for acquiring infection from nonsexual interpersonal contact.

14. How are hepatitis C and hepatitis E transmitted?

Transmission of **hepatitis C** is usually by parenteral exposure to HCV-infected blood or blood products. Other body fluids contaminated with infected blood can also cause infection, but not commonly. Even among monogamous couples, the rate of transmission to the uninfected partner is estimated at 1.5%. The rate of vertical (perinatal) transmission is also low (approximately 5%).

Hepatitis E is transmitted by the fecal-oral route.

15. Who is at risk for HAV infection?

- Susceptible travelers visiting countries with intermediate-to-high endemic rates of HAV infection
- Children living in communities with consistently elevated rates of HAV infection
- Men who have sex with men
- Intravenous drug users
- Patients requiring clotting factor concentrates
- People with occupational exposure to nonhuman primates born in the wild and those who handle HAV in laboratory settings

In addition, people with chronic liver disease are at increased risk for fulminant hepatitis in association with HAV infection.

16. List the groups at risk for HBV infection.

- Infants born to HBsAg-positive mothers, either perinatally (vertical transmission) or within the first 5 years of life (horizontal transmission)
- Adolescents and adults with high-risk behavior, including intravenous drug use, multiple heterosexual partners, and men who have sex with men
- People whose occupational activities include contact with blood or body fluids or those who staff institutional facilities for the developmentally disabled
- Household or sexual contacts of people with acute or chronic HBV infection
- Patients undergoing hemodialysis and those who receive clotting factor concentrates

17. Who is at risk for HCV infection?

- Intravenous drug users
- Patients who received blood products before 1987, especially those that received clotting factor concentrates or intravenous immune globulin products

18. For which hepatitis viruses is postexposure prophylaxis recommended?

Hepatitis A. Immunoglobulin is recommended for postexposure prophylaxis if the time since exposure is less than 2 weeks. HAV vaccines are currently not recommended for postexposure prophylaxis unless future exposure is likely, but this is an area of ongoing study.

Hepatitis B. Hepatitis immunization and hepatitis B immune globulin (HBIG) are recommended for perinatal exposure, sexual partners of a person with acute HBV infection, and percutaneous or permucosal exposure to blood from an HBV-infected person or a person whose infection status is unknown. Hepatitis immunization alone is recommended for household contacts of an HBsAg-positive person and sexual partners of a person with chronic HBV infection.

19. What vaccines are available for the prevention of hepatitis?

HAV and HBV vaccines.

20. What is the role of hepatitis B immune globulin?

HBIG provides short-term protection through passive immunization for high-risk exposure situations. Hyperimmunized donors are used to create HBIG, which contains high titers of anti-HBs. Standard IVIG is not effective because of the inadequate levels of anti-HBs-specific antibodies. The hepatitis vaccine series is uniformly initiated with administration of HBIG to add long-term protection. A HBV vaccine can be used alone or in conjunction with HBIG. The two vaccines produced in the U.S., Energix-B (SmithKline Beecham) and Recombivax HB (Merck), use recombinant DNA technology and are equally effective. These products are also interchangeable; the 3-dose series may be completed with any combination of the two vaccines.

21. Should everybody receive the hepatitis B vaccine?

Universal immunization with hepatitis B vaccine is recommended for all susceptible people. Routine childhood immunizations are recommended for all infants, and previously unimmunized children should complete the series by age 11–12 years.

22. What about hepatitis C, D, and E?

No vaccines are available at this time. IVIG has no role in hepatitis C, because eligible donors are tested specifically to be negative for anti-HCV antibodies. IVIG has not been shown to be effective in preventing HDV or HDE infection.

23. What are the current recommendations for prevention of perinatal transmission of HBV for full-term infants?

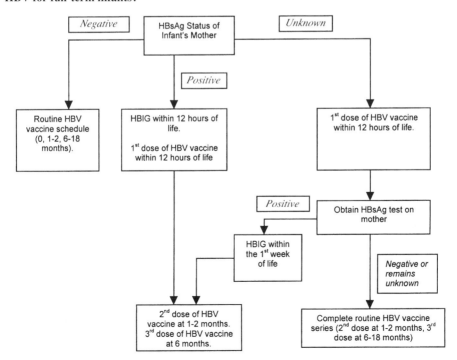

Special considerations and recommendations for preterm infants are outlined in the Red Book.

24. Match the serologic results with the correct clinical interpretation?
1. Anti-HBs– and anti-HBc–positive
2. Anti-HBs–positive, anti-HBc–negative
3. HBsAg-negative, anti-HBs–negative, IgM anti-HBc–positive
4. Anti-HCV–positive
5. IgM anti-HAV–negative, IgG anti-HAV–positive
6. IgM anti-HAV–positive, IgG anti-HAV–negative
7. HBeAg- and HBsAg-positive.
   a. Acute or recent HBV infection ("window phase" where HBsAg has become undetectable before anti-HBs can be detected).
   b. Protection from future infection from either past HAV infection or HAV vaccination.
   c. Positive screening test for HCV infection, but confirmation of infection by recombinant immunoblot is required.
   d. HBV infection with increased risk for transmission of the virus.
   e. Acute or recent HAV infection.
   f. Acute, resolved, or chronic HBV infection
   g. Immunity after HBV immunization
   h. Confirmation of HCV infection
   Answers: 1, f; 2, g; 3, a; 4, h; 5, b; 6, e; 7, d.

25. Why is the hepatitis B vaccine series routinely initiated in the newborn period?
1. The goal of universal immunization to eventually eliminate HBV transmission is best achieved by incorporating hepatitis B vaccination into the routine childhood immunization program.
2. Young children are at highest risk for acquiring the infection from household contact with an infected person.
3. Alaskan Native and Asian-Pacific Islander children and children of immigrants from HBV endemic countries are at especially high risk.
4. In the U.S., HBV infection is most often acquired during adolescence or adulthood when high-risk behavior is more common. However, these groups are more difficult to capture for completion of the 3-dose hepatitis vaccine series.

26. When should the hepatitis B vaccine series be initiated for children not vaccinated in the newborn period?
Children should complete the vaccine series before 11–12 years of age. Compliance after this age is more difficult.

27. Name three drugs that may be useful for the treatment of viral hepatitis.
Lamuvidine, interferon, and ribavirin.

BIBLIOGRAPHY

1. American Academy of Pediatrics, Committee on Infectious Diseases. 2000 Red Book. Elk Grove, IL, American Academy of Pediatrics, 2000.
2. Jonas MM: Treatment of chronic hepatitis in pediatric patients. Clin Liver Dis 3:856–867, 1999.
3. Ng VL, Balistreri WF: Hepatitis B: Clinical perspectives in pediatrics. Clin Liver Dis 3:267–291, 1999.
4. Rosenthal P, Lightdale JR: Labaratory evaluation of hepatitis. Pediatr Rev 21, 2000.

VII. Genitourinary Tract Infections

25. URINARY TRACT INFECTIONS

Daniel M. Ingram, M.S.P.H., Karen R. Beasley, B.S.,
and David Lane Ingram, M.D.

1. Which of the following are considered risk factors for urinary tract infections (UTIs): (a) wiping back to front, (b) pinworm infestation, (c) use of bubble bath, (d) tight clothing and underwear, or (e) all of the above?

(e) All of the above.

2. In children 2 months to 2 years old with fever of no apparent source, what per cent will be found to have a UTI: (a) 0.5–1%, (b) 5%, or (c) 10%?

(b) Approximately 5% overall, but UTIs are twice as prevalent in girls as in boys.

3. In what age group are boys more likely to have a UTI than girls?

In the newborn period boys are 5–8 times more likely to have a UTI than girls.

4. How much more likely is a UTI in uncircumcised compared with circumcised boys: (a) 2 times, (b) 5 times, or (c) 10 times?

(c) 10 times more likely. It is estimated that 7–14/1000 uncircumcised male infants will have a UTI during the first year of life compared with 1–2 /1000 circumcised male infants.

5. The most commonly found organism in the urine of a child with a UTI is (a) *Escherichia coli*, (b) *Klebsiella* species, (c) *Staphylococccus saprophyticus*, or (d) *Enterococcus* species.

(a) *E. coli* causes 70-90% of UTIs. Other gram-negative rods such as *Klebsiella* species are the second most common cause, followed by *Enterococcus* species and other gram-positive organisms. *S. saprophyticus* is a rare pathogen before puberty but causes 15% of UTIs in females in later adolescence and may be found in males and females. Sexual intercourse is an important risk factor for this agent.

6. True of false: An important but uncommon clinical presentation of a UTI in a newborn is cholestatic jaundice.

True. Infants in the first few weeks of life with a UTI may present with cholestatic jaundice, particularly infections in male infants and those caused by *E. coli*.

7. What is the chance that a child with a UTI will have a positive urine reagent slide test (dipstick)?

A positive test is defined as the presence of leukocyte esterase, nitrites, or 5 or more white blood cells (WBC)/ml in the urinalysis microscopy. Overall, tests are positive in 99.8% of children with UTIs.

Sensitivity and Specificity of Components of the Urinalysis, Alone and in Combination

TEST	% SENSITIVITY (RANGE)	% SPECIFICITY (RANGE)
Leukocyte esterase	83 (67–94)	78 (64–92)
Nitrite	53 (15–82)	98 (90–100)

Continued. on next page.

Sensitivity and Specificity of Components of the Urinalysis, Alone and in Combination (Cont'd.)

TEST	% SENSITIVITY (RANGE)	% SPECIFICITY (RANGE)
Leukocyte esterase *or* nitrite positive	93 (90–100)	72 (58–91)
Microscopy: WBCs	73 (32–100)	81 (45–98)
Microscopy: bacteria	81 (16–99)	83 (11–100)
Leukocyte esterase *or* nitrite *or* microscopy positive	99.8 (99–100)	70 (60–92)

8. Is bag urine (urine collected by placing a sterile bag over the genital area) an acceptable method for obtaining a urine sample for culture in a young child?

No. Contamination from surrounding tissues, even if the genital area has been cleaned, produces 85% false-positive cultures. In febrile boys, the overall false-positive rate is 93%; the rate rises to 99% in circumcised boys. According to some experts, a sterile culture (if the sample is not contaminated with the cleaning solution) rules out a UTI.

9. If a catheterized urine specimen is not possible in an infant, is it still acceptable to do a suprapubic bladder aspiration with needle and syringe to obtain a urine sample for culture?

Yes.

10. In a catheterized urine specimen culture, what concentration of bacteria per milliliter of urine has a 95% probability of indicating a UTI?

- According to some experts, > 100,000 colonies/ml has a 95% probability of indicating UTI.
- 10,000–100,000 colonies/ml indicates likely UTI.
- 1,000–10,000 colonies/ml is suspicious and requires repeat culture.
- < 1,000 colonies/ml is unlikely to be a UTI.

11. Single-dose oral therapy for UTIs is not recommended for prepubertal children. How long is the shortest duration of therapy recommended by the American Academy of Pediatrics (AAP)?

The shortest course of oral therapy recommended by the AAP is 7 days. Most uncomplicated UTIs are eliminated with a 7- to 10-day antimicrobial course, but many experts prefer 14 days for ill-appearing children with clinical evidence of pyelonephritis, regardless of the antibiotic.

12. Which antibiotics are *not* contraindicated in treating UTIs in pregnant adolescents: (a) amoxicillin, (b) cephalexin, (c) nitrofurantoin, (d) trimethoprim/sulfamethoxazole, or (e) all of the above?

(e) if the patient is not allergic to the drug.

13. Do any consensus statements recommend the use of ciprofloxacin for treating UTIs caused by *Pseudomonas* species in children?

Yes. The consensus statement by the International Society of Chemotherapy recommends ciprofloxacin for this purpose and states that no data support the concern that the cartilage damage caused by ciprofloxacin in young animals occurs in children.

14. According to the AAP guidelines, how should children with UTIs, aged 2 months to 2 years, be initially evaluated for urinary tract abnormalities?

(a) Ultrasonography	**(d) Renal cortical scintigraphy**
(b) Fluoroscopic voiding cysto-	**(e) (a) and (b)**
urethrography (VCUG)	**(f) All the above**
(c) Intravenous pyelogram	

(e) Initial evaluation after the first UTI should be done with renal ultrasound and VCUG.

15. In what situation or situations after resolution of UTIs should prophylactic antibiotic therapy be started to prevent recurrences?
  (a) Between the end of therapy and performance of VCUG
  (b) Until vesicoureteral reflux is no longer present
  (c) In children with frequent UTIs
  (d) All the above

(d) Prophylactic regimens with trimethoprim/sulfamethoxazole or nitrofurantoin at one-third the normal daily dose at bedtime is recommended.

16. Is the finding of 100,000 colonies/ml of *Lactobacillus* species, *Corynebacterium* species, or alpha hemolytic streptococci in a urine culture considered indicative of a UTI?

Usually not. Under most circumstances such findings are indicative of periurethral flora contamination.

17. How should you interpret the result of a urine culture with 50,000-100,000 colonies/ml obtained from an adequately performed clean-void urine specimen?

The culture should be treated as suspicious for a UTI and repeated.

18. How should you interpret the result of a urine culture with 10,000-50,000 colonies/ml obtained from an adequately performed clean-void urine specimen?

If the child is symptomatic, the culture is suspicious for a UTI and should be repeated. If the child is asymptomatic, a UTI is unlikely.

19. An adolescent boy has dysuria and 5 or more white blood cells/ml in the urinalysis, but the routine urine culture is sterile. What is the most likely cause of his symptoms?

The most likely cause is a sexually transmitted disease, such as gonorrhea or chlamydial infection, that resulted in urethritis. Neither organism will grow on culture plates used to evaluate UTIs.

20. Should you treat bacteriuria in an asymptomatic child with a neurogenic bladder due to spinal injury, spina bifida, or cerebral palsy?

No. Treatment is not warranted unless the child is symptomatic.

21. Cefixime has been recommended for oral treatment of cystitis and pyelonephritis in young children. Which organism causing UTIs is uniformly resistant to cefixime: (a) enterococci, (b) *E. coli*, (c) *Klebsiella* sp., or (d) *Citrobacter* sp.?

(a) Enterococci are not sensitive to cephalosporins (including cefixime). Enterococci should be treated with amoxicillin while awaiting sensitivity results

22. Which of the following is *not* a contradiction to using oral cefixime as treatment for UTI in a child over the age of 1 month: (a) vomiting, (b) allergy to cefixime, (c) lethargy, or (d) possible pyelonephritis?

(d) Cefixime may be used to treat pyelonephritis as long as the child is able to take oral medicines well and is not allergic to it.

23. If oral cefixime is used to treat a child over 1 month of age for UTI or possible pyelonephritis, how is it dosed?

The first daily dose is 16 mg/kg orally, followed by 8mg/kg/day for 13 more days. Treatment outcomes are equal to those with initial use of cefotaxime sodium for 3 days followed by oral cefixime for 11 days. Oral cefixime can be recommended as safe and effective treatment for children with fever and a UTI.

24. Can a once-daily regimen with intramuscular (IM) or intravenous (IV) gentamicin be used in neonates with a UTI caused by gentamicin-sensitive organisms?

Yes. Gentamicin, 4–5 mg/kg/day IM or IV, may be used in neonates with normal renal function for treatment of a UTI.

25. Is nitrofurantoin an acceptable antibiotic for treatment of a febrile UTI in children?

No. Nitrofurantoin does not achieve adequate renal tissue levels. It may be used for prophylaxis to prevent recurrent UTIs.

26. What is the recommended postcoital prophylactic treatment for adolescent girls who frequently develop UTIs after intercourse (honeymoon cystitis)?

If the girl is not allergic to the drug, one oral dose of trimethoprim/sulfamethoxazole (20/200 mg), cephalexin (250 mg), or nitrofurantoin (50–100 mg) may be used soon after intercourse to prevent UTIs.

27. Should a repeat urine culture be done after 2 days of antibiotic therapy for a UTI to determine adequacy of treatment?

No. A repeat culture at this time is generally not necessary if the infant or child has had the expected clinical response and the uropathogen is determined to be sensitive to the antimicrobial being administered.

28. Approximately what percent of children are found to have vesicoureteral reflux after their first UTI: (a) 5–10%, (b) 20–30%, or (c) 30–50%?

(c) 30–50%.

29. List risk factors for renal scarring in the absence of structural abnormalities of the urinary tract.

- First episode of pyelonephritis before 3 years of age
- Grades IV and V vesicoureteral reflux in conjunction with bacteriuria
- Delay in instituting therapy after the establishment of pyelonephritis

30. When is a VCUG indicated?

- All children less than age 5 years old with UTI
- Any child with febrile UTI
- Any male child with UTI
- School-aged girls with 2 or more UTIs

31. Is it necessary to wait 2–6 weeks after cessation of antibiotic therapy for a UTI before doing VCUG?

No. The incidence of finding reflux is the same whether the VCUG is done during therapy or some time after therapy.

32. What is the indication for using radionuclide cystography (RNC) in children?

RNC may be preferable to VCUG in follow-up examinations of children with vesicoureteral reflux because it has a lower radiation dose. However, VCUG with fluoroscopy shows reflux better than RCN and should be used for the initial examination.

33. Do any controlled studies show that antimicrobial prophylaxis reduces renal scaring in children with vesicoureteral reflux?

No.

34. Is a UTI a possible cause of failure to thrive in an otherwise asymptomatic infant?

Yes. Urinalysis and catheterized or suprapubic urine specimen for culture are appropriate in evaluating failure to thrive.

BIBLIOGRAPHY

1. American Academy of Pediatrics, Committee on Quality Improvement, Subcommittee on Urinary Tract Infections: Practice parameter: The diagnosis, treatment and evolution of the initial urinary tract infection in febrile infants and young children. Pediatrics 103:843–853, 1999.
2. Chon CH, Lai FC, Shortlife LM: Pediatric urinary tract infections. Pediatr Clin North Am 48:1441–1459, 2001.
3. Downs SM: Diagnostic strategies in childhood urinary tract infections. Pediatr Ann 28:670–676, 1999.
4. Elder JS: Urinary tract infections. In Behrman RE, Kliegman RM, Jenson HB (eds): Nelson Textbook of Pediatrics, 16th ed. Philadelphia, W.B. Saunders, 2000, pp 1621–1625.
5. Hoberman A, Wald E, Hickey RW, et al: Oral versus intravenous therapy for urinary tract infections in young febrile children. Pediatrics 104:79–86, 1999.
6. Lohr JA, Downes SM, Schlager TA: Urinary tract infections. In Long SS, Pickering LK, Prober CG (eds): Principles and Practice of Pediatric Infectious Diseases. New York, Churchill Livingstone, 1997, pp 370–377.
7. Pennington DJ, Zerin JM: Imaging of the urinary tract in children. Pediatr Ann 28:678–686, 1999.
8. Roberts KB, Akintemi OB: The epidemiology and clinical presentation of urinary tract infections in children younger than 2 years of age. Pediatr Ann 28:644–649, 1999.
9. Schaad UB, Salam MA, Aujard Y, et al: Use of fluoroquinolones in pediatrics: Consensus report of an International Society of Chemotherapy commission. Pediatr Infect Dis J 14:1–9, 1995.
10. Schlager TA: The pathogenesis of urinary tract infections. Pediatr Ann 28:639–642, 1999.

26. SEXUALLY TRANSMITTED DISEASES

Daniel M. Ingram, M.S.P.H., and David Lane Ingram, M.D.

1. What three agents in children are highly associated with sexual transmission?

Neisseria gonorrhoeae after 1 month old, *Chlamydia trachomatis* after 3 years old, and *Treponema pallidum* (syphilis), if not congenitally acquired.

2. What adult sexually transmitted diseases (STDs) may be acquired by sexual or nonsexual contact in children?

Trichomonas vaginalis, herpes simplex, human papillomavirus (HPV), human immunodeficiency virus (HIV), and bacterial vaginosis.

3. What is the only acceptable test to diagnose infection with *N. gonorrhoeae* or *C. trachomatis* in children?

Culture. DNA probes, enzyme-linked immunosorbent assays (ELISAs), and ligase chain reactions are not accurate enough for use in children.

4. How often should a sexually active female adolescent be screened for chlamydial vaginal infections with tests such as a DNA probe or ligase chain reaction?

According to current recommendations, every 6 months, whether or not she has vaginitis.

5. In the acute evaluation of an adolescent who has been raped, for which STDs should you screen?

Cultures for *N. gonorrhoeae* and *C. trachomatis* at the involved anatomic sites and acute serologies for syphilis, HIV, and hepatitis B virus.

6. What initial antibiotic treatment should be given to a rape victim?

- Ceftriaxone, 125 mg intramuscularly (IM); ciprofloxacin, 500 mg orally; or cefixime, 500 mg orally for gonorrhea
- Azithromycin, 1 gm orally for possible chlamydial infection
- Metronidazole, 2 gm orally for possible trichomonal infection

Although children and adolescents who have been raped are potentially at risk for HIV, there is no consensus for postexposure prophylaxis.

7. Describe an acceptable inpatient antibiotic treatment for an adolescent with pelvic inflammatory disease (PID).

- Cefoxitin, 2 gm intravenously (IV) every 6 hours, and doxycycline, 100 mg IV or orally 2 times/day until 24–48 hours after significant clinical improvement; then doxycycline alone to complete 14 days of treatment

    or

- Clindamycin, 900 mg IV every 8 hours, and 2-mg/kg loading dose of gentamicin, followed by 1.5 mg/kg IV or IM every 8 hours for 24–48 hours after significant improvement; then switch to clindamycin, 600 mg orally 3 times /day for a total of 14 days

According to some experts, all cases of adolescent PID should be treated on an inpatient basis. Outpatient oral therapy should not be used.

8. Which STD is most commonly associated with cervical tumors: (a) herpes simplex type 1, (b) herpes simplex type 2, (c) HPV, or (d) *T. vaginalis*?

(c) HPV DNA is detected by polymerase chain reaction (PCR) in 93% of invasive cervical tumors; 50% of cases are due to HPV type 16.

9. In male adolescents, are urethral chlamydial infections usually symptomatic or asymptomatic?

They are usually asymptomatic.

10. In prepubertal females, is vaginal gonorrhea usually asymptomatic or associated with a vaginal discharge?

Eighty-seven percent of prepubertal females with vaginal gonorrhea have a vaginal discharge.

11. Is a cervical culture needed to detect chlamydial or a gonococcal vaginal infections in prepubertal girls? Or is a vaginal culture acceptable?

A vaginal culture rather than a cervical culture should be done. In prepubertal girls, *C. trachomatis* and *N. gonorrhoeae* infect the vaginal tissue, making it a good site to culture. A speculum examination should not be done on a prepubertal girl to obtain these cultures.

12. Are chlamydial vaginal infections usually asymptomatic or symptomatic in prepubertal girls?

Sixty percent of girls are asymptomatic. Symptoms may include a vaginal discharge, which also may be caused by a coexisting gonococcal infection.

13. Are rectal gonococcal or chlamydial infections usually asymptomatic or symptomatic in prepubertal children?

They are almost always asymptomatic.

14. What is the chance that an adolescent female will acquire HIV from one act of vaginal intercourse with an HIV-positive male: (a) 0.1%, (b) 10%, (c) 20%, or (d) 30%?

(a) The risk is about 0.1 %.

15. What percent of adolescent males with urethral gonorrhea infection are asymptomatic?

Only 2.5% are asymptomatic by 14 days of infection.

16. What is the chance that an adolescent female with genital gonorrhea also has a chlamydial vaginal infection: (a) 1–2%, (b) 10–20% , or (c) 20–30%?

(c) For this reason, female adolescents with gonorrhea are automatically treated for presumed chlamydial infection.

17. Which rash is *not* consistent with secondary syphilis: (a) macular, (b) maculopapular, (c) vesicular, or (d) pustular?

(c) All of the other types may be seen in secondary syphilis, especially on the hands and feet.

18. Is the chancre of primary syphilis described as painful or painless?

Classically, the ulcer (chancre) of primary syphilis is described as painless.

19. How is bacterial vaginosis diagnosed in adolescent females? In prepubertal females?

(a) **Presence of "clue cells" in a wet mount of vaginal fluid**
(b) **Fishy odor when 10% potassium hydroxide (KOH) is added to the discharge on a glass slide ("whiff" test)**
(c) **pH of vaginal fluid > 4.5**
(d) **All of the above**

(d) In adolescent females; (a) and (b) in prepubertal females.

20. In a patient with syphilis, which serologic tests usually become negative after appropriate treatment?

The nontreponemal serologic tests, such as the rapid plasma reagin (RPR) or Venereal Disease Research Laboratory (VDRL) test, usually become negative. A small percentage of patients may have persistent low levels for years. The treponemal serologic tests, such as the microhemagglutinin (MHA-TP) or fluorescent treponemal antibody absorbed (FTA-ABS) test, remain positive for life, even if the patient is adequately treated.

21. Which is the appropriate treatment of primary or secondary syphilis in patients not allergic to penicillin: (a) oral penicillin VK , (b) oral penicillin G, or (c) intramuscular benzathine penicillin?

(c) Benzathine penicillin is the appropriate treatment.

22. Is *T. vaginalis* becoming more resistant to metronidazole?

Yes. Resistant infections may require a more prolonged treatment than the usual regimen of one 2-gm dose orally. The one-dose treatment fails in 5% of patients and sexual partners. Adequate treatment requires 500 mg twice daily for 7 days. Rare patients may require 500-750 mg 3 times /day for 7 days.

23. After an episode of vaginal fondling, an adolescent male develops a painful blister filled with clear fluid at the base of his fingernail. What is the most likely cause?

The boy has developed a whitlow caused by herpes simplex.

24. What medical treatment may be used to suppress recurrences of genital herpes simplex?

Acyclovir, 200 mg 4 times/day or 400 mg 2 times/day orally.

25. Approximately what percentage of mothers whose infants develop neonatal herpes simplex infections have a history of vaginal infection with herpes simplex or a sexual partner reporting a genital vesicular rash?

Only about 20–40%.

26. What is Fitz-Hugh–Curtis syndrome?

Perihepatitis (inflammation of the liver capsule), which usually is caused by *N. gonorrhoeae* or *C. trachomatis* and presents with severe pleuritic right upper quadrant abdominal pain in females or males (rare). Often perihepatitis is associated with PID. Perihepatitis is observed by laparoscopy in 5–15% of patients with acute salpingitis. Sedimentation rate, liver function tests, and white blood count are in the ranges seen in acute salpingitis. A small amount of basal pleural fluid may be seen on chest x-ray.

27. What rash may develop with gonococcemia and gonococcal polyarthritis: (a) macular (b) papular, (c) vesicular, or (d) all of the above?

(d) Small macules or papules are the most common lesions, but all forms of skin lesions have been seen, including pustules, vesicles, bullae, erythema multiforme, and erythema nodosum. The rash most frequently occurs on the extremities and sometimes on the trunk. The papules are usually painless, appear pustular, and resemble vasculitis.

28. What prophylactic regimen of anti-HIV drugs may be used after an adolescent has been raped by a person with HIV?

The U.S. Public Health Department does not recommend for or against the use of antiretroviral agents to reduce HIV transmission after possible nonoccupational exposure because of lack of efficacy data. Zidovudine, 200 mg 3 times/day, with or without lamivudine, 150 mg 2 times/day, for 4 weeks in adults and adolescents may be tried.

29. An adolescent boy has a painful ulcer on the penis with painful inguinal lymphadenopathy. How should you evaluate him for possible chancroid, an infection due to *Haemophilus ducreyi*?

Direct examination of clinical material by Gram stain may strongly suggest the diagnosis if large numbers of gram-negative coccobacilli are seen. The material from the ulcer or lymph node may be cultured. Special culture media and conditions are required for isolation; if chancroid is suspected, the microbiology laboratory should be informed.

30. What pattern of organisms is seen on Gram-stain of the specimen from the patient in question 29: (a) school of fish, (b) spaghetti and meatballs, (c) gaggle of swans, or (d) plaid.
(a) School of fish.

31. What STD is most likely to account for the most cases of asymptomatic PID: (a) *N. gonorrhoeae*, (b) *C. trachomatis*, or (c) HPV?
(b) *C. trachomatis* infections are a common cause of pelvic PID and are more likely than infections caused by *N.gonorrhoeae* to result in asymptomatic disease. The problem may be discovered years later when a woman is evaluated for sterility. HPV does not cause pelvic inflammatory disease.

32. What is the chance that an adolescent girl will become sterile after one episode PID?
Twelve percent of women become sterile because of fallopian tube damage after one episode of PID. This rate may increase to 40% if fallopian tubes are severely damaged.

33. Describe the most common clinical presentation of oral gonorrhea.
Seventy-five percent of children and adolescents with oral gonorrhea are asymptomatic. The rest may have a sore throat that does not respond to treatment for a group A streptococcal infection. Some patients may have a red swollen uvula.

34. How long after infection with HIV do 95% of patients have a positive ELISA test: (a) 6 weeks, (b) 3 months, or (c) 6 months?
Although the ELISA test may become positive by 3–4 weeks after infection, it takes about 6 months for 95% or more of patients to develop a positive test.

35. Is hepatitis B easily spread through vaginal intercourse?
Yes. This is one reason why children should receive the hepatitis B vaccination series before the onset of sexual activity (preferably before 11–12 years of age).

36. Can poison ivy contact dermatitis on the penis be acquired through sexual contact?
Yes. There is one report of a woman who was hiking with her boyfriend and inadvertently wiped herself with poison ivy leaves after urinating. A few hours later she had unprotected vaginal intercourse with her boyfriend. Both developed genital contact dermatitis presumably due to poison ivy.

37. What is the difference between true love and a herpes simplex genital infection?
A herpes simplex genital infection is forever.

38. Match the disease with the commonly associated vaginal discharge.

1. *Candida* species	**(a) Yellow-green discharge**
2. *C. trachomatis*	**(b) White frothy discharge**
3. N. gonorrhoeae	**(c) Thin, white fishy-smelling discharge**
4. Bacterial vaginosis	**(d) White cheesy discharge**
5. *T. vaginalis*	

Answers: 1 (d), 2 (a), 3 (a), 4 (c), 5 (b).

BIBLIOGRAPHY

1. American Academy of Pediatrics: Sexually transmitted diseases in adolescents and children. In Pickering LK (ed): 2000 Red Book: Report of the Committee on Infectious Diseases, 25th ed. Elk Grove, IL, American Academy of Pediatrics, 2000, pp 138–147.

2. American Academy of Pediatrics: Syphilis. In Pickering LK (ed): 2000 Red Book: Report of the Committee on Infectious Diseases, 25th ed. Elk Grove, IL, American Academy of Pediatrics, 2000, pp 547–559.
3. American Academy of Pediatrics: *Trichomonas vaginalis* infections. In Pickering LK (ed): 2000 Red Book: Report of the Committee on Infectious Diseases, 25th ed. Elk Grove, IL, American Academy of Pediatrics, 2000, pp 588–589.
4. Gutman LT: Sexually transmitted diseases. In Feigan RD, Cherry JD (eds): Textbook of Pediatric Infectious Diseases, 4th ed. Philadelphia, W.B. Saunders, 1998, pp 548–561.
5. Ingram DL: *Neisseria gonorrhoeae* in children. Pediatr Ann 23:341–345, 1994.
6. Ingram DL, White ST, Occhiuti, AR Lyna PR: Childhood vaginal infections: Association of *Chlamydia trachomatis* with sexual contact. Pediatr Infect Dis 5:226–229, 1986.
7. MacDonald NE, Gully PR: Sexually transmitted disease syndromes. In Long SS, Prober CG (eds): Principles and Practice of Pediatric Infectious Diseases. New York, Churchill Livingston, 1997, pp 381–384.
8. McKinzie J: Sexually transmitted diseases. Emerg Med Clin North Am 19:723–743, 2001.
9. Mylonakis E, Paliou M, Lally M, et al: Laboratory testing for infection with the human immunodeficiency virus: Established and novel approaches. Am J Med 109:568–576, 2000.
10. Westrom L, Eschenbach D: Pelvic inflammatory disease. In Holmes KK, Sparling PF, Mardh P, et al (eds): Sexually Transmitted Diseases, 3rd ed. New York, McGraw-Hill, 1999, pp 783–809.

VIII. Central Nervous System Infections

27. MENINGITIS

Charles R. Woods, M.D., M.S.

1. What is meningitis?

Meningitis is inflammation, due to any cause, of the leptomeninges (the arachnoid and pia mater) and the cerebrospinal fluid (CSF) spaces between them (the subarachnoid space). Bacterial meningitis indicates bacterial infection of the subarachnoid space and adjacent leptomeninges. The leptomeninges are avascular but surround the major arteries and veins of the cerebral circulation. The inflammatory response around these blood vessels can lead to parenchymal infarcts and permanent neurologic sequelae. Aseptic meningitis indicates inflammation that is due to causes other than bacterial, mycobacterial, or fungal infections. Aseptic meningitis is caused most commonly by viruses. Viral meningitis rarely causes permanent neurologic sequelae.

2. What are the most common etiologic agents of bacterial meningitis in developed countries?

AGE GROUP	ORGANISMS
Birth to age 2 to 3 months	Group B streptococcus (*Streptococcus agalactiae*)
	Escherichia coli (especially K1 strains) and other gram-negative enteric organisms, such as *Klebsiella* and *Salmonella* spp.
	Listeria monocytogenes
	Enterococci
1 month to adulthood	*Streptococcus pneumoniae* (pneumococcus)
	Neisseria meningitidis (meningococcus)

The above organisms are the typical pathogens seen in bacterial meningitis of hematogenous origin. Pathogens seen in the first two months of life occasionally cause meningitis in older infants. Pneumococcal and meningococcal infections sometimes occur in the first month of life. In children under age 5 years who have not been vaccinated, *Haemophilus influenzae* type b infection should be considered a potential etiologic agent. Premature infants and immunocompromised hosts are subject to infection with a much broader range of microbes, including *Candida* species and cryptococci. Viral meningitis also can occur at any age.

3. Which antibiotics should be used as initial empirical treatment of bacterial meningitis in neonates?

Ampicillin and cefotaxime. Ampicillin plus gentamicin is a commonly used regimen for treatment of neonatal sepsis, but gentamicin does not penetrate the blood-brain barrier well. Many *E. coli* strains and other gram-negative enteric organisms are ampicillin-resistant. Third-generation cephalosporins provide excellent coverage for these microbes, achieve excellent concentrations in the CSF, and are highly active against Group B streptococci. However, ampicillin and gentamicin are preferred by many experts for the initial treatment of Group B streptococccal meningitis. If pneumococcal meningitis is suspected in a neonate, vancomycin should be administered in place of ampicillin, pending culture and antimicrobial susceptibility results.

4. Which antibiotics should be used as initial empirical treatment of bacterial meningitis beyond the neonatal period?

Vancomycin plus ceftriaxone (or cefotaxime). Because of the potential for penicillin- and cephalosporin-resistant pneumococci as a cause of meningitis, vancomycin is recommended as part of initial therapy. Addition of rifampin may be considered in cephalosporin-intolerant children with pneumococcal meningitis.

5. What are the potential neurologic sequelae of bacterial meningitis?

Sensorineural hearing loss, either unilateral or bilateral, is the most common permanent neurologic sequela of bacterial meningitis. Other sequelae include cranial nerve palsies, ataxia, hemiparesis and other motor impairments, cognitive delays (including mental retardation), language and other learning disorders, visual field deficits (cortical or optic nerve-related), seizure disorders, hydrocephalus (communicating and noncommunicating), diabetes insipidus, and behavioral disorders. Death occurs in about 5% of cases.

6. What symptoms and signs should raise suspicion about bacterial meningitis in the first few months of life?

Clinical findings in neonates and young infants with meningitis often are minimal and can be subtle. Fever, lethargy, irritability (lack of consolability), poor feeding, high-pitched or other abnormal crying, and emesis can be manifestations of meningitis. A bulging fontanelle is present in about one-third of cases in young infants. Seizures also are common and should raise suspicion for meningitis. Signs of sepsis also may be present. Abnormally early or late onset of jaundice may occur with meningitis or sepsis in the first weeks of life. Focal neurologic findings, including cranial nerve palsies, may be present. Absence of fever or meningeal signs does not rule out bacterial meningitis in young infants with other signs of illness.

7. What symptoms and signs should raise suspicion about meningitis beyond early infancy?

The presentation of bacterial or viral meningitis in children often is nonspecific and difficult to distinguish initially from minor viral or other nonspecific illnesses. Symptoms of meningitis include fever, confusion, lethargy or other alterations of mental status, headache, irritability, nausea, vomiting, respiratory tract symptoms (often from associated viral infections, but possibly from increased intracranial pressure), and photophobia. Signs may include nuchal rigidity and other meningeal signs, change in affect or altered mental status, seizures (generalized or focal), focal neurologic deficits (including cranial nerve palsies), ataxia, and acute hearing loss.

8. How helpful is the presence or absence of nuchal rigidity, Kernig's sign, or Brudzinki's sign in making the diagnosis of meningitis?

The presence of these signs indicates a high likelihood of meningitis or other inflammatory processes that cause meningeal irritation. However, the absence of these signs does not rule out meningitis, especially in infants. Other causes of apparent nuchal rigidity, or neck stiffness, include torticollis, deep neck space infections (e.g., retropharyngeal abscess), and cervical adenitis. Kernig's sign is present when pain is elicited on attempted extension of knee in a supine patient with the knee and thigh flexed toward the abdomen. Brudzinski's sign is present when passive flexion of the neck by the examiner results in spontaneous flexion of the hips and knees.

9. How useful is the peripheral white blood cell count (WBC) and differential in deciding whether a child may have bacterial meningitis?

The peripheral WBC and differential count usually are not overly helpful, although they may provide adjunctive information that tips the balance of clinical decision-making toward or away from performing a lumbar puncture. Most cases of bacterial meningitis have a degree of leukocytosis with a predominance of mature neutrophils (polymorphonuclear leukocytes) and/or neutrophil band forms. Many cases are associated with a frank left shift (which generally means that the percentage of neutrophils plus bands exceeds 85–90% of the total WBC or that the percentage of bands exceeds 15–20%). However, most children with leukocytosis or left shifts do not have bacterial meningitis, and bacterial meningitis can occur (on rare occasions) with lymphocyte predominance in the peripheral blood. In a young infant, leukocytosis and/or left shift without an alternative explanation may lead one to consider the possibility of meningitis, but these findings alone are not necessarily indications for lumbar puncture. In addition, an unremarkable total WBC count or differential cannot be used to exclude bacterial meningitis if the clinical setting is suggestive.

10. Should dexamethasone or other glucocorticoid agents be used as part of the initial treatment for suspected bacterial meningitis?

In general, no. Several randomized, controlled studies have suggested that dexamethasone, when administered shortly before or within a few hours of initiation of antibiotic therapy, reduces the rate of hearing loss and other adverse neurologic outcomes in childhood meningitis caused by *H. influenzae* type b (Hib). However, in the era of Hib vaccination, Hib meningitis virtually has been eliminated among vaccinated infants and children. Clinical studies of pneumococcal meningitis to date have not produced results that warrant administration of dexamethasone. Animal data also suggest that dexamethasone may decrease penetration of vancomycin into CSF, which may be important when cephalosporin-resistant pneumococcal strains are the cause of meningitis. No data support the use of dexamethasone for meningococcal meningitis, which has a lower rate of permanent neurologic sequelae than pneumococcal meningitis. Dexamethasone can mask fever from meningitis during its use, with rebound fever after it is discontinued.

11. What does hyponatremia indicate early in the course of bacterial meningitis?

Low serum sodium concentrations may occur early in the course of bacterial meningitis, primarily because of the capillary leak associated with concurrent sepsis or the secretion of inappropriate antidiuretic hormone (SIADH). Sodium concentrations may be normal at the time of presentation but fall during the next 24–48 hours from either cause. SIADH can occur in viral meningitis but is uncommon in this setting. The condition of cerebral salt wasting, which results from increased production of brain and/or atrial natriuretic peptide, has been reported in tuberculous meningitis but has not been described during acute bacterial or viral meningitis. Intravascular fluid volumes generally are decreased in sepsis and normal to increased during SIADH. Both causes can be present in patients with meningitis, however, with SIADH becoming apparent after initial correction of volume status. Significant vomiting or diarrhea due to concurrent viral illness or ileus associated with sepsis also can explain hyponatremia.

12. How is the diagnosis of SIADH confirmed?

SIADH exists when hyponatremia (with a correspondingly low serum osmolality) is present in association with inappropriate excretion of sodium into the urine (with a urine osmolality that is higher than otherwise expected with a low serum osmolality). High urine specific gravity (typically > 1.025), when associated with hyponatremia, suggests SIADH but does not reliably confirm the diagnosis. SIADH also can be present with lower urine specific gravity in infants. A urine sodium concentration that is > 10 mEq/L in the presence of hyponatremia (generally < 130 mEq/L), if measured before administration of appreciable amounts of sodium-containing fluids, is generally sufficient to make a presumptive diagnosis. Urine sodium concentrations generally are low when hyponatremia is the result of sepsis alone. In patients with meningitis, any measurable ADH in the face of hyponatremia probably indicates SIADH, but real-time measurement of ADH is generally not available in most clinical settings. Measurements of urine and serum sodium concentrations and osmolality remain the fastest way to make a presumptive diagnosis. Consultation with nephrologists or endocrinologists may be helpful.

13. Should fluid replacement be restricted early in the course of meningitis?

No, unless SIADH is clearly present and the intravascular volume status is normal. Fluid restriction is the primary treatment of SIADH. However, for patients with meningitis and hyponatremia, the first step is careful clinical assessment of intravascular volume status. In patients with hypotension or poor perfusion, volume status should be addressed before consideration of fluid restriction. Meningitis often leads to at least small-to-moderate increases in intracranial pressure and regional alterations in cerebral blood flow autoregulation. Restriction of fluids when intravascular volumes are too low to maintain cerebral blood flow in areas of disturbed autoregulation can result in ischemic strokes. In addition, overvigorous fluid resuscitation must be avoided to prevent iatrogenic increases in intracranial pressure. Strict measurements of fluids administered by all routes as well as urine and other body fluid outputs are frequently necessary during the early treatment of bacterial meningitis.

14. What are the consequences of SIADH?

SIADH leads to hyponatremia. If the serum sodium falls rapidly or reaches the low 120s (in mEq/L), seizures may occur. Serum sodium concentrations should be followed at least twice daily during the first 48 hours of treatment of bacterial meningitis, even when they are initially normal, to avoid the unrecognized development of SIADH after presentation.

15. What types of CSF studies should be requested in evaluating a child for possible meningitis?

CSF should be evaluated for clarity (clear or turbid) and color (colorless, xanthochromic, or bloody). Routine CSF studies should include bacterial culture and Gram stain, WBC and differential, red blood cell count, glucose concentration, and protein concentration. Bacterial antigen tests generally are unnecessary unless the child has received antibiotics in the hours to days preceding the lumbar puncture and cultures remain negative. A sample of the CSF can be saved for such testing if bacterial cultures are negative and the clinical and laboratory findings are suggestive of bacterial meningitis.

Viral cultures can be ordered if viral meningitis is suspected, but they generally are of low yield. In recent years, polymerase chain reaction-based tests for conserved genetic sequences of enteroviruses have become available, are more sensitive than culture, and can be useful when proof of a viral cause may allow shortening of the hospital or parenteral antibiotic course. Fungal culture may be appropriate in immunocompromised hosts. Mycobacterial culture should be ordered when tuberculosis is a possibility, although the yield is low.

16. What are the expected findings in studies of the CSF of normal children?

Normal results can vary with age. The generally expected normal ranges are presented in the table below. As a general rule, premature infants and full-term infants in the first month of life have higher WBC and protein concentrations in CSF than older full-term infants. Upper limits of normal for WBCs and neutrophils vary among different studies.

CSF STUDY	PREMATURE INFANTS	TERM NEWBORNS TO 7 DAYS OLD	TERM INFANTS 8–30 DAYS OLD	AFTER FIRST MONTH OF LIFE
WBC/μl	0–23 (up to 40?)	0–20 (up to 40?)	0–20 (up to 25?)	0–6
Neutrophils/μl	Up to 40–60% of WBCs?	Up to 50–60% of WBCs	0–2 (or up to 20% of WBCs?)	0
RBC/μl	??	0–2	0–2	0–2
Glucose (mg/dl)	30–100	35–80	40–80	40–80
Protein (mg/dl)	45–200	20–140	15–100	10–45

Traditionally, the WBC count in CSF has been performed using a hemocytometer, and the differential has been reported as polymorphonuclear cells (neutrophils) or mononuclear cells (lymphocytes and/or monocytes). In recent years, use of spun Wright-stained specimens to assess the WBC differential has led some laboratories to report specific percentages of neutrophils, bands, lymphocytes, and monocytes as well as other types of WBCs. The clinical correlates of CSF lymphocytes vs. monocytes remain unclear.

17. Describe the typical findings in spinal fluid in children with meningitis.

CSF STUDY	BACTERIAL MENINGITIS	VIRAL MENINGITIS	TUBER-CULOUS MENINGITIS	PARA-MENINGEAL MENINGITIS	HERPES MENINGO-ENCEPHALITIS
WBC/µl	1,000–10,000	50–500	10–1,000	20–500	5–1,000
% Neutrophils	> 70	>50 (variable)	Low	Variable	Low
RBC/µl	< 10	Normal	Normal	Normal	10-500
Glucose (mg/dl)	< 30	Normal	10–45	Normal	Normal
Protein (mg/dl)	> 100	40–100	> 100	50–400	Increased

These values presume nontraumatic lumbar puncture. Considerable overlaps occur between categories. WBCs in CSF may not be markedly elevated early in the course of bacterial meningitis. Meningococcal meningitis can be present in the absence of CSF pleocytosis. Children with overwhelming sepsis and severe leukopenia can have meningitis with low WBC count in CSF on this basis. Many cases of viral meningitis have > 50% neutrophils on the WBC differential count. Some viral infections, especially echoviruses and sometimes herpes simplex, can cause hypoglycorrhachia.

18. Can the results from a traumatic (bloody) spinal fluid specimen be interpreted?

Yes, in some circumstances—but always with caution. A traumatic lumbar puncture is defined as a CSF with > 1000 RBC/mm^3 (in the absence of suspected intracranial hemorrhage). Many bloody specimens actually consist of > 95% CSF, even with RBC counts of 100,000/mm^3. Many experts allow 1 WBC/mm^3 in the CSF for every 500 or 1000 RBC/mm^3. An estimate of the upper limit of WBCs that can be allowed in a blood-contaminated CSF specimen can be calculated with the following formula:

$$\text{WBC (CSF) due to blood} = \text{WBC (blood)} \times [\text{RBC(CSF)/RBC (blood)}]$$

This estimate should be viewed as an upper limit; it may allow too many WBCs on the basis of the RBC count in the specimen, so that the presence of meningitis is missed. Marked differences in the proportions of neutrophils and mononuclear cells (lymphocytes plus monocytes) between the CSF and peripheral blood also should raise concerns about the presence of meningitis. When the WBC count in CSF exceeds 1000/mm^3 in a bloody specimen, especially with a predominance of neutrophils, the presence of bacterial meningitis should be suspected. The presence of a low glucose concentration also suggests meningitis in such situations. Elevated CSF protein concentrations in this setting are difficult to interpret and are of little diagnostic assistance.

19. When should cranial imaging be performed before lumbar puncture in patients with suspected bacterial meningitis?

In general, lumbar punctures can be performed without prior imaging of the central nervous system in an infant with an open anterior fontanelle. Cranial imaging before lumbar puncture is necessary only when patients are comatose, have papilledema or other signs of increased intracranial pressure, or present with focal neurologic findings. In such settings, the altered CSF fluid dynamics that result from removal of CSF during lumbar puncture may lead to or exacerbate impending brain herniation. When imaging studies are need before lumbar puncture, blood culture(s) should be obtained before administration of empirical antibiotic therapy. Lumbar puncture should be performed as soon as possible after imaging if no mass lesions or other contraindications are found on the imaging study.

20. What is the preferred imaging modality for children with suspected bacterial meningitis?

When imaging results are needed emergently, computed tomography (CT) scanning generally is preferred. Noncontrast CT scans generally do not reveal the presence of meningeal inflammation or cerebritis but can be used to rule out intracranial bleeding and midline shifts or other signs of cerebral edema. Magnetic resonance imaging (MRI) typically is better for evaluation of the posterior fossa and delineation of extra-axial fluid collections. When feasible, use of contrast with either modality is preferred for the diagnosis of intracranial infection.

21. What is a parameningeal infection?
Parameningeal infections occur anatomically near the subarachnoid space; an inflammatory response can be seen in the CSF. Examples include brain abscesses, intracranial subdural empyema, and intracranial epidural abscess. In general, the CSF is sterile, but spread from these sites into the CSF can occur. Chronic sinusitis or otitis media is the most common origin of such infections. Spinal epidural abscesses also can be considered in the category of parameningeal infection.

22. Does the presence of petechiae or purpura suggest a particular cause of apparent bacterial meningitis?
Petechiae and purpura in a patient with apparent bacterial meningitis suggests meningococci as the cause. However, these skin findings can be seen in sepsis and meningitis caused by *S. pneumoniae* and *H. influenzae* type b as well as tick-borne diseases such as Rocky Mountain spotted fever and human ehrlichioses in certain geographic areas. In such clinical settings, empirical antimicrobial coverage should not be limited to meningococci alone.
Note: Do not assume that petechiae = meningococcemia

23. Can results of Gram stains of CSF be used to guide the choice of antibiotic therapy?
Gram stains can provide information that suggests a specific cause, but initial treatment decisions should not be based on Gram stain results alone. The two most common causes of bacterial meningitis beyond the neonatal period are pneumococci and meningococci, both of which appear as diplococci in stains. With overdecolorization of Gram-stained slides gram-positive pneumococci may appear as gram-negative cocci, whereas with underdecolorization gram-negative meningococci may appear as gram-positive cocci. Morphologically, pneumococci appear in pairs oriented with the long axes aligned "head to toe," whereas meningococci typically appear to lie "side by side."

24. What is the significance of seizures early during the course of bacterial meningitis?
Seizures occur before admission or during the first few days of meningitis in 20–30% of children with bacterial meningitis. Generalized seizures before the third or fourth day after initiation of treatment for bacterial meningitis usually reflect cortical irritation rather then permanent injury to an area of the brain. Permanent seizure disorders usually do not result. Focal seizures are more concerning than generalized seizures for localized brain injury. Early seizures also can be due to hyponatremia (from sepsis or SIADH) or hypocalcemia (from sepsis). Early seizures associated with depressed mental status are worrisome for the presence of severely increased intracranial pressure.

25. What is the significance of seizures late during the course of bacterial meningitis?
Focal seizures at any time or generalized seizures that begin or recur beyond the fourth day of treatment may indicate the development of cerebritis or brain abscess, extra-axial fluid collections (e.g., subdural effusion or empyema), vascular thrombosis, or cerebral edema with increasing intracranial pressure. Such focal or late seizures are more ominous than early seizures for the development of seizure disorders or other permanent neurologic sequelae in survivors of bacterial meningitis.

26. How can viral meningitis be distinguished from bacterial meningitis before culture results are available?
This distinction is often difficult early in the course of disease, especially when the WBC count in CSF is greater than a few hundred. Predominance of neutrophils, even higher than 80%, is frequent early in the course of viral meningitis. The most reliable clinical tool is the observation of rapid clinical improvement (resolution of headache and other symptoms) after lumbar

puncture in children with viral meningitis. Such improvement does not occur in all cases of viral or aseptic meningitis, but, when it does, it is highly suggestive of a viral rather than bacterial cause of the meningitis. In the past, it was believed that, in patients with viral meningitis and initial neutrophil predominance in the CSF, repeating the lumbar puncture in 12–24 hours would demonstrate a shift to mononuclear cell predominance, confirming the cause as viral. Recent studies have shown that such shifts in this time frame are uncommon.

27. How does prior oral or intramuscular administration of antibiotics affect the results of CSF studies?

The only significant effect of "partial" treatment is that cultures may be falsely negative. The WBC and differential count and the protein and glucose concentrations in CSF can be interpreted at face value. Partial treatment generally does not affect these indices. The one exception may be two or more doses of intramuscular ceftriaxone in the 48–72 hours before lumbar puncture, which can be construed as "actual" treatment and may lead to a decrease in WBC count and/or alteration of the differential count toward lymphocytes.

28. Does meningitis caused by *Listeria monocytogenes* have a mononuclear predominance in the CSF?

Usually not. Neutrophil predominance is typical, as in other types of bacterial meningitis. If the mononuclear cells in the CSF are differentiated, many of them usually are monocytes or macrophages instead of lymphocytes. Monocytosis (monocytes increased above normal but not necessarily the predominant type of WBC) may be present in the peripheral blood.

29. Should sterility of the CSF be documented early in the course of treatment?

In most cases, documentation of sterility is unnecessary, especially in patients who improve rapidly. Some experts recommend repeat lumbar puncture 24–36 hours into therapy when the causative organism is a pneumococcal strain that is (or is likely to be) intermediately or fully resistant to penicillin or third-generation cephalosporins. Others modify this recommendation by limiting it to children who do not substantially improve within this time frame. In such cases, addition of rifampin may be necessary if cultures or Gram stains of the CSF remain positive. In neonates with meningitis caused by gram-negative enteric bacteria, many experts recommend repeat lumbar punctures every 24–72 hours into treatment until sterility is documented. Persistently positive CSF cultures in this setting may indicate either a focus of infection that requires drainage or the need for administration of intraventricular antibiotics (typically amikacin). In either case, the course of therapy may be prolonged to 4 weeks or more. Some, but not all, experts also recommend repeat lumbar puncture in cases of group B streptococcal meningitis, especially when the course is complicated.

30. When should a lumbar puncture be performed at the end of therapy?

In most cases, an end-of-therapy lumbar puncture is unnecessary. The primary indications are (1) apparent recrudescence or relapse and (2) meningitis in young infants caused by *E. coli* or other gram-negative enteric bacteria. End-of-therapy lumbar puncture can be useful in the second setting to determine whether therapy has been adequate or needs to be prolonged. Some experts recommend treatment for 4 weeks or more if neutrophils comprise 30% or more of the WBC count in CSF at the apparent end of therapy. This approach may not be necessary when the infant has had a benign course, rapid CSF sterilization, and normalization of CSF indices early in the course. Consultation with a specialist is generally prudent in such cases.

31. When should a CT scan or MRI of the brain be obtained in patients with meningitis?

Imaging studies of the head should be performed for new onset of focal neurologic findings or focal seizures in any infant or child, with or without meningitis. However, imaging of the brain does not need to be performed as part of the routine management of all children with bacterial meningitis. In patients with rapid clinical recovery and resolution of symptoms and signs, imaging generally is not necessary and adds no useful prognostic information. Circumstances in which imaging should be performed include (1) prolonged obtundation or depressed mental status or continued excessive irritability; (2) occurrence of seizures of any type 72 hours or more after initiation of therapy; (3) expanding head circumference or other signs that suggest hydrocephalus or increasing intracranial pressure; (4) recurrence of fever and/or peripheral blood leukocytosis after initial defervescence or normalization, which may indicate development of suppurative intracranial complications (e.g., abscess, subdural empyema), unless there is a clear cut alternative explanation; (5) prolonged fever (≥ 7 days); and (6) relapse or recurrence after completion of therapy.

32. How long should meningitis be treated?

Length of treatment depends on the specific cause and the clinical course. The shorter durations in the table below may be used in cases with rapid recovery and uncomplicated courses. Some experts recommend treatment until the child has been afebrile for at least 5 days.

ETIOLOGY OF MENINGITIS	DURATION OF PARENTERAL ANTIBIOTICS
Group B streptococci	14–21 days
E. coli and other gram-negative enteric rods	21 days (or 14 days after sterilization of CSF, whichever is longer)
Listeria monocytogenes	14–21 days
Haemophilus influenzae type b	7–10 days
Streptococcus pneumoniae	10–14 days
Neisseria meningitidis	7 days*

* Some studies suggest that 3–4 days may be adequate.

33. Should subdural fluid collections that develop during meningitis be drained?

If the fluid collection is a subdural effusion, neurosurgical drainage is unnecessary unless there is evidence of increased intracranial pressure. If findings on imaging studies are suggestive of subdural empyema, drainage often is required. Small subdural empyemas that are not associated with increased pressure, effacement of the brain, or focal neurologic signs sometimes may be managed medically in consultation with a neurosurgeon. Longer courses of antibiotic therapy and follow-up with serial imaging studies of the brain are required in either case.

34. Can children with bacterial meningitis be safely managed on regular inpatient units during the first 24–48 hours of treatment?

Sometimes—but generally this approach is unwise, especially for infants. In the first 24–72 hours of hospitalization, children with bacterial meningitis are at significant risk of developing seizures, cerebral edema, hyponatremia (often from SIADH), and worsening manifestations of sepsis (e.g., disseminated intravascular coagulation, acute respiratory distress syndrome). Such complications should be anticipated, and the close monitoring and rapid clinical responses typically required usually are best achieved in an intensive care setting. In selected cases, children with normal mental status, otherwise unremarkable physical findings, and minimal abnormalities on CSF studies and other laboratory tests may be admitted to regular pediatric beds, if close and frequent monitoring can be ensured. In such cases, the capability for quick transfer to pediatric intensive care should be ensured.

35. Do children with bacterial meningitis require any special isolation precautions in the hospital?

Children with suspected bacterial meningitis should be placed in droplet isolation for the first 24 hours of hospitalization unless a nonmeningococcal cause has been confirmed. Nasopharyngeal colonization is either eradicated or so greatly reduced after 24 hours of parenteral antibiotic therapy that droplet or contact spread from the patient is no longer a concern.

This precaution is based on the moderately increased risk of invasive disease in contacts of patients with meningococcal infections. An increased risk also exists for contacts of patients with *H. influenzae* type b infections (although infections due to this microbe now are rare). Contacts of persons who have pneumococcal infection usually are not at increased risk of invasive disease.

36. Do family members and other contacts of children with bacterial meningitis need to be given prophylactic antibiotics?

The answer depends on the causative agent. Pneumococci are not considered highly contagious; close contacts of patients with pneumococcal infection do not appear to be at increased risk of developing invasive pneumococcal infection. Close contacts (e.g., family members, child care or school classmates) of persons with meningococcal infection are at increased risk of developing invasive meningococcal disease, especially in the first few days after onset of symptoms in the index case. Infants and children should be given rifampin orally (4 doses of 10 mg/kg every 12 hr if > 1 month of age; 5 mg/kg/dose if ≤ 1 month of age) or a single dose of ceftriaxone intramuscularly (125 mg if ≤ 12 years old or 250 mg if > 12 years old). Patients over age 18 years can be given a single oral dose of ciprofloxacin (500 mg).

37. Discuss the role of bacterial antigen tests of CSF in determining the etiology of infection.

Because such test are unnecessary and not cost-effective in the vast majority of cases, they need not be ordered routinely. Both sensitivity and negative predictive values are poor. Bacterial antigen tests may be useful in cases of partially or pretreated bacterial meningitis in which cultures may be falsely negative. Recent administration of conjugate pneumococcal or *H. influenzae* type b vaccines may lead to false-positive results.

38. What causes aseptic meningitis?

Enteroviruses (including coxsackie and echoviruses) account for 80–90% of episodes of aseptic meningitis. The list of other potentially causative agents is protean and includes herpes simplex virus (primarily type 2), human herpes virus 6, mumps, adenoviruses, influenza and parainfluenza viruses, rhinoviruses, cytomegalovirus, human parvovirus, varicella, and Epstein-Barr virus. Culture-negative CSF pleocytosis also can be caused by *Chlamydia*, *Rickettsia*, *Ehrlichia*, *Mycoplasma*, and *Bartonella* species; the agents of syphilis and Lyme disease; fungal infections and parasitic infections (including roundworms, cysticercosis, *Toxoplasma* sp., and amoeba); and noninfectious diseases such as leukemia, tumors of the central nervous system, and systemic lupus erythematosus. Kawaski disease, heavy metal poisoning, dermoid or epidermoid cysts, and idiosyncratic reactions to therapeutic agents, such as trimethoprim-sulfamethoxazole and intravenous gamma globulin preparations, also can cause CSF pleocytosis.

39. What is the role of hearing testing in children who have had bacterial meningitis?

All children with proven bacterial meningitis and culture-negative meningitis in which a bacterial origin is suspected should undergo evaluations for hearing loss. Up to 30% of children with pneumococcal meningitis and 5–10% of children with meningococcal or Hib meningitis suffer mild-to-severe sensorineural hearing loss. Ideally testing should be initiated before discharge from the hospital. Screening for otoacoustic emissions (OAE) is commonly done; follow-up should include more formal hearing tests when OAE screening is abnormal. Concurrent middle ear fluid from associated otitis media may make initial evaluations inconclusive. Studies should be repeated once the fluid has resolved. Hearing deficits detected early in the course of meningitis sometimes improve. Permanent hearing deficits usually occur during the first few days of bacterial meningitis. Children with normal hearing at the end of therapy seldom develop later hearing loss as a result of meningitis.

40. How do bacteria reach the meninges?

Most bacterial meningitis in children is hematogenous in origin, meaning that a bacteremia preceded the meningitis. Bacteria probably cross the blood-CSF barrier of the choroid plexus within the ventricular system of the brain. The choroid plexus consists of a fenestrated endothelium and cuboidal epithelium with tight junctions between epithelial cells. Bacteria may traverse this barrier directly or perhaps inside phagocytic white blood cells. Direct seeding of the CSF can occur from penetrating head trauma or neurosurgical procedures. Contiguous extension of infections of the paranasal sinuses or middle ear occasionally occurs, usually in association with intermediary epidural or subdural empyemas.

41. Why is the CSF glucose concentration low in some children with bacterial meningitis?

CSF glucose concentrations are normally 50–65% of those of blood. Most glucose in the CSF is derived from the bloodstream at the choroid plexus, where CSF is produced. Inflammation of the choroid plexus, which can occur in CNS infections, can alter glucose transport into the CSF. Glucose utilization by the bacteria and/or responding white blood cells may further reduce CSF glucose concentrations. Low glucose concentration in CSF is termed *hypoglycorrhachia*.

42. What is the risk of development of bacterial meningitis in a child with untreated occult bacteremia?

After the development of Hib conjugate vaccine but before the development of pneumococcal conjugate vaccine, the risk of pneumococcal bacteremia among children 3 months to 36 months of age, with fever ≥ 39°C and no identified source of infection, generally was estimated at about 1.5%. Some studies suggest rates of about 3%. About 4% of such patients develop pneumococcal meningitis (i.e., about 60 cases of meningitis per 100,000 episodes of occult bacteremia). Widespread use of conjugate pneumococcal vaccines may substantially reduce this rate.

43. How long is the usual febrile course of bacterial meningitis in children?

The number of days of fever varies with cause. Among children with pneumococcal or meningococcal meningitis, 70–80% are afebrile by the fourth day of treatment and 90% by the sixth day of treatment. The febrile course for *H. influenzae* type b meningitis typically is longer: 70% of patients are afebrile by the sixth day of treatment and 90% by the tenth day.

44. What are the most common causes of prolonged or secondary fevers in bacterial meningitis?

Fever can be considered **prolonged** if it persists beyond 5–7 days of treatment. Febrile courses without abatement of the daily maximal temperatures are of more concern than persisting fever with declining daily temperatures. **Secondary fever** recurs after an afebrile period of 24 hours or more. Subdural effusions are the most common cause of prolonged fever and second only to nosocomial infections as a cause of secondary fever in children with bacterial meningitis. They are less common in the Hib vaccine era. When dexamethasone is used as part of the initial therapy of bacterial meningitis, it can suppress fever in some patients. When the dexamethasone is stopped, fever may reappear and can be confused with secondary fever in some patients.

CATEGORY	POTENTIAL CAUSES
Prolonged fever	Subdural effusion (rarely subdural empyema or brain abscess)
	Suppurative infections at non-CNS sites due to the primary infection
	Pneumonia and arthritis are the most common infections; others include pericarditis and osteomyelitis
	Drug fever (diagnosis of exclusion)
Secondary fever	Nosocomial infections: viral infections, phlebitis, urinary tract infections
	Subdural effusion (rarely empyema)
	Immune complex-mediated arthritis, erythema nodosum (primarily meningococcal infections)
	Drug fever (diagnosis of exclusion)
	Antibiotic-associated diarrhea (includes pseudomembranous colitis)

45. How quickly should antibiotics be given to a child with suspected bacterial meningitis?

In general, antibiotics should be administered as soon as possible after the diagnosis of bacterial meningitis is suspected. It is reasonable to delay administration for 1–2 hours to obtain blood and CSF cultures. Several studies suggest that delayed sterilization of CSF 24 hours into therapy is associated with greater risk of permanent neurologic sequelae. However, this finding does not mean that a delay of a few hours will have a similar effect. If CNS imaging is needed before lumbar puncture is attempted and will result in more than a 1- to 2-hour delay in obtaining CSF cultures, it is better to give antibiotics before the imaging study. In a study in emergency departments, the median time from presentation until antibiotics were administered (after lumbar puncture) was 2 hours, and the 75th percentile was 3 hours, 20 minutes. Rapid diagnosis and therapy do not appear to prevent deafness as a consequence of bacterial meningitis.

46. When should the possibility of cryptococcal meningitis be considered?

Cryptococcal meningitis is rare in immunocompetent hosts. It should be suspected primarily in children with advanced HIV infection (with immunosuppression) or in other immunocompromised hosts (those on chemotherapy or other immunosuppressive therapies). Typical symptoms include progressively severe headaches, often without fever. Nausea, dizziness, and irritability also are common findings. Lymphocyte predominance in the CSF (with 40–400 WBC/mm^3) with elevated protein and depressed glucose concentrations are characteristic. Cryptococcal antigen tests of the CSF and serum are positive in over 85% of cases.

47. How long can a child have bacteria in the CSF before exhibiting overt signs of meningitis?

The exact answer is not known, but the time frame is more likely hours than days. Many cases of bacterial meningitis occur several days into what appears to have been a viral respiratory and/or gastrointestinal illness. Often such children have been to see a physician one or more times before the visit during which meningitis is diagnosed. The likely pathogenesis sequence in such cases is development of an initial viral infection that facilitates a transient (or in some cases septic) bacteremia that then seeds the CSF. The meningitis is most likely a late development rather than a subtle process that smolders for several days before becoming clinically apparent.

BIBLIOGRAPHY

1. Ahmed A, Hickey SM, Ehrett S, et al: Cerebrospinal fluid values in the term neonate. Pediatr Infect Dis J 15:298–303, 1995.
2. Kallio MJT, Kilpi T, Anttila M, Peltola H: The effect of a recent previous visit to a physician on outcome after childhood bacterial meningitis. JAMA 272:787–791, 1994.
3. Kanegaye JT, Soliemanzadeh P, Bradley JS: Lumbar puncture in pediatric bacterial meningitis: Defining the time interval for recovery of cerebrospinal fluid pathogens after parenteral antibiotic pretreatment. Pediatrics 108:1169–1174, 2001.
4. Klein JO, Feigin RD, McCracken GH Jr: Report of the task force on diagnosis and management of meningitis. Pediatrics 78(Suppl):959–982, 1986.
5. La Via WV, Marks MI: Prolonged and secondary fevers in childhood bacterial meningitis. Antibiot Chemother 45:201–208, 1992.
6. Lee GM, Fleisher GR, Harper MB: Management of febrile children in the age of the conjugate pneumococcal vaccine: A cost-effective analysis. Pediatrics 108:835–844, 2001.
7. Meadows WL, Lantos J, Tanz RR, et al: Ought 'standard care' be the 'standard of care'? Am J Dis Child 147:40–44, 1993.
8. Negrini B, Kelleher KJ, Wald ER: Cerebrospinal fluid findings in aseptic versus bacterial meningitis. Pediatrics 105:316–319, 2000.
9. Neuman HB, Wald ER: Bacterial meningitis in childhood at the Children's Hospital of Pittsburgh: 1988-1998. Clin Pediatr 40:595–600, 2001.
10. Wubbel L, McCracken GH Jr: Management of bacterial meningitis: 1998. Pediatr Rev 19:78-84, 1998.

28. ENCEPHALITIS

Charles R. Woods, M.D., M.S.

1. How is acute encephalitis different from meningitis and encephalopathy?

Encephalitis refers to any inflammatory or infectious process that involves the brain, whereas *meningitis* refers to an inflammatory or infectious process of the leptomeninges and cerebrospinal fluid (CSF). *Meningoencephalitis* is best conceptualized as encephalitis with associated meningeal inflammation (usually of low grade compared with that of bacterial meningitis). *Encephalopathy* refers to any alteration of mental status from any cause or any disease of the central nervous system (CNS). *Myelitis*, *radiculitis*, and *neuritis* refer to involvement of the spinal cord, nerve roots, and nerves, respectively.

2. Describe the typical clinical features of viral encephalitis.

Clinical features common to many viral causes of encephalitis include acute onset of fever, headache, altered states of consciousness, and behavioral disturbances. Seizures and focal neurologic findings such as hemiparesis also are common. Viral meningitis usually is associated only with fever and meningeal signs such as nuchal rigidity; changes in mental status are uncommon. Other manifestations may depend on the specific area of brain involvement, and different viruses have tropisms for different cell types as well. In viral meningoencephalitis, CSF pleocytosis initially can have mononuclear cell predominance or neutrophil predominance that gives way to mononuclear predominance during the course of illness.

3. What viruses most commonly cause acute encephalitis?

Other than rabies and slow viruses, viral infections involve the CNS only as part of a systemic, generalized infection. Clinically symptomatic CNS infection occurs in at most a few percent of infected persons. Herpes simplex viruses types 1 and 2 and the various arboviruses are most commonly viewed as encephalitis viruses, in the sense that CNS involvement is the most important or injurious part of their clinical manifestations. Other viruses that can cause encephalitis include enteroviruses (e.g., polio), adenoviruses, influenza A and B, parainfluenza viruses, respiratory syncytial virus (RSV), human parvovirus, rotavirus, and hepatitis A and B. The nonsimplex herpes viruses—Epstein-Barr virus (EBV), varicella, cytomegalovirus, and human herpes virus 6 (roseola)—also can cause encephalitis. Smallpox, measles, mumps, and rubella were relatively common causes of encephalitis before widespread childhood vaccination.

4. What are arboviruses?

The term *arbovirus* describes viruses that are transmitted from animals to humans, generally by mosquitoes or ticks (arthropod-borne). There are more than 500 such viruses, and multiple viral groups—primarily *Togaviridae* (alphaviruses), *Flaviviridae*, *Bunyaviridae*, and *Reoviridae*—are represented. Arboviruses can occur in epidemics, but encephalitis typically occurs in only a small minority of infected persons, so that disease from any single arbovirus often appears sporadic. The prevalence and biology of the transmitting vector determine the seasonality and geographic distribution of a given arbovirus. In addition to encephalitis, some arboviruses occasionally cause aseptic meningitis or meningoencephalitis.

Editor's note: If you can think of other interesting viral group names, please let us know.

5. How many arboviruses that can cause encephalitis are found in North America: (a) 1, (b) arboviruses are too small to be counted, (c) 7, or (d) 100?

The answer is (c).

6. What are the seven most common arboviruses in North America?

ARBOVIRUS (VIRUS GENUS)	VECTORS	GEOGRAPHIC DISTRIBUTION	INCUBATION PERIOD (DAYS)	PRIMARY AGE GROUPS	MORTALITY AND MORBIDITY
West Nile virus (flavivirus)	*Culex, Aedes, Anopheles* mosquitoes	Eastern seaboard of the U.S., ?spreading westward (previously in Europe, Asia, Africa)	2–15	Children, older adults	~10% case fatality, largely in adults; sequelae can occur in survivors
St. Louis encephalitis virus (EV) (flavivirus)	*Culex* mosquitoes	U.S.: central, southern, northeastern, western regions; Manitoba, southern Ontario; South America and Caribbean	4–14	Adults > 50 yr	2–20% case fatality (↑ ed w/age); sequelae in 20% of survivors
La Crosse virus, other California serogroup viruses (bunyavirus)	*Aedes* mosquitoes	Widespread in North America, especially central U.S.; La Crosse increasingly recognized in eastern U.S.	5–15	Children	Rarely fatal; 10–15% of survivors have neurologic deficits
Western equine EV (alphavirus)	*Culex, Culiseta* mosquitoes	Central, Western U.S., Canada, areas of South America	2–10	Infants, adults > 50 yr	~10% case fatality; fatality; severe sequelae are common in children
Eastern equine EV (alphavirus)	*Aedes, Culiseta* mosquitoes	Eastern and Gulf States of U.S., Canada, Central and South America	3–10	Children, elderly adults	50–75% case fatality; sequelae in 80% of survivors
Venezuelan equine EV (alphavirus)	*Aedes, Culex, Psorophora* mosquitoes	Florida, Mexico, Central and South America	1–4	Adults	Fatalities are uncommon; sequelae are rare
Powassan (flavivirus)	*Ixodes, Dermacentor* ticks	Canada and western, north central, and northeastern U.S.	4–18	Human disease is rare; children can be infected	10–15% case fatality; sequelae are common in adult survivors

7. What is Colorado tick fever?

Colorado tick fever, seen primarily in western regions, rarely causes encephalitis. The primary reservoirs are birds and small mammals; humans and domestic animals are infected incidentally via the arthropod vector. Person-to-person spread does not occur. Headache, altered consciousness, and seizures are common manifestations. Nonspecific febrile prodromes with myalgias and vomiting are common. Infections usually are asymptomatic or self-limited. These viruses also can cause aseptic meningitis and meningoencephalitis. Case to infection rates are often higher in children than adults, but case fatality rates usually are higher in older adults.

8. What nonviral infections can have encephalitis as part of their manifestation?

Many bacteria, fungi, and parasites sometimes may generate acute encephalitis as a manifestation of systemic or local infections.

Bacteria

- *Mycoplasma pneumoniae*
- *Neisseria meningitidis*
- *Bartonella henselae* (cat scratch disease)
- *Rickettsia rickettsiae* (Rocky Mountain spotted fever)
- Ehrlichiosis

- *Coxiella burnetii*
- *Mycobacterium tuberculosis*
- *Treponema pallidum*
- *Chlamydia psittaci* and *C. pneumoniae*
- *Borrelia burgdorferi* (Lyme disease)
- Typhoid fever (can mimic encephalitis)

Parasites

- Agents of malaria (especially cerebral malaria due to *Plasmodium falciparum*)
- *Baylisascaris procyonis* (raccoon roundworm; causes eosinophilic meningoencephalitis)
- Amoeba
- *Toxoplasma gondii*

Embolic lesions from bacterial endocarditis or expanding mass effects from brain abscesses and subdural or epidural empyemas can present with encephalopathy and fever, mimicking viral encephalitis.

9. What noninfectious causes should be considered in a patient with acute encephalopathy or encephalitis?

1. **Postinfectious encephalomyelitis** (PIEM) is a subset of **acute disseminated encephalomyelitis** (ADEM), which is a broad term used to describe the clinical syndrome of monophasic, acute or subacute, demyelination of various white matter tracts in the CNS. ADEM arises from the immune response to a preceding infection (e.g., measles, varicella, mycoplasma, EBV) or as an idiopathic autoimmune disease. PIEM and ADEM are difficult to distinguish from viral encephalitis clinically. CSF studies and magnetic resonance imaging, along with absence of evidence of specific infections, can be very helpful in making this distinction. Acute cerebellar ataxia is another postinfectious syndrome that can arise in association with varicella, EBV, human parvovirus, and probably other viral infections.

2. **Guillain-Barré syndrome** (GBS), or acute inflammatory demyelinating polyneuropathy, is usually a postinfectious state; some cases may have clinical involvement of the CNS. CSF protein concentrations typically are elevated, and low-grade pleocytosis (< 50 cells/mm^3) is common. Many infections, viral and bacterial, appear able to trigger GBS, but *Campylobacter* infections of the gastrointestinal tract have emerged as a frequent cause.

3. **Noninfectious diseases** that can cause or mimic encephalopathy include tumors, especially when expanding into or located in the brainstem; metabolic disorders, acute or acquired, that lead to hypoglycemia, uremia, or hyperammonemia; toxic effects of drugs (including trimethoprim); heavy metal poisoning; subarachnoid hemorrhage; status epilepticus or postictal states; acute confusional migraine; cerebral vasculitis due to systemic lupus erythematosus or other autoimmune diseases; and psychiatric disorders.

10. How do arthropod-borne encephalitis viruses typically reach the CNS?

After a tick or mosquito bite, the virus replicates locally in the skin at the site of the bite. A transient viremia then may seed the reticuloendothelial system (primarily liver, spleen, and lymph nodes). After further replication, a larger secondary viremia ensues, which seeds other organs, including the CNS.

11. Name a common childhood viral illness associated with secondary viremia.

Chicken pox

12. What are two viruses that reach the CNS directly through neurons from peripheral sites?

Herpes simplex viruses (HSV) and rabies virus. Such transmission of HSV typically occurs during the neonatal period from cutaneous or mucous membrane sites of primary inoculation. HSV also can reach the CNS by the viremia of disseminated disease in the neonate.

13. What are the three primary clinical syndromes of neonatal HSV infection?

1. Disease limited to the skin, eyes, and/or mouth (~40% of cases)
2. Disseminated with viremia (~25% of cases)
3. Encephalitis, with or without skin lesions (~35% of cases)

Most neonatal HSV infections are caused by HSV-2, and most are acquired during birth from exposure to the virus in the lower genital tract. Postnatal infection from parents or other caregivers can result in neonatal HSV as well. Intrauterine infections are less common but have been increasingly recognized in recent years.

14. How do the different clinical syndromes of neonatal HSV infection usually present?

	SKIN, EYE, AND/OR MOUTH DISEASE (SEM)	DISSEMINATED	ENCEPHALITIS
Usual time of onset	10–11 days of age	4–7 days of age	11–18 days of age
Clinical features	Vesicles occur on the skin in 90% of cases; clusters typically appear on the presenting part of the baby (often scalp); 1–2-mm vesicles arise on an erythematous base and may coalesce to form bullae. Eye involvement occurs as keratoconjunctivitis and/or chorioretinitis. Localized lesions in the mouth, tongue, or larynx also can occur.	Irritability, seizures, respiratory distress (diffuse pneumonitis in 50% that can become hemorrhagic), jaundice (hepatitis), shock (can mimic bacterial sepsis), bleeding, vesicular rash (80% of cases), and manifestations of encephalitis (⅔ of cases)	Lethargy, irritability, tremors, poor feeding, bulging fontanelle, fever, temperature instability, seizures (~60%, focal or generalized), skin vesicles (60% of cases), and sometimes mild manifestations of disseminated disease)
Laboratory and radiographic findings	Usually none unless disseminated disease develops or there is extension of infection to the CNS.	Elevated serum transaminases, direct hyperbilirubinemia, neutropenia, thrombocytopenia, coagulopathy, diffuse interstitial infiltrates on chest radiographs	CSF pleocytosis (usually mononuclear cell predominance) and proteinosis. EEG abnormalities (85%), abnormalities on brain MRI or CT (75%). Brain involvement is not limited to the temporal or frontal lobes in neonates.
Outcomes (with antiviral therapy)	> 90% can have normal neurologic outcomes. Recurrent outbreaks of vesicles are common during the first year of life, even with initial treatment. Untreated cases can progress to encephalitis and rarely disseminated disease.	60% mortality. Severe cases may not respond to therapy. Neurologic sequelae are the rule in survivors. Death usually results from pneumonitis and bleeding diatheses.	10–20% mortality (some deaths occur late after acute phase of illness). 20–30% may be normal neurologically (?HSV 1 less severe than HSV 2 CNS infection). 50% or more have severe impairments.

CSF = cerebrospinal fluid, EEG = electroencephalography, MRI = magnetic resonance imaging, CT = computed tomography, HSV = herpes simplex virus, CNS = central nervous system.

15. What are the characteristics of intrauterine HSV infections?

Intrauterine infection with HSV usually is evident at birth. A triad of findings is most common: (1) skin vesicles and/or areas of scarring from vesicles that erupted in utero; (2) chorioretinitis (with optic atrophy in severe cases); and (3) brain involvement, which may manifest as microcephaly, encephalomalacia, or areas of hemorrhage, depending on severity and gestational age at onset.

16. How common is neonatal HSV infection?

Neonatal HSV infection occurs in about 1 in every 3000 live births in the United States, resulting in about 2000 cases per year. The majority of infected infants are born to mothers with no known history of genital herpes. Among infants born vaginally to mothers with primary HSV infection during pregnancy, risk of neonatal HSV infection is estimated at 33–50%. Risk of neonatal HSV infection among infants born to mothers with genital shedding of HSV from reactivation is in the range of 0–5%. When mothers have active genital lesions, cesarean delivery, when membranes have been ruptured for less than 4–6 hours, greatly reduces the risk of HSV infection in the infant.

17. When should HSV infection of the CNS be suspected in neonates?

It can be difficult to distinguish between infants with bacterial sepsis and/or meningitis and HSV, but routine addition of acyclovir to antibiotics for suspected sepsis or meningitis is not recommended. Infants with HSV encephalitis usually have some combination of lethargy, fever, irritability, and seizures, but absence of fever is common. At a minimum, neonatal HSV encephalitis should be considered when the infant (1) is poorly responsive (altered mental status); (2) has seizures of any type; (3) has skin vesicles (or ulcerative or crusted skin lesions); (4) has CSF pleocytosis with mononuclear cell predominance; or (5) does not improve clinically and bacterial cultures are negative at 48–72 hours. Increased CSF red blood cells (RBCs) from a clearly nontraumatic lumbar puncture can indicate the presence of hemorrhagic necrosis due to HSV encephalitis. CSF proteinosis also is common. *Brain involvement is often diffuse; there is no predilection for the temporal lobes as in older children and adults.*

18. Describe the management of an infant born to a mother with active genital herpes lesions at the time of birth.

Some experts recommend empirical treatment of infants born to mothers with primary infection during pregnancy, but many others wait until there are positive cultures or other clinical manifestations before starting therapy. Viral cultures of the mouth, nasopharynx, urine, stool or rectum, and conjunctivae should be obtained between 24 and 48 hours after birth. (Positive cultures for HSV obtained less than 24 hours after birth may indicate colonization from intrapartum exposure rather than active viral replication.) Mode of delivery and maternal infection status (primary vs. recurrent disease) do not affect management. Parents of infants with negative cultures should be educated to observe carefully for skin vesicles or any signs of respiratory distress or sepsis during the first few weeks of life.

19. When should HSV encephalitis be suspected in older infants and children?

The possibility should be considered in any child who presents with altered mental status. The typical presentation of HSV encephalitis in older infants and children is a prodrome of fever, malaise, irritability, and headache for 1–7 days, followed by progressive signs of CNS involvement over several days (sometimes with a waxing and waning course). Various combinations of personality changes, dysphasia, autonomic dysfunction, altered consciousness, ataxia, hemiparesis, cranial nerve deficits, and seizures (focal or general) can be seen. Meningeal signs are rare. CSF pleocytosis > 50 white blood cells/mm³ is common, and 90% of patients have initial lymphocyte predominance (30–40% neutrophils also is common). Most patients have elevated red blood cell counts in the CSF, reflecting hemorrhagic necrosis. *Temporal and frontal lobe involvement is common.* Over 90% of HSV encephalitis cases beyond the neonatal period are due to HSV-1 strains. With antiviral therapy, more than half of children can be expected to recover without neurologic sequelae.

20. How can the diagnosis of HSV encephalitis be confirmed?

In the past, brain biopsy often was required for symptomatic cases. CSF polymerase chain reaction (PCR) for HSV DNA has now become the diagnostic standard, although false-positive and false-negative results can occur. In addition, viral cultures of skin lesions, oropharynx, conjunctivae, urine, blood, stool or rectum, and CSF should be ordered for symptomatic neonates. Positive cultures for HSV obtained more than 24 hours after birth indicate active viral replication rather than colonization from intrapartum exposure. CSF viral cultures for HSV are rarely positive among older children and adults with HSV encephalitis.

21. How should HSV encephalitis be treated?

In neonates, recent data suggest that intravenous acyclovir, 60 mg/kg/day administered in 3 doses for 21 days, may improve outcomes in infants with encephalitis and/or disseminated disease more than the 30-mg/kg/day regimen that was considered standard in the past. Skin, eye, and mouth disease without encephalitis should be treated with 60 mg/kg/day for 14 days. For older infants and children, a regimen of 30 mg/kg/day in 3 divided doses should be administered for 21 days. Some experts use 1500 mg/m²/day, which correlates more closely with 60 mg/kg/day. Because neutropenia is a potential side effect of acyclovir, it is appropriate to assess the white blood cell differential and absolute neutrophil count twice weekly during therapy. Attention should be paid to adequate hydration to prevent acyclovir crystallization in renal tubules with resultant (reversible) renal dysfunction.

22. How long does CSF remain positive for HSV DNA by PCR after initiation of antiretroviral therapy?

In up to 80% of patients with HSV encephalitis, the CSF remained positive for HSV DNA by PCR testing a week into therapy. By the end of a 3-week course of antiretroviral therapy, CSF PCR tests almost always were negative, so that the test does not need to be repeated at the end of therapy.

23. What approach should be used to determine the specific cause of encephalitis in a child?

In an attempt to narrow the diagnostic focus, a careful elucidation of exposure risks must be undertaken: illness in contacts; travel history; exposure to mosquitoes, ticks, or animals (especially equines); recent injections of any kind; and potential exposures to heavy metals, pesticides, or other chemicals. CSF should be obtained for routine studies and possibly for viral or fungal cultures, depending on the specific clinical setting. Viral cultures, however, are of generally low yield. PCR studies for HSV and enteroviruses in CSF are now widely available and can be ordered if either of these agents is suspected. PCR tests for *Mycoplasma* spp. and human parvovirus (HPV) may be available in some settings.

- Nasopharyngeal (or throat) and rectal (or fecal) viral cultures should be obtained early in the course of disease.
- Serum should be sent as an acute specimen for later pairing with convalescent samples drawn 2 or more weeks later, in case serologic testing for specific agents is necessary.
- It also is wise to save CSF from any spinal taps throughout the course of the disease in case additional or confirmatory tests are needed.

Many state laboratories run serum and/or CSF antibody detection tests for arboviruses endemic to their region.

- Assays for *B. henselae* and HPV IgM also may be considered.
- Rapid antigen tests for specific respiratory viruses (RSV, adenoviruses, and parainfluenza and influenza viruses) may be considered when these diseases are prevalent in the community. Other serologies may be obtained when the clinical illness resembles that of a specific agent (e.g., EBV panels when the patient appears to have mononucleosis as well as encephalitis).

24. What is the initial approach to treatment and management of a child with apparent encephalitis?

Acyclovir is administered in most cases of apparent encephalitis until HSV is reasonably ruled out as the cause. In addition, seizures, cerebral edema, respiratory insufficiency, cardiac or respiratory arrest of central origin, and fluid and electrolyte imbalances (e.g., syndrome of inappropriate antidiuretic hormone) require interventions and should be anticipated if not present at the time of admission. Steroids generally should not be used until an infectious cause has been largely excluded.

25. What is the usual prognosis for a child with acute encephalitis?

Outcomes generally depend on the specific cause, if identified. Many children recover fully. Postinfectious encephalitides may carry better outcomes than infectious encephalitides. Residual neurologic deficits are common but by no means universal after encephalitis caused by HSV, other herpes family viruses, and most arboviruses. Severity of CNS symptoms and signs during the acute illness and the pace of recovery can provide insights into prognosis, as can the results of serial CNS imaging studies.

26. What is the role of *Mycoplasma pneumoniae* in acute encephalitis of childhood?

In a recent series of 159 children with acute encephalitis in Canada, 11 cases (7%) probably were due to *M. pneumoniae* infection, based on results of acute and convalescent serologic data and/or positive PCR results on CSF or throat specimens. However, two of the 11 cases also had evidence of HSV-2 by PCR of the CSF, and 5 others had evidence of concurrent enterovirus, human herpes virus-6, influenza virus, or parainfluenza virus infections. Another 39 patients had some evidence of mycoplasmal infection, but in 30 there was more compelling evidence of another cause. Thus, *M. pneumoniae* may play a role in some cases of encephalitis in children, but it is prevalent enough in the population that it may represent an unrelated factor or a cofactor for another agent. Among the 11 probable cases, 7 (64%) had long-term neurologic sequelae. Whether treatment may impact the outcome, if *M. pneumoniae* is the cause of encephalitis, is unknown.

27. A 13-month-old boy had begun to walk and pick up small objects with a pincer grasp at 11 months of age. He now has difficulty in sitting and transferring objects from hand to hand. He has lost 3 pounds in the past month and has bilateral cervical and axillary lymphadenopathy. What infection probably accounts for this scenario?

Human immunodeficiency virus (HIV) infection with HIV encephalopathy. Infants with untreated perinatally acquired HIV infection can develop high viral loads that facilitate viral invasion of brain parenchyma. Loss of previously gained developmental milestones, wasting, and adenopathy, are common manifestations and should suggest the possibility of HIV infection if the diagnosis is not yet known. Antiretroviral therapy can lead to full recovery, although focal neurologic findings, such as spastic diplegia, may be permanent once established.

28. What is progressive multifocal leukoencephalopathy (PML)?

PML is caused by infection of oligodendroglial cells by JC papovavirus in immunocompromised hosts. It was rare until the HIV pandemic but now occurs in 2–5% of adults with AIDS and can occur in older children or adolescents with perinatally acquired HIV infection who have progressed to AIDS. Clinical manifestations include limb weakness, cognitive dysfunction, visual loss, headache, and gait disturbances. The typical findings on computed tomography (CT) or MRI are hypodense, nonenhancing lesions in the white matter. CSF is usually normal, although mild mononuclear pleocytosis and proteinosis can be seen. Unless immunosuppression can be reversed, mean survival is about 4 months after onset of symptoms. Treatment with newer antiviral agents such as cidofovir may prove useful in the future.

29. What is the most common epidemic viral infection of the CNS outside North America?

Japanese B encephalitis virus (JBEV). JBEV is mosquito-borne and endemic in China, northern Southeast Asia, India, Sri Lanka, the Philippines, Indonesia, and southern Russia. Incidence is greatly decreased now in Japan and Korea due to the availability of an inactivated virus vaccine that has an approximately 80% protective efficacy. The vaccine is recommended for residents of endemic or epidemic areas and travelers planning to stay in the rural regions of such areas for longer than 30 days. The vaccine is given as a 3-dose series (0, 7, and 30 days or 0, 7, 14, if needed) and can be given to children 1 year of age and older.

JBEV is a flavivirus (related to dengue and yellow fever), and 90% of cases are asymptomatic. The mortality rate with encephalitis is 2–10%. The typical prodromal phase lasts for 2–3 days and is associated with headache, anorexia, nausea, vomiting, and low-grade fever. An acute phase of 3–7 days with high fever and mental status changes ensues. Seizures occur in 20% of children. Cortical dysfunction progresses from confusion to coma. The CSF usually has 100–1000 white blood cells/mm^3, with early neutrophil predominance giving way to lymphocytes later in the course of the disease. CSF protein is also elevated. Death ensues within 10 days of the acute phase. Survivors become subacute, then convalesce over another 2–4 weeks. Permanent sequelae, such as spastic paresis and extrapyramidal signs, are common.

30. What is the epidemiologic importance of enterovirus 71 vs. other nonpolio enteroviruses?

CNS infection by nonpolio enteroviruses typically takes the form of aseptic meningitis in immunocompetent hosts. Enteroviral meningoencephalitis can occur but usually resolves without permanent neurologic sequelae. Enterovirus 71, however, can cause brainstem encephalitis and rhombencephalitis and, in rare cases, acute flaccid paralysis (like polio). Outbreaks of infection have been seen in different parts of the world, including Southeast Asia and Canada. This enterovirus, therefore, may be more akin to polioviruses in its clinical impact than coxsackie virus, echovirus, and other numbered enteroviruses. The frequency of such severe complications among persons infected with enterovirus 71, however, may be low.

31. A 15-year-old boy is brought to the emergency department with fever, headache and altered mental status. His family reports no unusual activities or trauma. He had been swimming with several friends in a neighbor's farm pond 2 days before. CT scan without contrast shows no mass effects. CSF is obtained, and the laboratory technician reports that, while he was trying to perform a cell count, the white cells were observed to be moving across the hemocytometer. What does the boy have?

Amebic meningoencephalitis. *Naegleria fowleri* is the likely cause when motile trophozoites are seen in fresh CSF. *Acanthamoeba* and *Balamuthia* species can cause subacute or chronic granulomatous amebic meningoencephalitis. Sporadic cases of amebic meningoencephalitis occur when persons swim in water containing the amebae. Boys are more commonly affected than girls (2:1 ratio for *N. fowleri* and 5:1 for *Acanthamoeba* sp.), perhaps in part reflecting differences in rates of swimming in high-risk waters. Amebae reach the CNS directly from the nasal cavity across the cribriform plate via extensions of the olfactory nerves. *Acanthamoeba* sp. also can cause primary keratoconjunctivitis, especially among wearers of contact lenses. Amphotericin B with adjunctive rifampin and/or tetracycline may be of some value for *N. fowleri* meningoencephalitis. Only a few survivors have been reported. *Acanthamoeba* infections also are difficult to treat and typically require surgical excision of infected areas, including corneal grafting or keratoplasty for keratitis.

32. What are Nipah and Hendra viruses?

Both are newly recognized paramyxoviruses that have caused cases of encephalitis among pig workers in Malaysia and Australia. The viruses cause respiratory illness in pigs that can be transmitted to humans, but human-to-human transmission does not appear common. Pigs acquire the infection from pteropid bats, which are the natural reservoir of the viruses.

33. What are two postinfectious CNS manifestations of group A streptococcal infections?

Sydenham chorea is one of the major criteria for acute rheumatic fever and can occur in isolation weeks to months after a group A streptococcal infection. Recently, a new association has been described—or, more likely, an old linkage finally has been recognized: pediatric autoimmune neuropsychiatric disorder associated with group A streptococcal infection (PANDAS). The disorder consists of obsessive-compulsive behaviors and/or tic behavior shortly after group A streptococcal infection. Antibiotic treatment may abolish the symptoms, which can recur with subsequent infection. Studies to further evaluate this apparent linkage are ongoing.

34. What are "slow virus" infections of the CNS?

Viral or prion-associated diseases that result in progressive dementia and often other neurologic manifestations. "Slow virus" infections include progressive multifocal leukoencephalopathy, AIDS dementia, and subacute sclerosing panencephalitis (due to measles). Prion diseases, also called transmissible spongiform encephalopathies, include kuru, Creutzfeldt-Jakob disease, scrapie, and bovine spongiform encephalopathy ("mad cow" disease).

BIBLIOGRAPHY

1. Bitnun A, Ford-Jones EL, Petric M, et al: Acute childhood encephalitis and *Mycoplasma pneumoniae*. Clin Infect Dis 32:1674–1684, 2001.
2. Cherry JD, Shields WD: Encephalitis and meningoencephalitis. In Feigin RD, Cherry JD (eds): Textbook of Pediatric Infectious Diseases, 4th ed. Philadelphia, W.B.Saunders, 1998, pp 457–468.
3. Hung K-L, Liao H-T, Tsai M-L: The spectrum of postinfectious encephalomyelitis. Brain Devel 23:42–45, 2001.
4. Kimberlin DW, Lin C-Y, Jacobs RF, et al: Natural history of neonatal herpes simplex virus infections in the acyclovir era. Pediatrics 108:223–229, 2001.
5. Kimberlin DW, Lin C-Y, Jacobs RF, et al: Safety and efficacy of high-dose intravenous acyclovir in the management of neonatal herpes simplex virus infections. Pediatrics 108:230–238, 2001.
6. Murphy ML, Pichichero ME: Prospective identification and treatment of children with pediatric autoimmune neuropsychiatric disorder associated with Group A streptococcal infection (PANDAS). Arch Pediatr Adolesc Med 156:356–361, 2002.
7. Whitley RJ: Arthropod-borne infections. In Scheld WM, Whitley RJ, Durack DT (eds): Infections of the Central Nervous System, 2nd ed. Philadelphia, Lippincott-Raven, 1997, pp 223–253.
8. Whitley RJ, Gnann JW: Viral encephalitis: Familiar infections and emerging pathogens. Lancet 359:507–514, 2002.
9. Whitley RJ, Kimberlin DW: Viral encephalitis. Pediatr Rev 20:192–198, 1999.
10. Whitley RJ, Stagnio S: Perinatal viral infections. In Scheld WM, Whitley RJ, Durack DT (eds): Infections of the Central Nervous System, 2nd ed. Philadelphia, Lippincott-Raven, 1997, pp 223–253.

IX. Skin and Soft Tissue Infections

29. COMMON SKIN INFECTIONS

Shirley P. Klein, M.D., and Monica Jain Snowden, M.D.

1. What is the differential diagnosis of a skin lesion with a black center (eschar)?

Anthrax comes to mind first, but other possibilities include primary cutaneous aspergillosis, cutaneous zygomycosis, and ecthyma gangrenosum (*Pseudomonas* sp.). A spider bite may also have central necrosis with surrounding erythema or blisters.

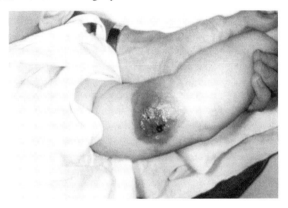

Cutaneous anthrax in a 7-month old infant.

2. What is ecthyma gangrenosum?

Ecthyma gangrenosum is an ulcerated lesion with a central eschar that often accompanies pseudomonal septicemia. Most patients are seriously ill and may have one or many lesions. Diagnosis is made by blood culture or Gram stain/culture of the ulcer. Treatment with systemic antibiotics is required.

3. Describe tinea corporis.

Tinea corporis is a fungal infection of the face, trunk, and limbs. It does not involve the hands and feet or hairy areas. The lesions are usually circular and slightly red, with a well-defined scaly, pustular, or vesicular border. The main causes include *Trichophyton*, *Microsporum*, and *Epidermophyton* spp. Tinea corporis is much more common in children than adults.

4. Can tinea corporis occur on the scalp?

Technically, no. By definition tinea corporis is a superficial infection of nonhairy skin. Tinea infections of the scalp are called tinea capitis.

5. Can tinea capitis be treated topically?

Some studies claim resolution with antifungal shampoos, but the recommended treatment is an oral antifungal agent that gets into the hair follicle. Antifungal shampoos such as ketoconazole (Nizoral) and selenium sulfide (Selsun), however, help clear the scalp lesions and may help prevent person-to-person spread, especially among asymptomatic family members.

6. What is the treatment of tinea capitis?

The treatment of choice remains oral griseofulvin, although higher and higher doses are required because of resistance. The dose of microsize griseofulvin is 20–25 mg/kg/day, given in one or two doses; the maximal dose is 500 mg to 1 gm per day. It is absorbed best with fatty foods such as whole milk, ice cream, or peanut butter or any greasy food that is bad for your health. The dose of the ultramicrosize griseofulvin is 10–15 mg/kg/day. If griseofulvin is not tolerated (rare) or not effective (occasional), other oral antifungals (fluconazole, ketoconazole, itraconazole, or terbinafine) may be used, although not all are approved in children or available in a suspension.

7. What is a kerion?

A kerion is a boggy, erythematous mass on the scalp, sometimes surrounded by pustules. Any purulent drainage is sterile, because a kerion is a hypersensitivity reaction to the fungus. It may lead to permanent hair loss.

8. What is an id reaction?

A rash occurring at a site that is not infected with the fungus or, in the case of contact dermatitis, a site that has not been in contact with the allergen is called autoeczematization or a dermatophytid ("id") reaction. It is believed to be a form of delayed hypersensitivity from absorption of parts of the fungus. It is uncommon and may occur with tinea pedis as well as tinea capitis. The rash is an erythematous vesicular or scaly eruption, mainly on the extremities, including palms and soles; in some children, it also appears on the trunk and face. Some lesions look fungal, but tests show no fungus in the lesions. Lesions resolve once the infection is treated. More severe cases may require treatment with systemic steroids.

9. Are steroids used to treat tinea capitis?

As a general rule, steroid treatment makes fungal infections worse. Exceptions to this rule in tinea capitis are the presence of a kerion or an id reaction, both of which represent an exaggerated inflammatory reaction to the fungus. Steroids speed recovery and may prevent permanent scarring from a kerion. The dose of prednisone is 0.5–1.0 mg/kg/day, tapered over 2–3 weeks.

10. Should children with any tinea infection be kept out of school?

Children with tinea infection may attend school as long as the infection is treated appropriately. They should avoid direct contact and sharing of clothing and hair accessories. Extreme measures such as shaving the head are not necessary.

11. The figure below shows the same patient in winter and summer. Identify the rash.

The rash is tinea versicolor, a skin infection caused by a form of *Pityrosporum orbiculare* (*Malassezia furfur*). This organism usually colonizes the skin by 6 months of age. Lesions are

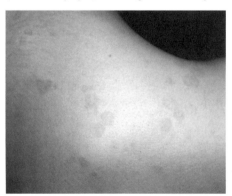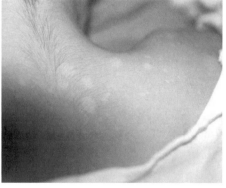

Tinea versicolor in winter (*left*) and in summer (*right*).

more likely to occur under certain conditions: adolescence, pregnancy, immunocompromised states, and warm, humid climates. The lesions are oval-shaped and macular, with scales around the borders. They may be reddish, brownish, light tan or white; hence the name "versicolor." They tend to be lighter in dark-skinned people and darker in light-skinned people. In winter, they tend to look darker as the pigment in tanned or darker skin fades.

12. List the differential diagnosis of tinea versicolor.

Vitiligo	Pityriasis alba
Seborrhea	Pityriasis rosea
Postinflammatory hypopigmentation	Melasma
Contact dermatitis	Secondary syphilis
Tinea corporis	

13. How is tinea versicolor diagnosed?

It is usually diagnosed by its characteristic appearance. Under Wood's light, it fluoresces to a golden, orange, or copper color. A potassium hydroxide (KOH) preparation of the scale shows hyphae and spores in clusters ("spaghetti and meatballs.") Culture is usually not helpful because the fungus is hard to grow.

14. How is tinea versicolor treated?

Although topical antifungals work well, they are not cost-effective for covering large areas. An antifungal lotion such as selenium sulfide (Selsun) may be applied using various regimens.

15. Match each of the following infections with the appropriate descriptor:

1. Tinea capitis	a. Herald patch
2. Tinea corporis	b. "Athlete's foot"
3. Tinea versicolor	c. Ringworm
4. Pityriasis rosea	d. Onychomycosis
5. Pityriasis alba	e. "Jock itch"
6. Tinea pedis	f. Kerion
7. Tinea cruris	g. Atopic
8. Tinea unguium	h. *Malassezia furfur*

Answers: 1, f; 2, c; 3, h; 4, a; 5, g; 6, b; 7, e; 8, d.

16. Describe the characteristics of candidal skin infections. Where are they most commonly found?

Candidal lesions are often bright (beefy) red and raised with sharp, irregular borders. Satellite papules, pustules, and/or vesicles may be present. The lesions have a predilection for intertriginous areas, such as the neck, axillae, inguinal, and diaper areas. Some infants also may have oral candidal lesions of thrush (white plaques on a red base).

17. Which topical antifungals work on which fungal infections of the skin?

Candidal infections: azoles such as clotrimazole (Lotrimin) work as well or better than nystatin; the allylamines (e.g., Lamisil) do not work well; tolnaftate (Tinactin) is ineffective.

Tinea corporis and athlete's foot: terbinafine (Lamisil) is best. All of the azoles (e.g., Lotrimin, Micatin, Nizoral, Spectazole) work well, and tolnaftate usually works. Nystatin is ineffective.

18. What is a Wood's lamp?

Also known as a Wood's light or Wood light, a Wood's lamp is an ultraviolet light with a filter that allows it to emit long-wave ultraviolet light rays (wavelengths from 320 to 400 nm). In 1925 it was discovered that hair infected by certain fungi would fluoresce under this light.

19. Is a Wood's lamp helpful in the diagnosis of tinea capitis?

The Wood's lamp is not as helpful as it used to be, because tinea capitis is now caused mainly by *Trichophyton tonsurans*. In the past, *Microsporum audouinii* and *Microsporum canis* were the most common causative agents. Both caused the hair to fluoresce bright green. The room must be dark, and the clinician must take care to examine the hair rather than the skin, scales, ointment, or lint, all of which fluoresce purple.

20. What is the difference between the two main organisms that cause tinea capitis?

	Microsporum canis	*Trichophyton tonsurans*
Fluorescence	Yellow-green	None
Source	Cats and dogs	Human (other children)
Contagious	No	Yes
Children infected	Rural and suburban	Primarily urban
Hair loss	Yes	Yes
Kerion	Yes	Yes
Clinical patterns	Thickened hairs	Dandruff-like, patches of alopecia, seborrhea-like, small pustules, and black dots

21. What causes pityriasis rosea?

The cause is unknown, but it is presumed to be viral because of the few recurrences, occasional cases in contacts, and seasonal (winter) peak incidence. In addition, prodromal symptoms may precede the onset of the rash.

22. What symptoms may precede the rash of pityriasis rosea?

The most common are headache, malaise, pharyngitis, rhinorrhea, swollen glands, and other vague constitutional symptoms.

23. In what age group does pityriasis rosea most commonly occur?

School-aged children and young adults, but cases have been described in patients as young as 3 months.

24. Describe a herald patch.

A large (3–5 cm), pink, oval-shaped patch with scales and often with central clearing. It is frequently misdiagnosed as ringworm, because it precedes the rest of the lesions by 1–2 weeks.

25. Where is the herald patch located?

Usually on the trunk or proximal lower extremity, but it can be anywhere.

26. Describe the rash of pityriasis rosea.

Most typical lesions are oval and about 1–2 cm with brownish or pinkish centers and slightly elevated scaly borders. Lesions may also be papular, bullous, vesicular, crusted, or purpuric and may be of any size.

27. Which shape describes the typical distribution of pityriasis rosea: (a) diamond, (b) star of David, (c) Christmas tree, or (d) star of Bethlehem?

The answer is (c). The typical distribution is mainly on the trunk, and lesions form a Christmas tree pattern on the back, following the lines of skin cleavage (lines of Blaschko). On the chest, it is more like an upside-down Christmas tree. Pityriasis rosea rarely involves the face and neck. In younger children and African-Americans, an atypical distribution may involve mainly the extremities and sometimes the neck and face.

28. How long does the rash of pityriasis rosea last?
From a few weeks to 2 or 3 months.

29. How is pityriasis rosea treated?
There is no treatment, but the rash always gets better. Many patients report itching at the onset of the rash and for the first week or so. The itching may be helped by topical or systemic antipruritics or by exposure to sunlight.

30. List the differential diagnosis for annular lesions.

Tinea corporis	Herald patch of pityriasis rosea
Nummular eczema	Impetigo
Granuloma annulare	Erythema migrans

31. What are the two main forms of impetigo?
1. **Bullous impetigo**, usually caused by phage group 2 *Staphylococcus aureus*.
2. **Vesicopustular impetigo**, usually caused by group A beta-hemolytic streptococci, with or without *S. aureus*.

32. Differentiate bullous impetigo from vesicopustular impetigo.
Bullous impetigo starts as superficial blisters that rupture and leave a scalded skin-like appearance. They occur mainly on the face, trunk, and extremities. There is no seasonal predilection.
Vesicopustular impetigo occurs mainly on the legs or any traumatized skin. It has a higher incidence in the summer and in tropical areas because of association with insect bites.
Both types are associated with red, weeping surfaces and honey-colored crusts.

33. How is impetigo treated?
Topical antibiotics are effective early, including bacitracin, polymixin, neomycin, and combinations. Mupirocin (Bactroban) is particularly effective and may be as effective as oral antibiotics. In younger children or in patients with more severe or extensive impetigo, oral antibiotics may be needed. Penicillin G or V is no longer recommended because of the likely presence of penicillin-resistant *S. aureus*. Effective drugs include cephalosporins, cloxacillin, clindamycin, and amoxicillin-clavulanic acid.

34. Compare cellulitis and erysipelas.

CELLULITIS	ERYSIPELAS
Subcutaneous	Superficial
Borders not elevated, borders not sharply defined	Distinct border
Follows trauma (break in skin)	Break in skin or hematogenous spread
Red, dusky red, or purplish	Bright red
Anywhere on the body	Anywhere, but mainly on face or scalp
Streptococci, staphylococci, *Streptococcus pneumoniae* (in past, *Haemophilus influenzae*)	Streptococci

35. Can impetigo caused by group A beta-hemolytic streptococci lead to rheumatic fever?
There are no recorded instances of rheumatic fever following skin infection. Acute glomerulonephritis and scarlet fever may follow skin infection with group A streptococci, depending on the strain involved.

36. List the complications of bacterial impetigo and their causative organism.

COMPLICATION	ORGANISM
Cellulitis	Streptococci or staphylococci
Lymphangitis	Streptococci
Lymphadenitis	Streptococci or staphylococci
Guttate psoriasis	Streptococci
Sepsis	Streptococci or staphylococci
Septic arthritis	Streptococci or staphylococci
Osteomyelitis	Streptococci or staphylococci
Endocarditis	Streptococci or staphylococci
Pneumonia	Streptococci or staphylococci
Scalded-skin syndrome	Staphylococci
Poststreptococcal glomerulonephritis	Streptococci
Toxic shock syndrome	Streptococci or staphylococci

37. Define impetigo of the newborn.

It is a bullous form of impetigo occurring in the first two weeks of life and caused by *S. aureus*, usually phage group 2.

38. How is impetigo of the newborn treated?

In a infant who is afebrile and not otherwise sick and has no other focus of infection, an oral antibiotic that covers *S. aureus* should be used. Mupirocin may be helpful but is not adequate treatment. A sick newborn obviously should be hospitalized for intravenous antibiotics.

39. What is the differential diagnosis of impetigo of the newborn?

Infectious rashes	**Noninfectious rashes**
Herpes simplex virus	Erythema toxicum neonatorum
Varicella	Neonatal pustular melanosis
Enterovirus	Incontinentia pigmenti
Congenital cutaneous	Epidermolysis bullosa
candidiasis	Pemphigus
Scabies	Pemphigoid

40. In what skin infections does autoinoculation occur?

Autoinoculation (spread by scratching, touching, or direct contact with another body part) occurs in impetigo, herpes simplex, molluscum contagiosum, smallpox, warts, and cutaneous tuberculosis.

41. What skin infections are spread by wrestlers?

Herpes gladiatorum (scrum-pox in rugby players) is primary inoculation with herpes simplex from direct contact with active lesions and abraded skin. Scabies and impetigo may be transmitted from person to person. The most common skin infection spread by wrestlers is tinea corporis, or tinea corporis gladiatorum. Nonskin infections spread by wrestlers are mainly upper respiratory infections, but HIV and hepatitis B could be transmitted through blood and secretions.

42. What is "hot tub dermatitis"?

It is a cutaneous infection caused by *Pseudomonas aeruginosa*. Other names include whirlpool dermatitis and pseudomonal folliculitis.

43. Describe the clinical course of hot tub dermatitis.
Papules and pustules develop within 1–2 days of exposure, primarily in areas covered by bathing suits. The lesions are pruritic. Most patients are otherwise asymptomatic, although some have systemic illness. Spontaneous regression occurs within 5–14 days, but recurrences may occur for up to 3 months.

44. What group of viruses is the most common cause of warts?
Human papillomavirus (HPV).

45. Are most warts benign or malignant?
Benign.

46. Where are most warts found in children?
Distal extremities: hands, feet, and digits.

47. How do children get warts?
The virus enters the skin via local disruption by trauma.

48. Match the virus with the wart.
1. HPV-1	(a)	Flat warts (verruca plana)
2. HPV-2,4	(b)	Anogenital warts (condyloma acuminata)
3. HPV-3	(c)	Common warts (verruca vulgaris)
4. HPV-6,11	(d)	Plantar warts

Answers: 1, d; 2, c; 3, a; 4, b.

49. In a child who presents with anogenital warts, what must the pediatrician consider in the differential diagnosis?
Anogenital warts are uncommon in children; one must consider sexual abuse. Most infections are acquired before or during birth or by other nonsexual means.

50. What is molluscum contagiosum?
Molluscum contagiosum is a viral skin infection most often described in young children. The lesions are grouped, pinpoint papules that increase in size. They are off-white or pinkish-tan and rounded; many have central umbilication.

51. What causes molluscum contagiosum?
A large poxvirus (DNA virus).

52. Where are the most common sites for molluscum contagiosum?
Lesions are often found on the trunk, face, axillae, and inguinal areas. Occasionally they are found in and around the mucous membranes of the mouth and genital areas.

53. How are the lesions spread?
The lesions are contagious (as the name suggests) and are spread by direct contact or auto-inoculation.

54. How is molluscum contagiosum treated?
Most cases resolve spontaneously without treatment. Multiple lesions or lesions in the conjunctiva or genital area may require treatment to prevent spread or scarring. Treatments include cryotherapy, curettage, various chemicals (e.g., cantharidin, podophyllin), and/or adhesive tape occlusion.

55. What other conditions should the clinician look for in a child with multiple or recurrent molluscum?
Immunodeficiency states, including HIV/AIDS.

56. Where are herpes simplex virus (HSV) lesions commonly found in infants and children?

Most lesions are found in the oral cavity, but they may occur on any skin or mucous membrane surface.

57. What are the most common types of HSV infections?

The traditional teaching is that HSV-1 infections are above the waist (e.g., gingivostomatitis) and HSV-2 infections are below the waist (e.g., genital herpes). These infections are so common and easily spread that both are found above and below the waist.

58. How is HSV diagnosed?

Diagnosis is usually clinical, but a Tzanck smear of the vesicle fluid may be helpful to differentiate viral from nonviral vesicles. A viral culture or a direct fluorescent antibody (DFA) test establishes the diagnosis.

59. What is herpetic gingivostomatitis?

It is the most common primary HSV infection in children. It usually occurs in toddlers and preschool children who present with fever, irritability, mouth pain, and blisters on the tongue, gingiva, and oral mucosa. Occasionally, some lesions may be perioral. The fever may last up to 1 week, and the oral lesions may last up to 2 weeks.

60. How is HSV spread?

HSV can be spread by direct contact or autoinoculation to fingers and other parts of the body (especially the genital area). It is especially contagious to neonates, immunocompromised people, and people with chronic dermatitis.

61. What is herpetic whitlow?

Localized primary herpes infection of the finger(s) usually occurs by cutaneous inoculation. It appears as clustered vesicles on a red base. Lesions tend to be quite painful and may be associated with local adenopathy and systemic symptoms. It is an occupational hazard in doctors, dentists, dental hygienists, and nurses from direct contact with oral or genital lesions. At present it is rare because most health professionals wear gloves.

62. How is HSV treated?

Most patients are treated symptomatically. Topical acyclovir is ineffective. Genital herpes in children is often treated with oral acyclovir. In severe cases or immunocompromised hosts, however, parenteral acyclovir is recommended. Newer oral antiviral agents currently used in adults may eventually replace parenteral acyclovir.

63. What is neonatal herpes? How is it treated?

Neonatal herpes is acquired at birth from the mother, who may or may not have active lesions. Most infections involve HSV-2, but HSV-1 is becoming increasingly common. Neonatal herpes is potentially life-threatening (up to 50% mortality rate), especially if encephalitis develops. If the disease is suspected, treatment should be started immediately with intravenous acyclovir for 2–3 weeks.

64. Describe the signs and symptoms of varicella (chickenpox).

Varicella is usually a harmless childhood infection. The incubation period is anywhere from 10 to 21 days. The illness begins with a prodrome of fever, malaise, and sore throat. It is followed by skin lesions that begin as pruritic papules and then progress within 24–48 hours to vesicles on an erythematous base. The vesicles then crust and dry up over the next several days. New crops of lesions appear over 3–4 days so that lesions in different stages are apparent at the same time. Varicella is contagious from a few days before the skin lesions appear to 5–7 days after the appearance of the lesions. Treatment is usually supportive, especially for the intense pruritus.

65. What are the major complications of varicella infection?

The more common complications of varicella infection include secondary infection of the lesions (usually caused by *S. aureus* or streptococci), cellulitis, and fasciitis (with group A beta-hemolytic streptococci). Rare complications include disseminated intravascular coagulation with purpura fulminans, viral or bacterial pneumonia, and encephalitis. Before introduction in 1995 of a preventive vaccine, varicella caused about 100 deaths per year in the United States. That number has now dropped significantly.

66. What is herpes zoster?

Also known as shingles, herpes zoster is due to reactivation of the chickenpox virus that has been inactive for years after the initial infection. The virus tends to hide in the sensory nerve root. Reactivation can occur following immunosuppression or other stress. The lesions are similar to other herpetic lesions and consist of clusters of vesicles on an erythematous base. Pain described as burning, stinging, and/or itching may precede or follow the rash.

67. What are the most common sites of herpes zoster lesions?

The skin lesions tend to follow a linear pattern along one or several dermatomes, especially in the head, neck, and thoracic regions, but they may occur in any dermatomal distribution. The lesions are unilateral but in rare cases may cross the midline.

68. How is herpes zoster treated?

Most children require no treatment except for supportive measures. Analgesics, topical antipruritics, and antihistamines may help. Immunosuppressed children or children with facial involvement, especially around the eyes, should be treated with parenteral acyclovir. Studies in adults show that oral antiviral agents may prevent postherpetic neuralgia.

69. Are steroids helpful for herpes zoster?

Studies in adults show some benefit from steroids at the onset of the illness, but this benefit has not been shown in infants and children.

70. Contact with zoster will result in which of the following condition(s): (a) chickenpox, (b) zoster, or (c) smallpox?

The answer is (a). Direct contact with lesions can transmit the varicella zoster virus to someone who has never had chickenpox. The person develops varicella rather than zoster.

71. Describe the characteristic rash of scabies.

Typical lesions are papules, vesicles, and burrows that tend to occur in a linear distribution. Most cases are not typical, and diagnosis is frequently not made at the first visit. A high index of suspicion is warranted.

72. What is the distribution of scabies in infants, children, and adults?

INFANTS	CHILDREN	ADULTS
Head/scalp	Trunk	Interdigital webs
Face	Extremities	Axillae
Trunk	Axillae	Genitalia
Palms	Groin	Waist
Soles	Elbows	Wrist/arm flexures, breasts/areolae

73. Describe the signs and symptoms of chronic scabies infection.

Because of itching and scratching, the rash becomes excoriated, crusted, eczematized, and secondarily infected. Norwegian scabies refers to a severe form of crusted scabies in debilitated patients, with hyperkeratotic, highly contagious lesions located mainly on the scalp, ears, elbows, knees, buttocks, and palms and soles.

74. How is scabies infection diagnosed?
Diagnosis is usually clinical (a high index of suspicion should be maintained) but can be confirmed by scraping one of the burrows and viewing the actual mite and her eggs or feces under the microscope.

75. Describe the treatment for scabies.
The treatment of choice for scabies is permethrin 5% cream, which is approved for infants as young as 2 months. In children under 2 years, it should be applied to the entire body, including the head and face, and left on the skin overnight. In older children and adults, it is applied from the neck down. Application of permethrin should be repeated in 1 week. Antihistamines and antipruritics may be helpful. Bedding and clothing should be washed in hot water. Itching may continue for weeks and may be treated with a mild topical steroid.

76. Who else should be treated when a member of the family has scabies?
For best results and eradication of the mite, the entire household should be treated simultaneously.

77. What is cutaneous larva migrans?
Also known as "creeping eruption," cutaneous larva migrans is a rash that results from invasion of the skin and migration by larval parasites, usually of the dog or cat hookworm. It forms a snake-like, winding path with some erythema and edema along the tract. It is usually seen on the feet, lower extremities, buttocks, and hands. Treatment consists of topical and, in rare cases, oral antiparasitic agents.

78. Describe the common skin manifestations of a spider bite and a bee sting.
Skin manifestations vary, depending on the arthropod or insect. They can range from pinpoint macular lesions to large hemorrhagic vesicles with necrosis. Most are pruritic and/or painful. Some arthropods are vectors for systemic diseases. All bites and stings can become secondarily infected with bacteria.

BIBLIOGRAPHY

1. Cohen BA (ed): Pediatric Dermatology, 2nd ed. St. Louis, Mosby, 1999.
2. Cohen BA: Pediatric dermatology: What's your Dx? Contemp Pediatr 18:36–44, 2000.
3. Eichenfield LF, Frieden IJ, Esterly, NB: Textbook of Neonatal Dermatology. Philadelphia, W.B. Saunders, 2001.
4. Hansen RC: Treating fungal infections. Contemp Pediatr Dermatol Update July(Suppl):6–10, 2001.
5. Hurwitz S: Clinical Pediatric Dermatology, 2nd ed. Philadelphia, W.B. Saunders, 1993.
6. Lobato MN, Vugia DJ, Frieden IJ: Tinea capitis in California children: A population-based study of a growing epidemic. Pediatrics 99:551–554, 1997.
7. Mancini AJ: Bacterial skin infections in children: The common and the not so common. Pediatr Ann 29:26–35, 2000.
8. Pickering LK (ed): 2000 Red Book: Report of the Committee on Infectious Diseases, 25th ed. Elk Grove Village, IL, American Academy of Pediatrics, 2000.
9. Roche KJ, Chang MW, Lazarus H: Cutaneous Anthrax infection. N Engl J Med 345:1611, 2001.
10. Weston Wl, Lane AT: Color Textbook of Pediatric Dermatology, 3rd ed. St. Louis, Mosby, 2002.

30. CELLULITIS AND PYOMYOSITIS

Kimberly J. Center, M.D., and Gail L. Rodgers, M.D.

1. Which organisms are commonly associated with cellulitis after skin injury?

The most common organisms associated with cellulitis are group A streptococci (*Streptococcus pyogenes*) and *Staphylococcus aureus*. They usually colonize the skin, and when a break occurs in the skin, they take the opportunity to invade and cause infection.

2. Name the causative agents of impetigo.

Group A streptococci and *S. aureus*.

3. What is bullous impetigo?

Bullous impetigo is usually secondary to a toxin-producing *S. aureus* strain (phage type 2), whereas nonbullous impetigo may be caused by either group A streptococci and *S. aureus* or a combination of the two.

4. List the treatment options for impetigo.

If few lesions are present and there are no underlying complications of cellulitis, topical therapy with mupirocin (Bactroban) can be applied. Numerous lesions, lesions covering extensive areas, and lesions complicated by deeper infection or systemic symptoms should be treated with an oral antibiotic. Agents should be active against group A streptococci and *S. aureus*. Examples include dicloxacillin, amoxicillin-clavulanate, clindamycin, erythromycin, cephalexin, cefuroxime axetil, cefadroxil, and cefprozil. Therapy is usually given for 7–10 days.

5. What are the complications of impetigo?

Complications of impetigo include cellulitis, lymphadenitis, and lymphangitis. Group A streptococcal infection can lead to scarlet fever and poststreptococcal glomerulonephritis.

6. After a dog or cat bite, which other organisms must be considered as causes of cellulitis?

In addition to group A streptococci and *S. aureus*, organisms that inhabit the animal's mouth must be considered. Examples include a wide variety of anaerobes, *Pasteurella multocida*, *Eikenella corrodens*, and *Capnocytophaga canimorsus*.

7. *C. canimorsus* is associated with the bite of which animal: (a) Mighty Mouse, (b) Rin Tin Tin, or (c) the Lion King?

The answer is (b)—a dog bite.

8. Prophylactic therapy is indicated for which animal bites?

Prophylactic therapy is controversial, but most experts agree that it should be given to patients who sustain high-risk wounds such as deep punctures (especially cat bites), injuries requiring surgical repair, and injuries involving the hands and/or face.

9. Name the best antibiotic therapy for prophylaxis and/or treatment of cellulitis after a dog or cat bite.

A penicillin combined with a beta-lactamase inhibitor (amoxicillin-clavulanate, ampicillin-sulbactam, ticarcillin-clavulanate and piperacillin-tazobactam).

10. In patients with penicillin allergy, which is the best antibiotic therapy for cellulitis after a dog or cat bite?

Trimethoprim-sulfamethoxazole and clindamycin, gentamicin and clindamycin, or a third-generation cephalosporin and clindamycin.

11. If cellulitis develops after a shark attack or bite or percutaneous injury from any other aquatic animal, which additional organisms must be considered?

Infections with *Aeromonas hydrophila*, *Plesiomonas shigelloides*, *Pseudomonas* spp., *Streptococcus iniae*, and *Vibrio* spp. have been associated with marine animal bites. The same organisms are associated with injuries in the aquatic environment.

12. List possible empirical antibiotic treatment of injury from aquatic animals.

In view of the diverse pathogens listed above, empirical therapy should include antibiotics active against *Pseudomonas* spp. Possible choices are ceftazidime and metronidazole or ciprofloxacin and metronidazole or a carbapenem (imipenem or meropenem). Antibiotic therapy should be tailored to the in vitro susceptibilities of organisms isolated from the wound.

13. An adolescent presents 12 hours after a fight at a local bar. He punched his adversary in the mouth and presents with swelling and erythema of the dorsum of his hand and tenderness over the third metacarpophalangeal joint. Movement of the finger is extremely painful. What are the most common complications associated with this type of injury?

Bone fractures, osteomyelitis, cellulitis, and tenosynovitis.

14. List the most common organisms associated with clenched-fist injuries.

Human mouth flora usually include streptococci, *S. aureus*, *E. corrodens*, and oral anaerobes, among others.

15. List empirical antibiotic choices for clenched-fist injuries.

A penicillin should be combined with a beta-lactamase inhibitor (amoxicillin-clavulanate, ampicillin-sulbactam). Clindamycin alone is not recommended because *E. corrodens* is universally resistant.

16. What is the most common organism responsible for soft tissue infections associated with leech therapy?

Aeromonas hydrophila.

17. A child whose symptoms of chickenpox are improving develops a high fever on day 5 of the illness. Some of her lesions are surrounded by erythema. What is the appropriate next step in diagnosis?

Obtain a culture of the lesion. The most common complication is skin superinfection with group A streptococci and/or *S. aureus*.

18. What initial antibiotic therapy is appropriate?

Antibiotics with activity against group A streptococci and *S. aureus* should be started. Examples include dicloxacillin, amoxicillin-clavulanate, clindamycin, erythromycin, cephalexin, cefuroxime axetil, cefadroxil, and cefprozil.

19. After a case of chickenpox a child develops high fever, systemic toxicity, and pain and edema of her left leg. The thigh area is mildly erythematous and exquisitely tender. She has full range of motion of the joints, and a magnetic resonance scan shows no indications of osteomyelitis. What are the possible diagnoses?

The diagnostic possibilities include cellulitis, pyomyositis, and necrotizing fasciitis. The clinical scenario of pain out of proportion to exam findings in a patient who is toxic-appearing make necrotizing fasciitis more likely.

20. What initial antibiotic therapy is appropriate?

Antibiotic therapy should be initiated after blood cultures are obtained. Antibiotics are aimed at group A streptococci and *S. aureus*. Usually nafcillin or oxacillin is used in combination with clindamycin. Clindamycin is added for the Eagle effect.

21. What is the Eagle effect?

Even though the authors are from Philadelphia, the answer has nothing to do with football. In experimental models of necrotizing fasciitis, the density of organisms is quite high, and often the organisms exhibit a stationary phase of growth in which beta-lactam agents are not effective because they act by inhibiting cell wall synthesis. Clindamycin may be effective because it inhibits protein synthesis, thus not requiring formation of cell wall for activity. This phenomenon is known as the Eagle effect. Thus, in experimental animal models, beta-lactam therapy alone resulted in increased mortality compared with clindamycin in addition to the Eagle effect. Clindamycin is theorized to inhibit toxins produced by the organisms. In areas with increasing prevalence of community-acquired methicillin resistant *S. aureus* (MRSA), most cases are susceptible to clindamycin.

22. What are the additional therapeutic options?

In addition to appropriate antibiotics, an essential part of treatment for necrotizing fasciitis is surgical evaluation for possible debridement.

23. A 3-week-old infant develops an abscess at the site of a scalp electrode. He is well-appearing but febrile. What are the likely causative agents?

A wide range of possible organisms may be responsible for scalp abscesses associated with scalp electrodes. Examples include group B streptococci, *S. aureus*, enteric gram-negative bacilli, *Neisseria gonorrhoeae*, and herpes simplex virus.

24. What diagnostic tests should be performed on this infant?

Most experts agree that a febrile 3-week-old infant with a focal infection should have a full evaluation for sepsis, including cultures of blood, urine, spinal fluid, and wound. In infections associated with scalp electrodes, special attention should be focused on testing for herpes simplex virus. Testing includes culturing of the mucosal sites, wound, and cerebrospinal fluid for virus as well as PCR of cerebrospinal fluid.

25. What antibiotics are appropriate for initial therapy?

Empirical therapy may include nafcillin and ceftriaxone. Addition of acyclovir should be considered.

26. Explain the differences between hospital- and community-acquired methicillin-resistant *S. aureus*.

One of the major differences between the two is that community-acquired MRSA usually causes soft tissue, bone, and joint infections in pediatric patients, whereas hospital-acquired MRSA classically is associated with bloodstream infections. Most community-acquired isolates are susceptible to clindamycin, whereas hospital strains usually are not. For serious infections with MRSA, consult an infectious disease expert.

27. What are the therapeutic options for community-acquired methicillin-resistant *S. aureus*?

Clindamycin, vancomycin, and linezolid.

28. List the differential diagnosis for necrotic purple lesions.

S. aureus and group A streptococci rarely cause purple discoloration of lesions. Necrotic purple lesions are often associated with *Pseudomonas aeruginosa* and enteric gram-negative bacilli, *Bacillus anthracis*, *Chromobacterium violaceum*, *Vibrio* spp., invasive fungi such as *Aspergillus* or *Mucor* spp., and nontuberculous mycobacteria.

29. What underlying conditions may predispose to ecthyma gangrenosum?

Ecthyma gangrenosum is a necrotic ulcer covered with a gray-black eschar. It is generally a sign of disseminated *P. aeruginosa* infection in immunocompromised patients.

30. What is a characteristic, distinguishing feature of the cutaneous lesions caused by *B. anthracis* (anthrax)?

Remember the three Ps: papule, purple, and painless.

31. A child with leukemia has a tunneled, totally implantable subcutaneous port for chemotherapy. He develops a tunnel infection with fever and cellulitis of the area. What organisms should be considered as the cause of the infection?

Virtually any organism can be a pathogen for device-associated bloodstream infections. Pathogens more likely to be associated with overlying cellulitis are *S. aureus*, gram negative bacilli, and fungi. Coagulase-negative staphylococci are more commonly associated with bloodstream infections without cellulitis.

32. List possible antibiotic choices for this patient.

Antibiotic choices should be based on prior knowledge of colonizing organisms in the patient and in the particular hospital/unit as well as severity of infection. Empirical therapy should be broad and include coverage for *S. aureus* and gram-negative bacilli.

33. Should the catheter be removed?

Although some studies have shown a lower risk of infection with totally implantable intravenous devices compared with tunneled or untunneled central catheters, when totally implantable devices become infected, the infection is usually more difficult to cure. Removal of the device is often necessary for cure.

34. A patient presents with fever, lower abdominal pain, and hip pain. Evaluation of bones, joints, and abdomen rules out infection in these areas. What other entity is possible?

Infection of the abdominal and pelvic muscles (psoas, obturator, and gluteal muscles).

35. What are the causative agents of pyomyositis?

The most common agents are *S. aureus* and group A streptococci. Gram-negative bacilli and anaerobes can be found with associated abdominal pathology.

36. What is the best imaging study to diagnose pyomyositis?

Magnetic resonance imaging (MRI).

37. What is the appropriate antibiotic therapy for pyomyositis?

Empirical therapy usually consists of an antistaphylococcal antibiotic such as nafcillin. An attempt should be made to make a microbiologic diagnosis by culture of blood (infrequently positive) or, if possible, aspiration of the involved area. Aspiration is usually difficult because of the unsuitable location.

38. What organisms are associated with toxic shock syndrome?

S. aureus and group A streptococci.

39. Describe the manifestations of toxic shock syndrome.

Toxic shock syndrome is caused by infection or colonization with strains of *S. aureus* and group A streptococci that produce toxins. The clinical manifestations include various mucocutaneous findings as well as shock with multisystem organ involvement. Common findings include conjunctival hyperemia without exudate, strawberry tongue, erythema of the oral mucus membranes and pharynx, and a rash. The rash associated with *S. aureus* is usually erythroderma. A scarlatiniform rash is often seen with group A streptococci.

40. What empirical antibiotic therapy should be initiated for toxic shock syndrome?

Typically a combination of nafcillin and clindamycin is used. In areas with high prevalence of methicillin-resistant *S. aureus*, vancomycin may be substituted for nafcillin. Clindamycin is added for theoretical reasons related to the Eagle effect (see question 21). Experts advise the use of intravenous gammaglobulin for patients with toxic shock based on anecdotal benefit and case reports; to date, no randomized controlled trials have been performed.

41. A patient has sustained a 20% partial-thickness scald burn. The burn is dressed, but the surgeons report that it is healing well. The patient is febrile, and *S. aureus* is cultured from the surface of the burn. Which of the following is the appropriate next step: (a) surgical debridement, (b) observation only, (c) antistaphylococcal therapy, or (d) steroid therapy?

The answer is (b).

42. How is an infected burn wound diagnosed?

Burn patients are often colonized with pathogens, and the fact that fever and leukocytosis are associated with burn injury makes it difficult to diagnose infections. The diagnosis of burn wound infection is made clinically. A biopsy should be performed for any wound that is not healing well or is associated with surrounding erythema or cellulitis, purulent discharge, or progression from a partial-thickness to full-thickness burn. A biopsy showing invasion of the organism into viable underlying tissue and/or $\geq 10^5$ organisms per gram of tissue is diagnostic for infection.

Case scenario: A previously healthy 10-year-old girl presents with a 3-week history of fevers up to 105°C and skin lesions. She has had no unusual travel or pet exposures. On examination she is not toxic-appearing. Lesions are large erythematous rings with a blue-gray central discoloration and surrounding edema. They are tender. Complete blood count with manual differential is normal. Blood cultures yield no growth. During this time, she has been treated for presumptive Lyme disease without improvement.

43. What is the next diagnostic step?

Lesion biopsy.

44. What is the likely diagnosis?

Sweet's syndrome, also known as acute febrile neutrophilic dermatosis, which is an uncommon, recurrent, dramatic skin disease characterized by painful plaque-forming inflammatory papules associated with fever. The cause of Sweet's syndrome is unknown, although it is thought to represent hypersensitivity to an unknown antigen.

45. What therapy is indicated?

Systemic corticosteroids.

46. A 2-year-old boy presents with high fevers for 4 weeks. He has developed two nodular lesions with surrounding edema and erythema on his fingers. On physical examination he is ill-appearing, and the lesions are tender. What are the next steps that should be performed for diagnosis?

Cultures of blood and lesion biopsy should be performed. Echocardiography of the heart to rule out endocarditis should be considered in view of the history and peripheral skin nodules.

47. *Burkholderia cepacia* is isolated from the lesions and blood. Which of the following immunodeficiencies is associated with this infection: (a) agammaglobulinemia, (b) HIV infection, (c) chronic granulomatous disease, or (d) Wiskott-Aldrich syndrome?

The answer is (c).

BIBLIOGRAPHY

1. Aebi C, Ahmed A Ramilo O: Bacterial complications of primary varicella in children. Clin Infect Dis 23:698–705, 1996.

2. Darmstadt GL: Subcutaneous tissue infections and abscesses. In Long SS, Prober CG, Pickering LK (eds): Principles and Practice of Pediatric Infectious Diseases. New York, Churchill Livingstone, 1997, pp 507–517.
3. Fleisher GR: The management of bite wounds. N Engl J Med 340:138–140, 1999.
4. Gubbay AJ, Isaacs D: Pyomyositis in children. Pediatr Infect Dis J 19:1009–1013, 2000.
5. Nizet VF: Myositis and pyomyositis. In Long SS, Prober CG, Pickering LK (eds): Principles and Practice of Pediatric Infectious Diseases. New York, Churchill Livingstone, 1997, pp 517–523.
6. Resnick SD: Toxic shock syndrome: Recent developments in pathogenesis. J Pediatr 116:321–327, 1990.
7. Talan DA, Citron DM, Abrahamian FM, et al: Bacteriologic analysis of infected dog and cat bites. N Engl J Med 340:85–92, 1999.
8. Viani RM, Bromberg K, Bradley JS: Obturator internus muscle abscess in children: Report of seven cases and review. Clin Infecct Dis 17:117–122, 1999.
9. Vugia DJ, Peterson CL, Meyers HB, et al: Invasive group A streptococcal infections in children with varicella in Southern California. Pediatr Infect Dis J 15:146–150, 1996.

X. Skeletal Infections

31. INFECTIOUS ARTHRITIS

Nizar F. Maraqa, M.D., and Ana M. Alvarez, M.D.

1. Which of the following represents the most common mechanism for developing infectious arthritis in childhood: direct organism inoculation, contiguous extension from an adjacent site of infection, hematogenous dissemination, overgrowth of skin flora, or none of the above?

In children, hematogenous dissemination is the most common mechanism for developing arthritis. The other listed mechanisms occur less frequently and in specific situations.

2. What is the most common infecting agent causing septic arthritis in patients of all ages?
Staphylococcus aureus.

3. Name the second and third most common infecting agents in children after the neonatal period.
Group A streptococci and *Streptococcus pneumoniae*.

4. Which joint is most commonly affected by infectious arthritis?
The knee joint is involved in 45% of cases of childhood septic arthritis. Other commonly involved joints include the hip (25%), ankle (13%), elbow (10%), and shoulder (5%). Approximately 2–5% of cases have multiple joint involvement.

5. An ill-appearing, febrile, 2-year-old boy lies supine in bed with his leg flexed, abducted, and externally rotated. Which diagnosis should be considered?
Septic arthritis should be ruled out before proceeding to other diagnoses (see question 10).

6. A 16-year-old girl presents with history of fever, shaking chills, transient skin rash, and sore throat a few days after the onset of menses. She has swelling and redness of both knee joints. What is the most likely causative organism?
Neisseria gonorrhoeae. This clinical scenario is typical of gonococcal arthritis. The blood culture is frequently positive, whereas synovial fluid cultures are rarely positive. The organism usually can be isolated from nasopharyngeal, rectal, and urethral/cervical cultures. Another form of gonococcal infection is a monoarticular suppurative arthritis, in which the organism is usually isolated from the joint aspirate. Gonococcal infections, especially when recurrent, should alert the physician to the possibility of an underlying deficiency of the complement immune system.

7. Match the following infectious etiologies in column A with the proper epidemiologic situation in column B:

A	B
1. Gram-negative bacilli arthritis	a. Sternoclavicular arthritis in heroin addicts
2. *Staphylococcus aureus* arthritis	b. Occurs 2 weeks after an upper respiratory infection in a 1-year-old child with delayed immunizations

(Continued. on next page.)

A	B
3. *Streptobacillus moniliformis* arthritis	c. Follows a tick bite
4. Lyme arthritis	d. Follows a rat bite
5. *Haemophilus influenzae* type B arthritis	e. Occurs adjacent to skin or soft tissue infection
6. *Pseudomonas aeruginosa* arthritis	f. Chronic monoarticular granulomatous arthritis
7. Brucella arthritis	g. Follows instrumentation of urinary or gastrointestinal tract

Answers: 1, g; 2, e; 3, d; 4, c; 5, b; 6, a; 7, f.

8. Formulate a differential diagnosis for hip pain in children.
- Septic arthritis of the hip
- Legg-Calvé-Perthes disease
- Slipped capital femoral epiphysis
- Fracture
- Toxic tenosynovitis
- Pelvic osteomyelitis
- Pyomyositis of pelvic muscles

9. What are the nonbacterial causes of infectious arthritis?
Viruses (e.g., varicella-zoster virus, rubella, parvovirus), mycobacteria, and fungal organisms can cause infectious arthritis but are far less common than bacteria in children.

10. List the differential diagnoses for infectious septic arthritis in children.
- Toxic synovitis
- Epiphyseal osteomyelitis
- Infective endocarditis
- Villonodular arthritis
- Leukemia and other malignancies
- Serum sickness
- Hemophilia
- Bursitis
- Osteochondritis
- Collagen vascular diseases
- Ulcerative colitis
- Henoch-Schönlein purpura
- Legg-Calve-Perthes disease
- Slipped capital femoral epiphysis
- Metabolic diseases (e.g., gout, ochronosis)

11. What laboratory tests are usually considered in cases of suspected septic arthritis?
A few tests can prove helpful in the etiologic diagnosis and management of septic arthritis: complete blood count and differential, erythrocyte sedimentation rate and C-reactive protein, and (before administration of antibiotics) blood culture and histochemical analysis and culture of joint aspirate. Accessory cultures (e.g., overlying wounds, cellulitis, infected skin lesions) or urethral/cervical cultures (gonorrhea in adolescents) may be helpful in the appropriate clinical situation.

12. For what should joint fluid aspirate be routinely tested?
Joint fluid should be tested routinely with Gram stain and aerobic/anaerobic cultures, leukocyte count and differential, glucose concentration (compared with concomitant blood glucose), ability to clot spontaneously, and mucin clot test. In specific situations, the fluid also should be tested for acid-fast stain and culture, fungal stain and culture, and uric acid crystals.

13. What is the average sensitivity of bacterial (aerobic and anaerobic) cultures of joint fluid in children with septic arthritis?
Most references agree that joint fluid cultures have a sensitivity of approximately 30% in children with septic arthritis. The sensitivity is low because the synovial fluid exerts a bacteriostatic effect.

14. How often is the blood culture positive in children with septic arthritis?

On average, blood cultures acquired before administration of antibiotics is positive in about one-third of all cases of septic arthritis in childhood.

15. How should joint fluid be collected for diagnostic studies?

Joint fluid should be collected in a heparinized syringe with an 18- to 20-gauge needle so that the large clot that forms does not preclude the enumeration of leukocytes. Fluid aspiration of the knee (the most commonly involved joint) can be performed by primary care physicians; however, aspiration of shoulder and hip joints should be performed by an experienced specialist (orthopedist or radiologist).

16. Describe the mucin clot test.

Glacial acetic acid is added to the joint aspirate while stirring; normal fluid reacts by forming a white precipitate that clings to the stirring rod with a clear supernatant. Refer to the next question for description of the mucin clot test in different causes of arthritis.

17. Compare the findings of joint fluid analysis in childhood arthritides.

	SEPTIC ARTHRITIS	RHEUMATIC FEVER ARTHRITIS	JUVENILE RHEUMATOID ARTHRITIS
Spontaneous clot	Large and rapid	Small to absent	Large
Mucin clot appearance	Curdled, milk-like	Tight, rope-like	Small, friable mass
Mean white blood cells mm (%PMN)	> 50,000	18,000	15,000
Glucose (joint fluid/ blood × 100%)	30%	75%	75%

Note: Do not be fooled. The joint fluid white blood cell count in Lyme arthritis, although typically high, can mimic the joint fluid from patients with juvenile rheumatoid arthritis.

18. What is toxic synovitis? How is it differentiated from septic arthritis?

Also referred to as irritable hip, reactive synovitis, and transient synovitis, toxic synovitis is a condition frequently seen in childhood. Patients are usually afebrile and have a minimally elevated or normal erythrocyte sedimentation rate (ESR). Prognosis is excellent, because the condition is self-limiting. The presence of fever, white blood cell count > 12,000 cells/µl, and ESR > 40 mm/hr best differentiate septic arthritis from toxic synovitis.

19. What is reactive arthritis?

It is a postinfectious joint inflammation, perhaps as a result of similarities between bacterial antigens and human proteins. It can follow a variety of infections, particularly those caused by *Chlamydia trachomatis* and *Shigella*, *Salmonella*, *Campylobacter*, and *Yersinia* species. The onset is usually a few days to several weeks after a transient mild episode of diarrhea. ESR is usually mildly elevated. Analysis of joint fluid helps differentiate reactive arthritis from septic arthritis. Spontaneous resolution is the rule within 7–10 days, regardless of therapy.

20. Name a few organisms that can cause either infectious or reactive arthritis.

Group A streptococci, *Neisseria gonorrhoeae*, and *Neisseria meningitides*.

21. List the possible empiric antibiotic therapy for childhood septic arthritis.

The choice of empiric agent should be based on efficacy against the most likely organisms as well as safety and cost. A semisynthetic penicillin (nafcillin or oxacillin) and a third-generation cephalosporin are recommended. Alternatively, cefuroxime may be used as single empiric therapy. A more specific therapy should be used as soon as an etiologic agent is identified. The following table illustrates the choice of initial antibiotic therapy for childhood septic arthritis.

		MOST COMMON ORGANISMS	INITIAL ANTIBIOTIC THERAPY
Neonate	Without meningitis	S. aureus, group B strepto-cocci (GBS), bacilli (GNB)	Oxacillin + gentamicin
	With meningitis	S. aureus, GBS, GNB	Oxacillin + 3rd generation cephalosporin
Children	Immunized	S. aureus	Semisynthetic penicillin
	Nonimmunized	S. aureus + H. influenzae	Cefuroxime
Adolescent		N. gonorrhoeae	Third generation cephalosporin

22. What is the recommended duration of therapy for uncomplicated childhood septic arthritis?

A minimum of 3 weeks and an average of 4 weeks of antibiotic therapy are accepted as sufficient duration of therapy. Shorter courses have been associated with clinical failure. In general, septic arthritis caused by S. aureus or Enterobacteriaceae is treated longer than that caused by *Haemophilus influenzae* type B or meningococci.

23. What follow-up is required in children with septic arthritis?

Follow-up should include serial weekly clinical examinations and measurement of acute phase reactants (ESR and C-reactive protein) until values are within normal limits. In addition, a radiograph at or near the end of therapy is performed to evaluate for the presence of osteomyelitis. If osteomyelitis changes are demonstrated, the duration of antibiotic therapy is extended.

24. When is surgical drainage of septic arthritis considered an emergency?

In all children with septic arthritis of the hip or shoulder joints, early surgical drainage can prevent bony destruction. The sun should never set on a septic hip.

25. What characteristics of the shoulder and hip make septic arthritis a surgical emergency?

The heads of the humerus and femur lie inside the joint capsule of both of these joints.

26. What factors are associated with poor outcome in childhood infectious arthritis?

• Prolonged duration of symptoms before initiation of therapy (typically more than 10–14 days)
• Infants younger than 1 year of age
• Infections caused by S. aureus or Enterobacteriaceae are associated with more sequelae than those caused by *H. influenzae*
• Persistently positive joint fluid culture after 7 days of appropriate therapy

27. What is the FABER maneuver?

It is a maneuver that elicits pain during **f**lexion, **ab**duction, and **e**xternal **r**otation of the hip joint. It is useful for the detection of pyogenic sacroiliitis, a condition that occurs without the classical external signs of redness, warmth, and swelling associated with typical infectious arthritis of other sites.

28. Which is the radiographic method of choice for diagnosing pyogenic sacroiliitis?

Computed tomography is more useful than plain radiography for delineation of changes of infectious arthritis affecting the sacroiliac joints.

29. Describe the characteristics of tuberculous septic arthritis.

Mycobacterium tuberculosis is a rare cause of septic arthritis in childhood. It occurs in 1–6% of tuberculosis infections. The joints most commonly involved are the knee and hip. The onset is insidious, and the course is chronic. The Mantoux skin test is usually positive. Synovial fluid analysis typically reveals white blood cell counts of 10–20 thousand cells/ml with predominance of neutrophils. Mycobacteria can be cultured from the synovial fluid in 75% of cases and from synovial biopsy in 90%.

30. What is Phemister's triad?

The triad of radiographic findings in mycobacterial infection of the joint: minimal joint space narrowing, marginal erosions, and extensive demineralization.

31. What is Pott's disease?

Pott's disease (tuberculous spondylitis) was first described by Percival Pott in 1779. It is characterized by paraplegia with an accompanying kyphotic deformity of the spine.

32. What is Poncet's disease?

This poorly understood polyarthritis accompanies tuberculosis infection without evidence of mycobacteria in the involved joints. It seems to respond well to anti-inflammatory and antituberculous medications.

33. Describe the course of parvovirus B19 arthritis in children. How is it different in adults?

In children, parvovirus B19 arthritis usually occurs 1–2 days after the onset of rash and involves multiple joints in an asymmetric fashion. In adults, by contrast, joint involvement is symmetrical. The arthritis is thought to be mediated by formation of immune complexes. It lasts 1–2 months and is self-limiting. A few patients may develop chronic persistent infection.

34. When does arthritis occur in relation to jaundice in hepatitis B infection?

Hepatitis B infection can be associated with arthritis that symmetrically affects multiple small joints of the hands. It usually precedes the onset of jaundice by 1 week.

35. Describe the arthritis associated with rubella virus infection.

Arthritis following rubella infection is less common in children than adults. It usually follows the rash and involves the small joints of the hand. It lasts several days and resolves without sequelae. The joint fluid has predominantly mononuclear cells. Another form of arthritis related to rubella occurs in 25% of young females 1-3 weeks after vaccination. This form is also self-limited.

BIBLIOGRAPHY

1. Dagan R: Management of acute hematogenous osteomyelitis and septic arthritis in the pediatric patient. Pediatr Infect Dis J 12:88–92, 1993.
2. Kocher MS, Zurakowski D, Kasser JR: Differentiating between septic arthritis and transient synovitis of the hip in children: An evidence-based clinical prediction algorithm. J Bone Joint Surg 81A:1662–1670, 1999.
3. Krogstad P, Smith A: Osteomyelitis and septic arthritis. In Feigin RD, Cherry JD (eds): Textbook of Pediatric Infectious Diseases, 4th ed. Philadelphia, W.B. Saunders, 1998, pp 698–704.
4. Shetty AK, Gedalia A: Septic arthritis in children. Rheum Dis Clin North Am 24:287–304, 1998.
5. Smith J, Hasan M: Infectious arthritis. In Mandell GL, Bennett JE, Dolin R (eds): Principles and Practice of Infectious Diseases, 5th ed. New York, Churchill Livingstone, 2000, pp 1175–1182.
6. Welkon CJ, Long SS, Fisher MC: Pyogenic arthritis in infants and children: A review of 95 cases. Pediatr Infect Dis 5:669–676, 1986.

32. OSTEOMYELITIS

Nizar F. Maraqa, M.D., and Ana M. Alvarez, M.D.

1. What is osteomyelitis?

In simplistic terms, osteomyelitis is inflammation of the bone. The clinical disease is an infectious process that eventually leads to microscopic bone death. The infection is most commonly bacterial; however, viruses, rickettsiae, mycobacteria, and fungi also may cause osteomyelitis.

2. How is acute osteomyelitis different from chronic osteomyelitis?

Clinically, osteomyelitis is classified as either acute or chronic based on the presumptive duration of infection at the time of presentation. It is generally agreed that osteomyelitis is chronic if symptoms have been present for more than 2 weeks at presentation.

3. Describe the age and gender distribution of osteomyelitis.

Osteomyelitis occurs more commonly in children than adults. In fact, more than half the cases of osteomyelitis occur in children less than 5 years of age. Osteomyelitis at all ages occurs more commonly in males, possibly because of their increased tendency for outdoor activity and trauma.

4. What is the most common mechanism by which microorganisms cause osteomyelitis in children?

The most common mode by which microorganisms reach the bone in children is hematogenous inoculation after bacteremia. Other mechanisms less commonly seen in healthy children include spread from a contiguous site of infection and direct inoculation from trauma or surgery.

5. What is the presumed sequence of events in acute hematogenous osteomyelitis of the long bones?

1. Thrombosis of the slow-flowing, sinusoidal metaphyseal vessels as a result of trauma or embolization
2. Inoculation of affected area from transient bacteremia
3. Proliferation of microorganisms and formation of an inflammatory exudate under pressure
4. Focal bone necrosis
5. Spread of infection to subperiosteal area after traversing the cortex

6. Which organisms are the most common causes of osteomyelitis in childhood?

Staphylococcus aureus is by far the most common agent, followed by group A streptococci and *Streptococcus pneumoniae*. Gram-negative organisms occur less frequently. *Salmonella* species are encountered in children with hemoglobinopathies who develop osteomyelitis. *Kingella kingae* (an upper respiratory tract commensal) has increasingly been isolated from osteoarticular infections in children. (Hold cultures for 7 days for optimal isolation of this organism). *Haemophilus influenzae* type B is rarely seen since the introduction of the vaccine. *Pseudomonas* species may be seen in cases of vertebral or pelvic osteomyelitis, especially in intravenous drug users. Anaerobes are uncommon causes of acute hematogenous osteomyelitis. However, they may be encountered as a result of spread from a contiguous site of infection or in cases of chronic osteomyelitis. Fungi, as causes of osteomyelitis, are seen almost exclusively in immunocompromised hosts.

7. Why is *S. aureus* well suited to cause osteomyelitis?

S. aureus has the ability to adhere to type 1 collagen of bone fibrils. It then proliferates, giving rise to microcolonies surrounded by a protective glycocalyx that allows the bacteria to escape host defenses.

8. **When do you expect to see polymicrobial osteomyelitis?**

Cases of subacute or chronic osteomyelitis may be polymicrobial. Acute osteomyelitis, on the other hand, is rarely polymicrobial except in certain clinical situations such as the spread of infection from contiguous infectious foci or the presence of vascular insufficiency or peripheral neuropathy (e.g., spina bifida) adjacent to the site of osteomyelitis. Staphylococci and streptococci remain the most common isolates. However, gram-negative rods are also frequently encountered.

9. **Describe the clinical signs and symptoms of childhood osteomyelitis.**

Variable constitutional symptoms may occur in children with osteomyelitis. They usually precede the onset of focal signs of bone pain, swelling, redness, focal point tenderness over the affected bone, and limited function. The clinical picture, however, may vary with the child's age (refer to following questions for more details about age-specific findings).

10. **Describe the clinical picture of osteomyelitis in neonates.**

Constitutional symptoms in neonates with osteomyelitis is are usually nonspecific. Fever occurs in only 30–50% of cases, and irritability may be present. As the infection progresses, it frequently manifests as pseudoparalysis of the affected limb. (*Note:* Syphilis also may cause pseudoparalysis.)

In contrast to older patients, osteomyelitis in neonates may affect multiple bones.

11. **Why is osteomyelitis in neonates different from osteomyelitis in older children and adolescents?**

The unique bone anatomy and structure (i.e., thin cortex and loose periosteum) in neonates allows the spread of infection outside the bone to surrounding muscle and subcutaneous tissues. The result is a widespread area of swelling and redness. In older infants and children, however, the periosteum is thick, limiting the spread of infection and producing highly focal signs. In addition, the vascular anatomy of the immature growth plate in neonates allows the infection to perforate into the adjacent joint cavity, causing a concomitant septic arthritis in 50–70% of cases.

12. **Which organisms most commonly cause osteomyelitis in neonates?**

S. aureus remains the most common cause. Gram-negative organisms account for a minority of cases, whereas *Streptococcus agalactiae* (group B streptococci [GBS]) is isolated at older ages (2–4 weeks) and usually affects a single bone. (Not to be funny, but think about GBS in osteomyelitis of the proximal humerus in newborns). Recently some centers in the United States have reported more cases of osteomyelitis in neonates caused by *S. agalactiae* than by *S. aureus*.

Premature infants, especially those with a long stay in the neonatal intensive care unit, very low birth weight, and exposure to broad-spectrum antibiotics, are at risk of osteomyelitis caused by *Candida* spp. in addition to the usual bacterial causes.

13. **What should be considered in the differential diagnosis of pseudoparalysis in the newborn?**

In addition to osteoarticular infections, pseudoparalysis may be seen in neurologic disease (e.g., polio), cerebral hemorrhage, trauma, child abuse, and scurvy.

14. **What special circumstances in neonates are associated with osteomyelitis?**

1. Osteomyelitis of the skull can be seen in newborns that have an infected cephalohematoma after delivery.

2. Osteomyelitis of the calcaneus may be seen after heel puncture in newborns, a procedure commonly done in place of venipuncture.

3. Osteitis involving the long bones can be a manifestation of syphilis infection in newborns. For this reason, plain radiographs of the skeleton are an integral part of the recommended work-up for newborns suspected to have congenital syphilis.

4. Maxillary osteomyelitis of the newborn has been described in the literature. It is by no means restricted to the newborns but can be seen throughout infancy and, to lesser extent, childhood. If not managed properly, the condition may be complicated by orbital cellulitis or brain abscess. Management includes antibiotics as well as surgical drainage, curettage, and sequestrectomy.

15. What are the focal signs of osteomyelitis in children and adolescents?

Osteomyelitis is characteristically a focal disease in children and adolescents. Point tenderness is found over the affected bone; tenderness also can be elicited at the site of infection by percussion of the affected long bone away from the area of maximal point tenderness. Patients may have a limp or restriction in mobility or function. Rarely, older children may present with signs of deep venous thrombophlebitis. A draining sinus or bony deformity is rare in acute disease and suggests subacute or chronic infection.

16. What bones are most commonly affected in acute childhood osteomyelitis?

Acute hematogenous osteomyelitis typically occurs in the tubular long bones of the extremities. The lower extremity is more commonly affected than the upper extremity.

17. What are nontubular bones? How commonly are they affected by osteomyelitis?

Nontubular bones include cuboidal bones (calcaneus, patella, tarsals, and phalanges), irregular bones (ilium, pubis, and ischium) and flat bones (ribs, skull, sternum, and scapulae). Nontubular bones are involved in less than 20% of cases of osteomyelitis. The calcaneus is most commonly affected.

18. Describe the characteristics of pelvic osteomyelitis.

Pelvic osteomyelitis typically involves the ischium and is caused most commonly by *S. aureus*. The diagnosis is difficult to establish. Patients may present with hip pain, abnormal gait, or pain and tenderness in the buttocks or sciatic notch. Local pain may be elicited by compressing the pelvis. The disease is more commonly seen in patients with inflammatory bowel disease. Antibiotic therapy alone may be sufficient; however, surgery is indicated in patients who do not respond to antibiotics. The prognosis is generally good.

19. What is peculiar about osteomyelitis in children with hemoglobinopathies (e.g., sickle cell disease)?

Osteomyelitis occurs with greatest frequency in children 18–24 months of age and has the propensity to affect multiple bones. It is caused most commonly by *Salmonella* spp., followed by staphylococci as well as other gram-negative bacilli (e.g., *Escherichia coli*, *Shigella* or *Serratia* spp.). In some series, *S. aureus* is more common in this setting than *Salmonella* spp. It appears that the relative frequency of *Salmonella* spp. has been decreasing compared with *S. aureus* in the past few decades. Both organisms are important considerations in this clinical setting.

20. How do you differentiate bone infarction from acute osteomyelitis in children with hemoglobinopathy?

It is difficult to differentiate osteomyelitis from bone infarction in children with hemoglobinopathies. Children with infarction usually have a history of multiple episodes of dactylitis and bone infarcts as well as a temperature of 39°C. Patients with osteomyelitis usually lack this history and have mild leukocytosis with immature neutrophils. In addition, radionuclide scans (e.g., gallium 67 or bone marrow scan with technetium sulfur colloid) may show increased uptake more frequently with infection than with infarction.

21. What is a Brodie abscess?

A Brodie abscess is a subacute or chronic form of osteomyelitis that results in the formation of intraosseous abscesses. The distal end of the tibia is most frequently involved. Patients are typically adolescents who have long bone pain and tenderness, a radiographic bony defect, and a normal erythrocyte sedimentation rate (ESR). Surgical debridement and culture-directed antibiotic therapy are often curative.

22. Define epiphyseal osteomyelitis.

Epiphyseal osteomyelitis is a rare form of hematogenous osteomyelitis of the epiphysis of tubular bones in children less than 15–18 months of age. It occurs before the disappearance of the transphyseal blood vessels that carry the organism to the epiphysis, causing an infection similar to that of the metaphysis. The presentation may be acute, resembling septic arthritis, or subacute, with indolent pain or limp.

23. List a differential diagnosis for osteomyelitis.

The differential diagnosis is broad. It includes but is not restricted to septicemia, septic arthritis, toxic synovitis, cellulitis, thrombophlebitis, bone infarction (hemoglobinopathies or Gaucher disease), benign or malignant tumors (e.g., Ewing sarcoma, osteosarcoma, neuroblastoma), leukemia or lymphoma, eosinophilic granuloma, histiocytosis X, rheumatic fever, polyarteritis nodosa, reflex neurovascular dystrophy, trauma (e.g., fracture) and child abuse.

24. Which laboratory tests may be useful in the diagnosis of osteomyelitis?

The definitive diagnosis of osteomyelitis is made by isolation of an organism from bone or from structures contiguous to the bone. These cultures are usually acquired by invasive methods (e.g., bone aspiration or biopsy) and are positive in 65-85% of cases.

Blood culture acquired before initiation of antibiotic therapy may be helpful in identifying the causative organism. The yield is variable and ranges between 20% and 70%.

Approximately one-half of patients have leukocytosis (> 15,000 cells/μl), and the majority have elevated acute phase reactants (e.g., ESR and C-reactive protein).

25. Name radiographic studies that may be helpful in the diagnosis of osteomyelitis in children and adolescents.

Radionuclide imaging (bone scan) is a highly useful modality in the diagnosis of osteomyelitis early in the disease process; however, it is less specific than other imaging modalities such as **magnetic resonance imaging** (MRI). MRI is especially useful in making the diagnosis and delineating the anatomy of the involved part of the skeleton. Although **plain radiographs** may show evidence of osteomyelitis, they are usually normal in the early stages of the disease and thus may not be as useful in making the diagnosis of acute osteomyelitis.

26. In which clinical situation is plain radiography of more benefit in the diagnosis of osteomyelitis than a radionuclide scan?

Plain radiography may be more useful in diagnosis of osteomyelitis in neonates because the ossification of bones is less than in older children, allowing earlier detection of osteomyelitis changes.

27. Match the radiographic finding (column A) with the typical time at which it appears after the onset of acute hematogenous osteomyelitis (column B).

A	B
1. Obliteration of interposed translucent fat planes	a. 3 days
2. Bone destruction and new periosteal bone formation	b. 3–7 days
3. Soft tissue swelling in the region of the metaphysis	c. 10–21 days

Answers: 1, b; 2, c; 3, a.

28. What is considered appropriate empiric antibiotic therapy for acute osteomyelitis?

A semisynthetic penicillinase-resistant penicillin (e.g., nafcillin) or cephalosporin may be used as initial empirical therapy targeting *S. aureus* or group A streptococci. However, when the patient is younger than 4 years, especially if immunizations have not been adequate, empiric therapy should provide coverage for *Haemophilus influenzae*. When treating neonatal osteomyelitis, consider a combination of nafcillin and an aminoglycoside or a third-generation cephalosporin to provide coverage for Enterobacteriaceae in addition to group B streptococci and *S. aureus*. Vancomycin should be considered only in communities with a high incidence of community-acquired methicillin-resistant *S. aureus*.

29. Match the epidemiologic factors in column A with the most appropriate antibiotic regimen in column B.

A	B
1. A 3-year-old with osteomyelitis caused by *H. influenzae*	a. Ceftazidime plus an aminoglycoside
2. A 2-year-old with sickle cell disease and osteomyelitis	b. Cefuroxime
3. A 15-year-old with osteomyelitis caused by *P. aeruginosa*	c. Ceftriaxone

Answers:
1, b: Cefuroxime has adequate coverage for gram-positive organisms (e.g., *S. aureus*) and *H. influenzae*.
2, c: Empirical therapy should cover *Salmonella* species.
3, a: Dual-agent therapy is recommended until susceptibilities of the organism are identified and the patient shows good clinical response.

30. What is the recommended dose and frequency of administration of semisynthetic penicillinase-resistant penicillins?
Semisynthetic penicillinase-resistant penicillins (e.g., nafcillin, oxacillin) recommended for treatment of osteomyelitis should be administered at 200 mg/kg/day intravenously every 4–6 hours. The recommended minimal duration of therapy for acute osteomyelitis is 4–6 weeks; shorter courses have been associated with failures and recurrences. However, even with adequate therapy 5–10% of patients may experience a recurrence.

31. Describe the impact of outpatient parenteral antibiotic therapy (OPAT) on the management of osteomyelitis in childhood.
OPAT has been shown to be both safe and effective in the management of osteoarticular infections in children. It has allowed shorter hospital stay and improved patient and family quality of life. On the other hand, OPAT is not without complications related either to the antibiotic used or the vascular access device. However, strict patient selection and close follow-up by a dedicated medical team can decrease the occurrence of such complications.

32. List the appropriate conditions that allow switching from parenteral to oral antibiotic therapy in the treatment of children with osteomyelitis.
1. The etiologic agent is established.
2. The patient has shown good response to intravenous antibiotic therapy and considerable reduction in local signs and symptoms of infection.
3. The patient has demonstrated adequate caloric and fluid intake by the oral route.
4. The hospital or clinic has the ability to perform serum-cidal assays (Schlichter test) to monitor degree of antibiotic absorption. This controversial prerequisite is not universally practiced in clinical settings.
5. Oral antibiotic agents used for treatment of osteomyelitis must be administered at doses 2–3 times the recommended doses (in package inserts) for routine childhood infections.

33. How is the child with osteomyelitis followed as an outpatient?

It is recommended that children with osteomyelitis have weekly serial physical examinations and measurement of acute phase reactants (i.e., ESR and C-reactive protein).

34. A 13-year-old boy presents to the emergency department 3 days after stepping on a nail. He has low-grade fever and local signs of swelling, erythema, and tenderness of the foot over the puncture wound entrance. The white blood cell count is 11,000 cells/µl, and the sedimentation rate is 29 mm/hour. Specify the most likely diagnosis, pathogen, and therapy.

The patient most likely has osteochondritis of the foot secondary to a penetrating nail puncture wound. The most common organism (over 90% of cases) is *Pseudomonas aeruginosa*, especially when the nail penetrates through sneakers because *Pseudomonas* sp. grows favorably in the soles of shoes.

The most important aspect of management is adequate surgical debridement and drainage, which may be followed by a relatively short course of 10–12 days of antibiotics. An aminoglycoside and either an antipseudomonal penicillin or ceftazidime may be used initially. Agent-specific therapy may be used after the organism is identified. Although not approved for children less than 18 years of age, ciprofloxacin should be considered as an outpatient treatment option.

35. What is diskitis? How does it present?

Diskitis, an infection of the intervertebral disk, occurs predominantly in children younger than 5 years of age. The lumbar disks are most frequently affected. Patients are unable to walk or have a limp; they also have back pain, loss of lordosis, and hip pain or stiffness. Nonambulatory children may refuse to sit and are usually irritable. Percussion of the spine commonly elicits tenderness. Fever is generally absent or low-grade. ESR rate is usually elevated, and leukocytosis is seen in one-third of patients. Thoracic diskitis may present with abdominal pain, ileus, and vomiting. (*Caution:* Back pain in children should not be ignored; unlike adults, they are not trying to avoid work.)

36. Describe the radiographic progression of diskitis.

Narrowing of the intervertebral disk space is apparent on lateral spine plain radiography 2–4 weeks after the onset of infection. This finding is followed by destruction of the adjacent cartilaginous vertebral endplates and, finally, by herniation of the intervertebral disk into the vertebral body.

37. Describe the management of diskitis.

Most experts recommend culture-driven antibiotic therapy for 4–6 weeks. Some experts argue that because of the low yield of biopsy or aspiration, empirical antistaphylococcal antibiotic therapy may be used.

38. List the differential diagnoses of diskitis.

Noninfectious disk necrosis, vertebral osteomyelitis, and spinal or paraspinal tumors.

39. Describe the pathogenesis of vertebral osteomyelitis.

Because of valveless venous anastomotic connections, vertebral osteomyelitis usually begins with septic thrombophlebitis that involves two adjacent vertebral bodies supplied by a single nutrient vessel and then extends to involve adjacent structures. Extension of infection may lead to an epidural abscess or paraspinous mass (when it involves the lumbar vertebrae—most common), mediastinitis (when it involves the thoracic vertebrae), or retropharyngeal abscess (when it involves the cervical vertebrae—least common).

40. How do patients with vertebral osteomyelitis usually present?

They are typically older than 8 years and have an indolent course of low-grade fever and backache for months.

41. What is the most common cause of vertebral osteomyelitis?

S. aureus is the most common organism isolated from biopsy specimen in vertebral osteomyelitis. However, other agents are encountered in specific settings. For example, *P. aeruginosa* is seen in intravenous drug users, *Brucella* sp. in areas of the world where brucellosis is endemic, mycobacteria and *Coccidioides* sp. in endemic areas, and *Candida* sp. in immunocompromised hosts.

42. What is the earliest change on plain radiographs in a patient with vertebral osteomyelitis?

Plain radiography of the spine may reveal localized rarefaction of one vertebral body. Later changes include anterior osteophytic reactions and bone sclerosis.

43. What is the modality of choice for the radiologic diagnosis of vertebral osteomyelitis?

MRI is the imaging modality of choice for vertebral osteomyelitis. It can differentiate clearly between the vertebral disk and vertebral body as well as detect evidence of osteomyelitis earlier than radionuclide imaging.

44. How is tuberculosis of the spine different from pyogenic vertebral osteomyelitis radiographically?

It is quite difficult to tell the two conditions apart radiographically. However, tuberculosis causes less bone destruction, less bone proliferation, and less sclerosis than pyogenic vertebral osteomyelitis. In addition, osteophytic bridging between vertebrae is extremely rare in spinal tuberculosis.

45. Describe the management of vertebral osteomyelitis.

Management of vertebral osteomyelitis usually includes spinal immobilization, antibiotic therapy (for at least 4–6 weeks), and surgical drainage (when indicated).

46. Describe the typical clinical presentation of chronic osteomyelitis in children.

Typically, children with chronic osteomyelitis present with a painful nonfunctional extremity and a chronically draining sinus. Patients may have low-grade fever or no fever at all. They usually have a normal or mildly elevated sedimentation rate. In most children, chronic osteomyelitis follows a surgical procedure, major trauma, or inadequately treated acute hematogenous osteomyelitis.

47. How is chronic osteomyelitis treated?

Treatment involves aggressive surgery to achieve adequate drainage; to remove necrotic debris, sequestra, or foreign bodies; and to obliterate dead spaces. Surgery is followed by long-term parenteral, then oral antibiotic therapy (4–6 months). Shorter courses of antibiotic therapy are usually associated with a high failure rate.

Many adjunctive therapies have been studied, including local irrigation with antibiotic solutions, hyperbaric oxygen therapy, and surgically implanted acrylic beads impregnated with an antibiotic (used to sterilize and temporarily maintain a dead space). More studies are required to prove the additional benefit of such therapies.

48. What are some of the potential complications of chronic osteomyelitis?

Secondary amyloidosis, local sarcomatosis, and carcinomatous changes at the site of infection are extremely rare complications of chronic osteomyelitis in childhood.

49. What is chronic recurrent multifocal osteomyelitis (CRMO)?

CRMO is an ill-defined disease of uncertain etiology. Patients tend to be adolescent girls who present with low-grade fever and bone swelling. Flat bones are frequently involved. Bone scan reveals increased uptake in several bones. The course usually consists of remissions and recurrences over months to years. Antibiotics are not helpful. Steroids and nonsteroidal anti-inflammatory drugs may provide some benefit but are controversial. The differential diagnosis includes but is not limited to histiocytosis X, leukemia, and neuroblastoma.

BIBLIOGRAPHY

1. Burnett MW, Bass JW, Cook BA: Etiology of osteomyelitis complicating sickle cell disease. Pediatrics 101:296–297, 1998.
2. Gomez M, Maraqa N, Alvarez A, et al: Complications of outpatient parenteral antibiotic therapy in childhood. Pediatr Infect Dis J 20:541–543, 2001.
3. Jacobs RF, Adelman L, Sack CM: Management of *Pseudomonas* osteochondritis complicating puncture wounds of the foot. Pediatrics 69:432–435, 1982.
4. Krogstad P, Smith A: Osteomyelitis and septic arthritis. In Feigin RD, Cherry JD (eds): Textbook of Pediatric Infectious Diseases, 4th ed. Philadelphia, W.B. Saunders, 1998, pp 683–698.
5. Kumar A: Osteomyelitis. eMed J 2(10), 2001 (available at www.emedicine.com).
6. Mader JT, Calhoun J: Osteomyelitis. In Mandell GL, Bennett JE, Dolin R (eds): Principles and Practice of infectious Diseases, 5th ed. New York, Churchill Livingstone, 2000, pp 1182–1196.
7. Maraqa NF, Rathore MH: Outpatient parenteral antimicrobial therapy in osteoarticular infections in children. J Pediatr Orthop [in press].
8. Wong M, Isaacs D, Howman-Giles R: Clinical and diagnostic features of osteomyelitis occurring in the first three months of life. Pediatr Infect Dis J 14:1047–1053, 1995.

33. REACTIVE ARTHRITIS

Carlos D. Rosé, M.D.

1. What is the difference between infectious and reactive arthritis?

This question used to be an easy one until researchers began to look for infectious agents in synovial membranes with increasingly sensitive techniques. Classically, **infectious arthritis** is a condition in which viable microorganisms can be isolated from synovial fluid and membrane, whereas **reactive arthritis** is a sterile arthritis secondary to a remote (intestinal or urogenital) infection. Recent work has shown that synovial tissue in patients with early oligoarthritis is a rich source of chlamydial particles, *Yersinia* sp. antigen, and *Borrelia burgdorferi* DNA; furthermore, up to 20% of the samples are positive for broad-range universal 16S ribosomal RNA (bacterial genetic material). The classification is still useful because infectious (bacterial and parasitic) arthritis responds to antimicrobials, whereas reactive arthritis responds only marginally, if at all (highly controversial).

2. Is Lyme arthritis infectious or reactive?

It is both. Pretreatment synovial fluid harbors borreliar DNA according to polymerase chain reaction (ospA probe) in about 75% of the samples, whereas only 7% are positive after treatment. Because about 10% of patients with Lyme arthritis continue to show antibiotic-resistant synovitis beyond 6 months, it is suggested that the arthritis of Lyme disease is infectious at onset but becomes "reactive" in a small but distinct subset of patients. Perhaps such patients are genetically predisposed, as suggested by the disproportionate high number of HLA-DR4 carriage in this group.

3. What are the most important viral agents capable of producing arthritis in humans?

• Human Parvovirus B19	• Mumps	• Hepatitis C
• Varicella-zoster	• Epstein-Barr virus	• Chikungunya
• Rubella	• Hepatitis B	• Ross-River Valley fever

4. Which of the following can cause prolonged or recurrent arthritis: varicella-zoster, mumps, rhinovirus, coronavirus, rubella, or parvovirus?

Wild rubella virus infection has been associated with recurrent episodes of a "dry" (mild swelling, severe contractures), painful, symmetrical polyarthritis that may continue for years. Episodes last days and affect knees and finger joints. Human parvovirus B19, the agent of fifth disease, produces a symmetrical, small-joint polyarthritis in adolescents and a large-joint oligoarthritis in preschool children that lasts for about 1–3 months. Chronic disease has been described in adults for up to 4 years. As a matter of fact, a definable subset of rheumatoid factor (RF)-negative rheumatoid arthritis (RA) in adults is caused by parvovirus B-19. Positive polymerase chain reactions in bone marrow red-cell precursors have been found in two adult women with chronic arthritis years after onset of the acute infection.

5. Describe the clinical pattern for most cases of viral arthritis.

Except for chickenpox, which tends to cause monoarticular knee arthritis 1 week to 10 days after the decline of the rash, all other viral arthritides tend to present with the following characteristics:

- Acute onset
- Symmetrical "dry" polyarthritis
- Very painful and erythematous joints with para-articular involvement
- Self-limiting course (weeks)
- Good response to anti-inflammatory drugs
- Moderately abnormal acute-phase reactants

6. Which of the following vaccines can be associated with arthritis: diphtheria-pertussis-tetanus (DPT), mumps-measles-rubella (MMR), oral polio vaccine, hepatitis B, or varicella?
MMR, hepatitis B, and varicella.

7. What is the catcher's crouch?
Seven to 10 days after MMR vaccination, the toddler presents with low-grade fever, faint macular rash and painful knee flexion contracture with mild swelling ("catcher's crouch"). Hepatitis B vaccination also has been associated with transient knee arthritis 1–2 weeks after the second dose. Unsettled issue: Can MMR vaccination cause a chronic arthritis that resembles juvenile RA?

8. Match the infection with the rheumatologic syndrome.

Syndrome	Infection
1. Erythema multiforme	a. Herpes simplex virus type 1
2. Erythema nodosum	b. Group A streptococci
3. Reiter's syndrome	c. *Yersinia enterocolitica*
4. Henoch-Schönlein purpura and hypersensitivity vasculitis	
5. Acute rheumatic fever	

Answers: 1, a; 2, b; 3, c; 4, b; 5, b.

9. Name two mechanisms for viral arthritis and the viruses involved.
1. Synoviopathic: rubella, mumps, and varicella-zoster.
2. Hypersensitivity to virus-coded protein: parvovirus B19 and hepatitis B.

10. Of the reactive arthritides, which are important in pediatrics?
In adults, chlamydial infection is by far the most common form of reactive arthritis. In some instances, it is associated with clinical urethritis; in others, the genitourinary symptoms are absent. In children, most reactive arthritides are postdysenteric. In the United States, the most common agents are *Salmonella* and *Yersinia* species. On rare occasions a child may present with the extra-articular manifestations of Reiter's syndrome: conjunctivitis, urethritis, uveitis, aortic valvulitis, stomatitis, and keratoderma blennorrhagica.

Whether the name of Hans Julius Conrad Reiter (1881–1969) should continue to be used as an eponym is controversial. He was an ardent Nazi supporter and a firm believer in eugenics. He personally approved large number of medical experiments conducted among prisoners. In addition, he was not the first to recognize the condition carrying his name.

11. How do reactive arthritides present?
Onset of acute gastroenteritis is followed 1–3 weeks later by acute monoarthritis or asymmetrical oligoarthritis of the lower extremities. Onset also can be followed by enthesopathy (inflammation at the insertion site of the tendon) and become chronic, particularly in those who carry HLA-B27. Reactive arthritis is in fact classified with the spondyloarthropathies.

12. Which of the following bacteria are not associated with postinfectious arthritis?

Group A streptococci	*Escherichia coli*
Staphylococcus aureus	*Streptobacillus moniliformis*
Streptococcus viridans	*Neisseria meningitidis*
Mycoplasma pneumoniae	*Neisseria gonorrhoeae*
Clostridium tetani	*Borrelia burgdorferi*
Haemophilus influenzae	*Clostridium difficile*

C. tetani, H. influenzae, and *E. coli*.

13. Describe the arthritic syndrome associated with the other bacteria in question 12.

Bacteria	Clinical manifestation
Group A streptococci	Acute rheumatic fever; poststreptococcal arthritis (consideration should be given to obtaining an antistreptolysin O [ASO] titer in a child with unexplained reactive arthritis)
S. aureus	Sterile arthritis following septic arthritis
S. viridans	Polyarthritis during subacute bacterial endocarditis
M. pneumoniae	Vasculitis and polyarthritis, hemolysis
S. moniliformis	Rat bite fever (pustules and polyarthritis)
N. meningitides	Polyarthritis and vasculitis in chronic meningococcemia
N. gonorrhoeae	One joint with septic arthritis with multiple acutely inflamed and sterile joints
B. burgdorferi	Persistent synovitis after bacteriologic eradication
C. difficile	Arthritis following pseudomembranous colitis

14. In what regions of the world is *Brucella* sp. a common cause of arthritis?

Middle East and Spain. Brucellosis is acquired by contact with infected animals (especially goats) or ingestion of unpasteurized milk products.

15. Name a common parasitic infection associated with arthritis.

Giardia lamblia.

16. What is gardener's hand?

Flexor tenosynovitis secondary to infection with *Sporothrix schenckii*. This fungus is commonly found on rose thorns. Be careful when you stop to smell the roses.

17. What is desert rheumatism?

Polyarthritis in people infected with *Coccidioides immitis*. This fungus is found in the soil and is endemic in the Southwestern United States.

BIBLIOGRAPHY

1. Nocton JJ, Dressler F, Rutledge BJ et al: Detection of *Borrelia burgdorferi* DNA by polymerase chain re-action in synovial fluid from patients with Lyme arthritis. N Engl J Med 330:229, 1994.
2. Naides SJ, Scharosch LL, Foto F, et al: Rheumatologic manifestations of human parvovirus B19 infection in adults: Initial 2 years' clinical experience. Arthritis Rheum 33:1297, 1990.
3. Rose CD, Eppes SC: Infection-related arthritis. Rheum Dis Clin North Am 23:677, 1997.

XI. Fever

34. FEVER WITHOUT LOCALIZING SIGNS AND OCCULT BACTEREMIA

James Jeffrey Malatack, M.D., and Deborah M. Consolini, M.D.

1. Define fever without localizing signs.

Fever is a common presenting symptom in pediatric outpatient practices and emergency departments. When the duration of fever is less than 1 week and the initial history and examination fail to reveal a cause, the condition may be termed fever without localizing signs (FWLS).

2. How does FWLS differ from fever of unknown origin?

Fever of unknown origin (FUO) is defined as prolonged fever (> 2 weeks) without apparent cause after performance of repeated physical examinations and routine screening laboratory tests and cultures. Despite some overlap in final diagnosis with FUO, most children with FWLS require more urgent evaluation.

3. What is the differential diagnosis of FWLS in the infant or young child?

- Self-limited viral infection
- Bacterial meningitis
- Aseptic meningitis
- Pneumonia
- Urinary tract infection
- Bone or joint infection
- Gastrointestinal infection
- Occult bacteremia

4. Define occult bacteremia.

One category of illness included in FWLS is occult bacteremia, which is defined as the presence of bacteremia in a child 3–36 months of age that is not anticipated on clinical grounds.

5. For a cranky infant with fever to 40°C and no signs of focal infection on exam, which of the following is the most appropriate approach to diagnosis and management?

- **a. Admission, full sepsis work-up (including cerebrospinal fluid, blood, and urine cultures), and empiric therapy with IV antibiotics**
- **b. Administration of antipyretics and reevaluation**
- **c. Screening with complete blood count, urinalysis, and blood culture to help guide response**
- **d. Discharge home with close follow-up**
- **e. Admission for observation**

Management of the infant with FWLS must incorporate knowledge of patient risk factors (e.g., age), a careful clinical evaluation, appropriate use of laboratory tests, sound judgment, and close follow-up. Depending on the given situation, any one of these approaches may be right or wrong.

6. Is the infant or young child with FWLS at high risk for serious bacterial infection?

Although the risk of serious bacterial infection varies with age, the vast majority of children with fever and no apparent focus of infection on exam have self-limited viral infections that resolve without treatment or significant sequelae.

7. If the majority of children with FWLS have self-limited illnesses, what is the big concern?

A small number of apparently well-appearing young children with FWLS may be seen early in the course of a serious bacterial infection. The clinician faces the difficult challenge of attempting to separate the vast majority of children who have self-limited illnesses from the few who require medical intervention.

8. What is the presumed pathogenesis of invasive bacterial infections after the newborn period?

Following asymptomatic nasopharyngeal colonization, invasion of the bloodstream may occur in susceptible children. This bacteremia occasionally disseminates to distant sites, resulting in serious focal infections.

9. What is the adverse outcome of most concern in infants and children with FWLS?

Because many focal infections following bacteremia (e.g., pneumonia) can be treated when they become apparent and are usually not associated with significant sequelae, the outcome of most concern is bacterial meningitis.

10. Why has medical research failed to develop clear guidelines for identifying the febrile child with a serious bacterial infection or for preventing serious sequelae?

Clinical variables such as how "sick" or "toxic" a child appears to be are difficult to quantify objectively. In addition, the rarity of the outcome of most concern (meningitis) makes it difficult to study preventive interventions.

11. If meningitis is the major concern, why has medical research focused on occult bacteremia?

Because rare outcomes such as meningitis are difficult to study, medical research has focused on more common outcomes that are known, albeit occasional, antecedents of meningitis. Occult bacteremia is one such antecedent, as are a number of other laboratory tests. Unfortunately, in practice, these alternative outcomes do not reliably predict which patients will develop meningitis.

12. List the clinical signs and symptoms that have been used to assess febrile infants for "toxicity."

- Responsiveness to environment
- Activity
- Irritability (uncharacteristic or paradoxical)
- Consolability
- Quality of cry
- Color
- Hydration
- Social responses

13. What information and skills must the clinician possess to assess adequately the infant with FWLS?

- An understanding of risk estimates of serious bacterial illness for different age groups
- The ability to extract from the physical exam the most pertinent and predictive information for serious illness
- An understanding of the most useful diagnostic tests in assessing potential risks and when to use them
- Knowledge of when, if ever, it is appropriate to use expectant antimicrobial treatment

14. In the infant with FWLS, which clinical or laboratory factors are most predictive of higher risk for serious bacterial infection?

- Age
- High peripheral white blood cell count
- Positive blood culture
- Cerebrospinal fluid pleocytosis
- Pyuria

Although a high peripheral white blood cell count increases the risk of a positive blood culture in patients with FWLS, the positive predictive value of this test is low for bacteremia and lower still for serious focal infection. (Reminder: Positive predictive value means the number of positive test results in patients with the disease.)

15. How does age influence the assessment of risk for serious bacterial infection in infants with FWLS?

The risk of serious bacterial infection varies with age. Only 1–2% of all children are brought to medical attention for fever in the first 3 months of life. However, a greater proportion of young febrile infants will have serious bacterial infections compared with older children with FWLS. The risk is greatest during the immediate newborn period and through the first month of life.

16. List clinical factors other than age that may increase the susceptibility to invasive bacterial infection.

- Functional or anatomic asplenia
- Abnormalities of the complement system
- Immunodeficiencies, acquired (e.g., human immunodeficiency virus, systemic lupus erythematosus) or congenital (e.g., severe combined immunodeficiency syndrome, De George syndrome)
- Chronic immunosuppressant therapy (e.g., steroids)
- Abnormalities of opsonization or phagocytosis
- Specific antibody deficiencies
- Viral respiratory tract infections (which may potentiate bacterial invasion)

17. What age-related organisms are responsible for serious bacterial infection in young children with FWLS?

< 1 month old	1–3 months old	3–24 months old
Group B streptococci	*S. pneumoniae*	*S. pneumoniae*
Escherichia coli (and other gram-negative) enteric organisms)	Group B streptococci	*N. meningitidis*
	N. meningitidis	*Salmonella* spp.
Listeria monocytogenes	*Salmonella* spp.	
Streptococcus pneumoniae	*L. monocytogenes*	
Staphylococcus aureus		
Neisseria meningitidis		
Salmonella species		

A few points should be kept in mind in interpreting the above information:

1. Some viruses can cause serious infection in neonates and at the onset can present as FWLS (e.g., herpes simplex virus, enterovirus).

2. The division of responsible organisms by age is not absolute. For example, *E. coli* can cause meningitis in a child older than 1 month.

3. In the 3–24 month age range, the listed organisms usually cause FWLS (*Salmonella* spp. often but not always has GI symptoms), whereas other bacterial infections (e.g., *S. aureus*) usually present with a focus on exam.

4. *Haemophilus influenzae* type b, formerly an important cause of occult bacteremia, has become extremely rare since the almost universal administration of the conjugate *H. influenzae* type b (HIB) vaccines.

18. A 24-month-old, fully immunized boy presents with a temperature of 40.1°C. He has meningismus, irritability, and inactivity. What organisms are you most concerned about?

S. pneumoniae and *N. meningitidis*.

19. In a well-appearing febrile infant less than 3 months of age, what constellation of clinical and laboratory factors has been shown to be associated with low risk of serious bacterial infection?

In a prospective study conducted at the University of Rochester to identify factors associated with a low risk of serious bacterial infection, 233 non–toxic-appearing infants less than 3 months of age with FWLS were hospitalized and treated expectantly for suspected septicemia. Infants were considered to be at low risk of serious bacterial infection if they met the following criteria:

- No clinical evidence of infection of the ear, skin, bones, or joints
- White blood cell count of 5,000–15,000/mm^3
- Fewer than 1,500 band cells/mm^3
- Normal urinalysis

Of the 144 infants meeting these criteria, only 1 (< 1%) had a definable bacterial infection (*Salmonella* gastroenteritis). In contrast, 22 (25%) of the 89 infants who failed to meet one or more of these criteria were found to have a serious bacterial infection.

20. In the Rochester study, were the risk estimates for serious bacterial infection defined only for an inner city population?

No. The population was mixed, and analysis by location of the patient's home revealed no difference in risk between suburban and urban children.

21. Name the organisms associated with occult bacteremia.

- *S. pneumoniae*
- *N. meningitides*
- *H. influenzae* type b (rare since the almost universal administration of the conjugate HIB vaccines)

22. Does the risk of occult bacteremia differ according to organism?

Yes. Data from the Children's Hospital of Pittsburgh and Yale-New Haven Hospital, predating the conjugate HIB vaccines, showed that 44% of bacteremias due to *S. pneumoniae* met criteria for "occult" infection, whereas 20% of bacteremias due to *N. meningitidis* and only 8% due to *H. influenzae* type b could be considered occult.

23. What is the major concern about occult bacteremia?

Some febrile children 3–36 months of age who do not appear to be toxic and have no apparent focus of infection on exam have bacteremia, most often due to *S. pneumoniae*, but occasionally to *N. meningitidis* or rarely to *H. influenzae* type b. The vast majority of children with occult bacteremia (particularly *S. pneumoniae* occult bacteremia) have transient infection that resolves without treatment or significant sequelae. However, a small number of children with occult bacteremia develop a serious focal infection such as meningitis.

24. Is high fever alone associated with an excessive risk of bacteremia?

High fever alone significantly increases the risk of bacteremia in neonates but not in infants older than 3 months. In the largest study of children 3–36 months of age with fever ≥ 39°C, the incidence of bacteremia was approximately 3%.

25. How does the total white blood cell (WBC) count influence the risk estimate for bacteremia in highly febrile children?

In a study by Bass et al., the risk of bacteremia was greater when high fever was associated with high total white blood cell count:

Total WBC Count/mm^3	Proportion with Bacteremia (%)
< 10,000	0/99 (0)
10,000–14,999	5/83 (6)

Continued on next page.

Total WBC Count/mm³	Proportion with Bacteremia (%)
15,000–19,999	16/182 (8.8)
20,000–29,999	30/127 (23.6)
30,000–34,999	4/13 (30.8)
> 35,000	5/8 (62.5)
> 15,000	55/330 (16.7)

26. The total WBC count is the most commonly used laboratory test in assessing young children with FWLS for risk of serious illness. How good a test is it in this clinical setting?

Children with high fever, no focus of infection on exam and WBC counts $\geq$ 15,000/mm³ have an approximately three times greater risk of bacteremia than those with WBC counts $\leq$ 15,000/mm³. However, because of the low incidence of occult bacteremia, the positive predictive value of the total WBC count for bacteremia is low. Thus, the great majority of highly febrile children with WBC counts $\geq$ 15,000 or more do not have bacteremia. In addition, the outcome of concern is not occult bacteremia but meningitis.

27. Does a high total WBC count accurately distinguish children with occult bacteremia who develop bacterial meningitis from children who do not?

No. In one study, children with occult bacteremia who did not develop meningitis had a significantly higher mean total WBC count at presentation than children who developed meningitis. This apparent paradox is due to the association of specific bacteria (e.g., *S. pneumoniae*) with leukocytosis. Although pneumococcal bacteremia is associated with a higher total WBC count, it is also associated with a lower risk of bacterial meningitis than bacteremia with *N. meningitidis* or *H. influenzae* type b.

28. What diagnostic tests other than the total WBC count have been evaluated as potential predictors of serious bacterial illness in children with FWLS?

- WBC count differential
- Erythrocyte sedimentation rate
- C-reactive protein
- Morphologic changes in peripheral blood neutrophils
- Microscopic examination of buffy coat of blood
- Quantitative blood cultures

No test, however, has been found to have sufficient sensitivity and positive or negative predictive value to be clinically useful for an individual patient.

29. How useful is a blood culture in the outpatient assessment of children with FWLS?

The practice of obtaining blood cultures in the infant or young child with FWLS developed as an attempt to identify patients with bacteremia so that they could be scrutinized more closely or treated to prevent the evolution of bacteremia to meningitis. Recent studies argue that blood cultures in children with FWLS fail to accomplish the intended purpose. Most children with occult bacteremia who develop focal complications return for care before the blood culture results are known, whereas in most children asked to return because of positive culture results bacteremia has cleared spontaneously and hospitalization or additional care is not warranted. In the final analysis, nothing supplants good follow-up with a concerned parent for timely intervention (when it is necessary).

30. A 12-month-old infant is seen in the emergency department for fever. Examination reveals no source of infection. A blood culture is drawn, and the child is sent home based on a nontoxic exam. Forty-eight hours later the laboratory informs you that the blood culture is positive for *S. pneumoniae*. You reevaluate the child, who is now afebrile and well-appearing. No focus of infection is apparent on exam. What is the most appropriate management?

Discuss with the family the likely benign nature of the bacteremia but arm them with the necessary information to recognize the rare case of a complicating outcome. Ensure willing and easy access to follow-up.

31. List signs that a parent should be instructed to look for in a child with FWLS as indicators of a more serious problem.

- Persistent or paradoxical irritability
- Lethargy
- Inattentiveness to environment
- Alteration in breathing pattern
- Bulging fontanelle
- Color change
- Cool hands and feet
- Poor urine output
- Nonblanching rash (petechiae and/or purpura)
- Refusal to move extremity or joint
- Localized redness, pain, or swelling

32. What is the risk of bacterial meningitis in children with occult bacteremia?

The risk of meningitis complicating occult bacteremia varies depending on the particular organism. In a study conducted at Yale-New Haven Hospital and the Children's Hospital of Pittsburgh, only 1.8% of children with occult pneumococcal bacteremia subsequently developed bacterial meningitis. The risk of developing meningitis was 15 times greater for occult *H. influenzae* type b bacteremia and 81 times greater for *N. meningitidis* bacteremia. Since occult bacteremia due to *H. influenzae* type b has become rare, the risk of meningitis among children with occult bacteremia has decreased significantly.

33. What is the current estimated risk for bacterial meningitis in patients 3–36 months of age with FWLS?

Currently, it is estimated that bacterial meningitis will develop in approximately 1 of 1,000 untreated children with FWLS.

34. Is it reasonable to obtain blood tests and treat 1000 children with FWLS with parenterally administered, broad-spectrum antimicrobial agents to prevent one case of bacterial meningitis?

The answer to this question leaves the secure confines of science and resides in the murky waters of value judgments. On the one hand, we have chosen as a society to screen all newborns to find the 1 in 5,000 with hypothyroidism, the 1 in 20,000 with phenylketonuria (PKU), and the 1 in 50,000 with galactosemia so that intervention may prevent the rare child with one of these inborn errors of metabolism from developing mental retardation. Why should we not hospitalize and treat 1000 at-risk children to prevent one from developing bacterial meningitis and its accompanying sequelae, including death? On the other hand, the financial cost of newborn screening is not prohibitive compared with expectant hospitalization and parenteral antibiotic treatment. An additional cost to consider in the febrile child is the psychosocial disruption of expectant management, which can be difficult to calculate.

35. Does expectant antimicrobial therapy for febrile children in the outpatient setting prevent serious complications such as meningitis?

No definitive data confirm that ceftriaxone or any antibiotic prevents the rare occurrence of meningitis in children with occult bacteremia. In one clinical trial, 6,733 children with FWLS, aged 3–36 months, were randomized to receive one dose of ceftriaxone (50 mg/kg) or amoxicillin (60 mg/kg/day for 2 days). Among children with bacteremia, there was no statistically significant difference in the frequency of complications between the two groups. Neither drug prevented meningitis. Do you now feel better about question 34?

36. List the risks of routine antimicrobial treatment of children with FWLS in the outpatient setting.

- Substantial cost
- Increased potential for adverse drug reactions
- Selection of resistant organisms
- Potential for decreased vigilance in following-up "treated" children

37. How will widespread use of the conjugate pneumococcal vaccine change the management of children with FWLS?

The use of the conjugate pneumococcal vaccine decreases the risk of occult bacteremia. The current strategy, followed by some clinicians, of obtaining WBC counts and blood cultures and starting empirical antibiotics may become obsolete in vaccinated children.

38. What is the most important factor to consider in the initial assessment and management of the child with FWLS?

Age. Although there is no single correct approach to the management of children with FWLS, there is general agreement that very young children should be managed differently from older children.

39. Because of the substantially greater risk of serious infection in young infants with fever, the newborn remains a special patient in assessing fever. What factors justify a more conservative approach to the management of the febrile infant younger than 1 month?

Infants younger than 1 month exhibit few early signs of illness. They have a limited repertoire of symptoms, most of which are nonspecific. Subtle changes in feeding habits or behavior are common manifestations of infection. Although fever is a hallmark of infection, it is a variable manifestation in the first few weeks of life. Temperature instability rather than fever can be the sole indicator of illness. Physical exam findings also may be unreliable, making it difficult to assess degree of wellness. In addition, the immaturity of the neonate's host defenses results in a relatively immunocompromised state. Neonates are also unimmunized.

40. A 21-day-old infant living at home is brought to your office with a fever of 38.5°C and poor feeding. What should you do?

Admit the infant to the hospital; order cultures of blood, urine, and CSF; and give empirical antibiotics until culture results are known.

41. What is the appropriate empirical antibiotic treatment for the neonate (infant < 1 month old) with FWLS?

The most likely bacterial pathogens in this age group include group B streptococci, *E. coli* and other gram-negative organisms, and *L. monocytogenes*. Thus, appropriate antibiotic choices for empirical therapy are ampicillin, 50 mg/kg/dose IV every 6 hours, and gentamicin, 2.5 mg/kg/dose IV every 8 hours. Alternatively, a third-generation cephalosporin can be substituted for gentamicin.

42. A 2-month-old infant is seen in the emergency department with a temperature of 38.5°C. What issues are important in deciding what to do next?

Before studies attempted to identify factors associated with a low risk of serious bacterial infection in febrile infants younger than 3 months, cultures of blood, CSF, and urine, followed by admission and empiric antimicrobial treatment, were the standard of care for this age group. A reasonable alternative to that aggressive approach is now recommended for infants 1–3 months of age. The lynchpin of the alternative approach is that the infant looks well. In addition, nothing in the history should raise concern (no change of behavior, such as decreased eating, increased sleeping, or uncustomary irritability). Physical examination must reveal no focus of infection and be reassuring. The author cannot emphasize strongly enough that the child must appear well. The alternative approach includes a laboratory evaluation to establish low risk with assessment of CSF, complete blood count with differential, and urinalysis. If the evaluation results are not concerning, no hospitalization or treatment is indicated. The physician must ensure close follow-up, and the parents must be armed with the information needed to react appropriately to changes in the infant's clinical course.

43. A-14 month-old infant is seen in a free clinic where you volunteer 1 night per week. The child has had tactile fever, as reported by the mother, since the previous day. In the clinic he is febrile (38.6°C) and somewhat fussy but consolable by the mother. The shelter at

which the mother lives has no phone and no transportation. You are clearly unable to ensure follow-up. What should you do?

If it is impossible to ensure follow-up, hospitalization for observation without treatment is an alternative. Since this alternative is offered in an authoritative text, you can argue your case with third-party payors.

44. Why not simply treat all febrile infants with empiric IV antibiotics after performing blood, CSF, and urine cultures and avoid all this follow-up worry?

1. Empirical treatment is not without associated risks.

2. Studies of parental opinion reveal that parents are willing to assume a small risk to avoid hospitalization and IV antibiotics.

3. The outcome of concern is not bacteremia but meningitis, which rarely occurs in a well-appearing infant.

45. What risks are associated with hospitalization and empirical treatment pending culture results?

1. Costs
2. Iatrogenic complications:
   - Error of drug type
   - Error of drug dose
   - Injury from venous cannulation
   - Nosocomial infection
3. Psychosocial disruption

46. What is the most important factor to consider in the evaluation of the child older than 24 months who presents with FWLS?

By 24 months of age, the physical examination is a reliable indicator of the site and severity of infection. Consequently, the 2-year-old child should be viewed and managed like an older child.

47. A 36-month-old child has a fever of 40.5°C. She had a brief (5-minute) seizure at home that ended before the 10-minute ride to the hospital. On arrival in the emergency department, the triage nurse informs you that the child is sleepy and appears postictal. The mother had given the child an acetaminophen suppository before leaving home. Your evaluation 25 minutes later reveals an afebrile, alert, and interactive toddler. Physical examination reveals no focus of infection, including meningismus. What is the most appropriate management?

a. The "works": admission; culture of blood, urine, and CSF; and empirical IV antibiotics until cultures are demonstrated to be negative.

b. The "works," hold the chili: complete blood count, blood culture, CSF studies (including cells, protein, glucose, and culture), urinalysis, and urine culture to assess risk. If the risk is low, give intramuscular ceftriaxone and send home.

c. Send home with close follow-up, relying on the accuracy of your physical exam findings in a child older than 24 months. Ensure that the family is armed with the necessary information to recognize a deteriorating clinical condition.

d. Obtain a complete blood count, urinalysis, and urine culture. If results are unremarkable, prescribe a 10-day course of amoxicillin and discharge home.

The correct answer is c. Keep in mind, however, that it is natural for families to relax their vigilance after the medical community deems the child free of serious disease. This principle applies for children of any age. The experience of having a sick child has probably already exhausted the parents. As a counter to the parents' desire to let down their guard, one must stress that continued vigilance is necessary to detect potential complications.

48. What facets of the management strategy for 3- to 24-month-old children with FWLS remain unclear?

There is less consensus about the correct management strategy for 3- to 24-month-old children with FWLS than for either older or younger children. It remains unclear if all patients in this age group need to have tests done as part of the initial evaluation. If tests are to be done, it remains unclear which tests should be ordered. It also remains unclear whether any of these children deserve expectant antibiotics. Finally, if antibiotics are given, which antibiotics should be used? The following four cases illustrate factors that should be taken into account to help guide management decisions.

49. An 18-month-old presents with fever of 40°C. He is cranky but consolable and has acute otitis media (AOM) in the right ear. What is your approach to management?

The preceding discussion of FWLS is not applicable in the setting of a febrile child with a focal infection, including AOM. The presence of one focal infection is associated with a reduced likelihood of developing a subsequent focus of infection, regardless of antimicrobial treatment. Management of a highly febrile child with AOM who appears well should focus on the AOM. Keep in mind that, although the above patient may have a decreased risk of adverse outcome compared with patients with FWLS, close and careful follow-up remains necessary.

50. A 21 month-old boy presents with fever of 39.5°C. Exam reveals bilateral AOM. The child appears ill, significantly distressed and uninterested in the environment. Acetaminophen treatment to ameliorate the otalgia reduces the fever but does not change the child's toxic appearance. What care is indicated?

A toxic child should be managed without consideration of the presence of a first focus of infection (AOM in this patient). Although a first focus of infection may reduce the likelihood of a second focus of infection, it does not immunize the infant against a secondary focus. If a child is ill-appearing, the appropriate response is based on the ill appearance—not on the presence of an obvious source for the fever. AOM does not "bail you out" and allow routine treatment, as in the prior example. A sick infant warrants cultures, hospitalization, and empirical IV antibiotics pending culture results—inflamed tympanic membranes or not.

51. A 15-month-old, previously healthy boy presents with temperature of 39.3°C. He is listless and irritable when disturbed. Aside from the expected fever-related increase in heart rate and respiratory rate, his exam is normal. How should you proceed?

The degree of the child's toxicity dictates the cadence of your response. The extremely ill-appearing infant demands a rapid response to assess and treat expectantly. In the less ill-appearing child, you have more time for assessment. Often the fever itself rather than its underlying cause is responsible for the child's ill appearance. Antipyretic therapy with reevaluation when and if the fever decreases allows assessment of the impact of the infection rather than the fever on the child's well-being.

52. In the case above, antipyretics are administered with a resultant decrease in temperature to 37.9°C. The child now appears well. He is playing with a stuffed animal and laughing with his father. How do you proceed?

No further evaluation is indicated. The child may go home as long as you are able to ensure reliable follow-up and have given the parents the necessary information to recognize deterioration in the child's clinical status. Remember to take the stuffed animal away from the child because it belongs to the emergency department.

53. After a telephone call from a mother who reports that her 9-month-old daughter has been grunting and moaning since being put to bed and is "burning-up" to touch, you agree to meet the child in the emergency department. The child is febrile (39.6°C), lethargic, and irritable. She has been febrile for about 48 hours but did not look "this sick" to her mother until this evening. The mother's attempts to console the infant by picking her up are met with increased though feeble protests. What needs to done?

The infant is ill with FWLS. You should be concerned that the earlier fevers may have been due to bacteremia and that the patient may now have a serious focal infection, such as meningitis.

The child needs a full sepsis evaluation with blood, CSF, and urine cultures and initiation of empirical antimicrobial therapy with ceftriaxone, pending culture results. If CSF pleocytosis is found and gram-positive infection is suspected by Gram stain, vancomycin should be added to cover penicillin-resistant pneumococci.

54. In light of the multifaceted and varied responses to the febrile infant, as discussed in this chapter, what underlying principles may be used to guide your approach to young children with FWLS?

As an overall strategy, the infant with FWLS requires a thoughtful assessment, individualized management, and close follow-up.

55. Summarize the management approach for infants and young children with FWLS.

Decisions need to be based on the age of the affected child.

1. The neonate (< 1 month old) should receive cultures of urine, blood, and CSF as well as parenteral antibiotics under hospital observation.

2. The alternative to routine hospitalization and empirical IV antibiotic treatment pending culture results may be considered in infants older than 1 month and younger than 3 months who look well, meet the Rochester low-risk criteria, and are likely to have excellent follow-up.

3. For infants and children older than 3 months, routine laboratory tests are generally not useful. Parents of the child with FWLS who is sent home must be armed with the necessary information to recognize a deteriorating medical condition.

4. Children greater than 24 months of age may be managed like older children.

Conjugate vaccines are changing the landscape of the clinical problem of the infant with FWLS. The HIB vaccine has virtually eliminated *H. influenzae* type b infections, and it appears that Prevnar is having a significant affect on invasive *S. pneumoniae* infections. The care of the febrile infant without localizing signs has evolved in the past 20 years as clinical research continually redefines the issues of concern. Continued close assessment of the pediatric infectious disease literature is necessary to maintain currency in such a rapidly changing field.

BIBLIOGRAPHY

1. Alpern ER, Alessandrini EA, Bell LM, et al: Occult bacteremia from a pediatric emergency department: Current prevalence, time to detection, and outcome. Pediatrics 106:505–511, 2000.
2. Baraff LJ, Oslund SA, Schriger DL, et al: Probability of bacterial infections in febrile infants less than three months of age: A meta-analysis. Pediatr Infect Dis J 11:257–265, 1992.
3. Bass JW, Steele RW, Wittler RR, et al: Antimicrobial treatment of occult bacteremia: A multicenter cooperative study. Pediatr Infect Dis J 12:466–473, 1993.
4. Dagan R, Powell KR, Hall CB, et al: Identification of infants unlikely to have serious bacterial infection although hospitalized for suspected sepsis. J Pediatr 107:855–860, 1985.
5. Fleisher GR, Rosenberg N, Vinci R, et al: Intramuscular versus oral antibiotic therapy for the prevention of meningitis and other bacterial sequelae in young, febrile children at risk for occult bacteremia. J Pediatr 124:504–512, 1994.
6. Kramer MS, Lane DA, Mills EL: Should blood cultures be obtained in the evaluation of young febrile children without evident focus of infection? A decision analysis of diagnostic management strategies. Pediatrics 84:18–27, 1989.
7. Long SS: Antibiotic therapy in febrile children: "Best-laid schemes..." J Pediatr 124:585–588, 1994.
8. Malatack JJ, Long SS: Fever of unknown origin. In Long SS, Pickering LK, Prober CG (eds): Principles and Practice of Pediatric Infectious Diseases. New York, Churchill Livingstone, 1997, pp 124–134.
9. McCarthy PI, Jekel JF, Dolan TF Jr: Temperature greater than or equal to 40°C in children less than 24 months of age: A prospective study. Pediatrics 59:663–668, 1977.
10. Offit PA, Offit BF, Bell LM (eds): Breaking the Antibiotic Habit: A Parent's Guide to Cough, Cold, Ear Infection and Sore Throat. New York, John Wiley & Son, 1999.
11. Shapiro ED: Fever without localizing signs. In Long SS, Pickering LK, Prober CG (eds): Principles and Practice of Pediatric Infectious Diseases. New York, Churchill Livingstone, 1997, pp 119–124.
12. Shapiro ED, Aaron NH, Wald ER, et al: Risk factors for development of bacterial meningitis among children with occult bacteremia. J Pediatr 109:15–19, 1986.

35. RASH AND FEVER

Terry Yamauchi, M.D.

1. On what criteria is the diagnosis of Kawasaki disease based?
1. Fever greater than 101°F, lasting 5 or more days without other diagnoses
2. At least four of the following unexplained symptoms:
   • Bilateral conjunctival injection
   • Mucous membrane changes
   • Extremity involvement, such as erythema of the palms and soles, edema of hands or feet, or generalized/periungual desquamation
   • Polymorphous rash (primarily truncal) without vesicles, crusting, or scarring
   • Cervical lymphadenopathy

2. What is the therapy of choice for Kawasaki disease?
High-dose intravenous gammaglobulin and aspirin.

3. The childhood disease roseola is also known by what other names?
Roseola infantum, exanthem subitum, and sixth disease.

4. Describe the typical clinical presentation of roseola.
Fever of 102–106°F, suboccipital adenopathy, periorbital edema with rash (macular or maculopapular) that involves the trunk and extends to the neck, extremities, and face. The rash typically lasts 2 days. The causative agent of roseola is human herpesvirus 6 (HHV-6). It is the most common identifiable cause of febrile seizures in children under the age of 2 years.

5. What is the most common life-threatening diagnosis in a child with a petechial rash and fever?
Meningococcemia (caused by *Neisseria meningitidis*).

6. What are the manifestations of varicella infection (chickenpox) in unvaccinated children?
After an incubation period of 11–21 days, a maculopapular rash starts on the trunk and scalp; crops of new lesions appear centrifugally. The rash progresses from maculopapular to vesicles and pustules, which umbilicate and crust. Varicella is contagious until all lesions have crusted and no new lesions are appearing.

7. What are the prognostic indicators for meningococcemia in infants and children?
   • Shock
   • Hyperpyrexia
   • Rapid progression of petechial skin lesions
   • Leukopenia
   • Absence of cerebrospinal fluid pleocytosis

8. What is the characteristic rash of Lyme disease?
Erythema migrans, usually at site of the tick bite. Lyme disease is spread by the deer tick, which is very small and often not noticed.

9. List the initial symptoms of Rocky Mountain spotted fever.
Abrupt onset of severe headache, shaking rigors, prostration, muscle aches, and high fever (103–104°F).

10. Describe the initial lesions of Rocky Mountain spotted fever. How do they progress?
Initially, the lesions are macular, rose-colored, and blanching and appear on wrists, ankles, palms, and soles. The rash spreads to the trunk, neck, and face.

11. Describe the characteristic appearance and cause of erysipelas. How is it treated?
The characteristic appearance of erysipelas is a painful, hot, rapidly enlarging lesion with an erythematous, raised border. The lesion frequently involves large areas of skin. . The etiologic agent is group A beta-hemolytic streptococci, and the treatment of choice is penicillin.

12. What is the initial manifestation of erythema infectiosum?
The initial manifestation is bilateral erythema of the cheeks ("slapped-cheek" appearance of the face).

13. What are the five childhood exanthems?
Rubella, measles, scarlet fever, Filutov-Duke disease (form of scarlet fever), and erythema infectiosum.

14. What specific viral syndrome causes ulcerative lesions in the anterior mouth, skin lesions of the hands and feet, and occasionally skin lesions of the trunk and face?
Hand, foot, and mouth disease.

15. What virus most commonly causes hand, foot, and mouth disease?
Coxsackievirus A16.

16. Match the following diseases with their characteristic rash.
Disease	Characteristic rash
a. Varicella	1. Crops of new lesions in a centrifugal pattern
b. Scarlet fever	2. Erythema migrans
c. Kawasaki disease	3. Sandpaper rash
d. Lyme disease	4. polymorphous rash

Answers: a, 1; b, 3; c, 4; and d, 2.

17. List four viruses that may cause petechial rashes with fever.
1. Adenovirus	3. Enterovirus
2. Epstein-Barr virus	4. Rubeola virus

18. What microorganism is most often associated with Stevens-Johnson syndrome?
Mycoplasma pneumoniae.

19. List the differences between chickenpox (varicella) and smallpox (variola) rashes.
Smallpox	Chickenpox
Ill 2–4 days before rash	No symptoms until rash appears
Lesions most numerous on face, arms, and legs	Lesions most numerous on trunk
Lesions on palms and soles	Lesions on palms and soles are rare
Scabs from 10–14 days after rash appears	Scabs from 4–7 days after rash appears
Scabs fall off 14–28 days after onset of rash	Scabs fall off within 14 days after onset of rash

20. What is the most common manifestation of cutaneous herpes simplex virus infection in children?
Herpetic whitlow.

21. List the characteristic findings when a herpetic lesion is scraped, stained and observed under a microscope.

Multinucleated giant cells and atypical keratinocytes with large nuclei. These classic findings are seen on Tzanck preparation, although direct fluorescent antibody tests, culture, or polymerase chain reaction is more commonly used.

22. What is the etiologic agent of erythema infectiosum?

Parvovirus B19

23. With which of the following diseases is parvovirus B19 associated: aplastic crises, non-immune fetal hydrops and fetal death, or mad cow disease?

Aplastic crises in patients with chronic hemolytic anemia and immunodeficiencies and non-immune fetal hydrops and fetal death.

24. What are the initial symptoms of scarlet fever?

Fever, vomiting, and sore throat.

25. Describe the rash of scarlet fever.

The rash is coarse, red, sandpaper-like, and centrally distributed. Look for Pastia's lines, which are accentuation of the rash in the axillary and inguinal regions.

26. Describe the classic enanthem of measles.

Koplik spots, which are 1- to 2-mm papules on an erythematous base on the buccal mucosa.

27. Describe the classic exanthem of measles.

Measles begins with a discrete maculopapular rash on the upper trunk and face. The lower trunk and extremities follow, and the rash becomes confluent.

28. What are the other names for rubella?

German measles and third disease.

29. Which of the following agents should be included in the differential diagnosis of petechiae and fever?

Neisseria meningitidis	*Streptococcus pyogenes*
Neisseria gonorrhoeae	*Staphylococcus aureus* (endocarditis)
Pseudomonas aeruginosa	*Chlamydia pneumoniae*
All but *C. pneumoniae* .	

30. Name two microbial causes of fever and petechiae for which a positive blood culture cannot be obtained.

Rickettsia rickettsii (Rocky Mountain spotted fever) and *Rickettsia prowazekii* (louse-born typhus).

31. One specific antibiotic can cause a rash in patients infected with one specific virus. Name the virus and the antibiotic.

Epstein-Barr virus, which causes infectious mononucleosis, and ampicillin.

32. What infectious agent causes classic "diaper rash" in infants?

Candida albicans.

33. Describe the classic appearance of diaper dermatitis.

The classic candidal diaper dermatitis has an erythematous border with isolated ("satellite") lesions on the advancing edge.

34. What infectious agent is associated with the petechial gloves-and-socks syndrome?
Parvovirus B19.

35. What two bacteria commonly cause secondary infection in patients with varicella-zoster viral infections?
Streptococcus pyogenes and *Staphylococcus aureus.*

36. Match the infectious agent with the disease that it causes.

Infectious agent	Disease
a. Parvovirus	1. Roseola infantum
b. Human herpes virus 6	2. Smallpox
c. Varicella-zoster virus	3. Chickenpox
d. Variola	4. Erythema infectiosum
e. *Rickettsia tsutsugamushi*	5. Scrub typhus

Answers: a, 2; b, 4; c, 3; d, 1.

37. Which disease characterized by fever, chills, headache, and maculopapular and petechial rash usually occurs in the summer?
Rocky Mountain spotted fever is usually a summer disease. Because ticks are the carriers of the infectious agent, the disease is seen during tick season.

38. What is the main differentiating feature between ehrlichiosis and Rocky Mountain spotted fever?
The rash of ehrlichiosis generally spares the palms and soles.

39. The classic symptoms of staphylococcal scalded-skin syndrome are fever, irritability, and erythematous (tender) skin. What is the Nikolsky sign?
The Nikolsky sign is wrinkling of the upper layer of the epidermis with sloughing by light rubbing.

40. What is the best way to distinguish staphylococcal scalded-skin syndrome from toxic epidermal necrolysis?
Skin biopsy.

41. List the clinical criteria that define toxic shock syndrome (TSS).
The diagnosis is established by the presence of three major and at least three minor criteria, with negative cultures (blood, throat, and cerebrospinal fluid). Serologic testing must rule out Rocky Mountain spotted fever, leptospirosis, and rubeola.

Major criteria
• Temperature > 38.9°C
• Hypotension (shock or orthostatic)
• Macular erythroderma with late desquamation within 1–2 weeks

Minor criteria
• Mucous membrane inflammation (conjunctival or pharyngeal)
• Gastrointestinal system (vomiting, diarrhea)
• Musculoskeletal system (myalgia, elevated creatine phosphokinase)
• Central nervous system (altered consciousness)
• Hepatic signs and symptoms (elevated bilirubin, elevated transaminase)
• Renal signs and symptoms (elevated blood urea nitrogen, > 5 white blood cells/high-power field, decreased platelet count)

42. What causes TTS?
TTS was previously associated with tampon use, but in children it often occurs with inapparent staphylococcal and streptococcal infections.

43. Which of the following diseases causes a "sunburn-like" rash (erythroderma): cutaneous larva migrans, malaria, TSS, or histoplasmosis?
  TSS.

44. List the complications of varicella.
  Pneumonia (more common in adults), zoster (also more frequent in adults), otitis media, hepatitis, encephalitis, cerebellar ataxia, transverse myelitis, Reye's syndrome, and secondary bacterial infection.

45. Ataxia is the most common central nervous system manifestation of varicella-zoster infection. When in the course of the disease does it occur?
  Oddly enough, near the resolution of the illness, approximately 7–10 days after onset.

46. Match the maculopapular exanthem disease with the infectious agent.

Disease	Agent
a. Meningococcemia	1. *Streptococcus pyogenes*
b. Bartonellosis	2. *Rickettsia rickettsii*
c. Rocky Mountain spotted fever	3. *Ehrlichia canis*
d. Ehrlichiosis	4. *Neisseria meningitidis*
e. Scarlet fever	5. *Bartonella bacilliformis*

  Answers: a, 5; b, 3; c, 4; d, 1; e, 2.

47. Describe the typical lesions of erythema nodosum.
  Erythema nodosum lesions are raised, erythematous, and painful to touch. Their usual size is about 2–4 cm, and their duration is 2–6 weeks.

48. What are the most common infectious agents associated with erythema nodosum?
  In the past, streptococci and mycobacteria were the most common agents. Currently, erythema nodosum is most often associated with respiratory infection with *Histoplasma capsulatum*, *Cryptococcus neoformans*, and *Coccidioides immitis*.

49. Describe Gianotti-Crosti syndrome.
  This distinct clinical entity is characterized by a papular exanthem, generalized lymphadenopathy, hepatomegaly, and acute anicteric hepatitis.

50. Which virus is most often associated with Gianotti-Crosti syndrome?
  Hepatitis B virus.

BIBLIOGRAPHY

1. Castellano A, Schweitzer R, Tong MJ, et al: Papular acrodermatitis of childhood and hepatitis B infection. Arch Dermatol 114:1530–1532, 1978.
2. Chapman SW, Daniel CR: Cutaneous manifestations of fungal infection. Infect Dis Clin North Am 8:879–910, 1994.
3. Cherry JD: Cutaneous manifestations of systemic infections. In Feigin RD, Cherry JD (eds): Textbook of Pediatric Infectious Diseases, vol. 1, 4th ed. Philadelphia, W.B. Saunders, 1998, pp 713–737.
4. Cherry JD: Contemporary infectious exanthems. Child Infect Dis 16:199–207, 1993.
5. Cherry JD. Roseola infantum (exanthem subitum). In Feigin RD, Cherry JD (eds): Textbook of Pediatric Infectious Diseases, vol. 1, 4th ed. Philadelphia, W.B. Saunders, 1998, pp 738–741.
6. Hall CB, Long CE, Schnabel KC, et al: Human herpesvirus-6 infection in children: A prospective study of complications and reactivation. N Engl J Med 331:432–438, 1994.
7. Puig L, Diaz M, Alexandre RC, et al: Petechial glove and sock syndrome caused by parvovirus B19. Cutis 54:335–340, 1994.
8. Yoto Y, Kudoh T, Haseyama K, et al: Human parvovirus B19 infection in Kawasaki disease. Lancet 344:58–59, 1994.

36. FEVER OF UNKNOWN ORIGIN

Robert N. Tiballi, D.O.

1. Define fever of undetermined origin.

Fever of undetermined origin (FUO) is one of the most challenging of all medical evaluations. Strict criteria established in 1961 by Beeson and Petersdorf include fever > 101°F for longer than 3 weeks and failure to establish a diagnosis despite 1 full week of intensive evaluation. Criteria for true FUO are more commonly met in the adult population. Most pediatricians apply the term FUO after 1 continuous week of fever without focus or diagnosis.

2. What are the causes of FUO in children?

Classically, one-third of pediatric cases of FUO are due to infection, whereas about 10% are due to malignancy. Collagen vascular disease is present in 10–20% of published reviews, and 5–10% of cases are due to inflammatory bowel disease. Although no diagnosis is found in one-third of cases, 10–15% of pediatric cases of FUO resolve spontaneously without a diagnosis. In most cases, children with FUO are not overwhelmingly ill. They have episodic fever but are able to maintain their usual daily activities. Fulminantly ill children with fever are excluded from this category despite the possible lack of diagnosis.

3. True or false: FUO may be caused by medications, even by antibiotics.

True. Although FUO due to medications is not a regular occurrence, neither is it unusual. Beta-lactam antibiotics such as penicillin and cephalosporins may cause fever even in the absence of rash or urticaria. The fevers resolve quickly when the offending agent is discontinued. Often the complete blood count (CBC) shows progressive eosinophilia until the offending agent is removed. In addition, liver enzymes such as aspartate aminotransferase (AST) and alanine aminotransferase (ALT) are frequently elevated.

4. What drugs are most often associated with FUO?
- Phenytoin
- Sulfa drugs
- Metoclopramide
- Phenothiazines
- Benzodiazepines

5. True or false: Most children who have FUO without a diagnosed etiology develop a malignancy.

False. Roughly 10% of children with FUO are later found to have a malignancy. In adults, the rate of FUO due to malignancy is approximately 20%. Collagen vascular diseases and inflammatory bowel disease are more common causes of FUO in children than malignancy.

6. True or false: Sinusitis should be excluded in pediatric patients with FUO.

True. Sinus infections may be asymptomatic, even when radiographic changes are dramatic. Computed tomography (CT) scans of the sinuses are highly sensitive for sinusitis and should be performed rather than plain x-rays. In patients with chronic, recurrent otitis media, CT of the mastoids may be helpful in diagnosing mastoiditis, which may be present in the absence of classic signs such as mastoid tenderness and cutaneous erythema.

7. True or false: An echocardiogram should be performed on every child with FUO to exclude endocarditis.

False. Although endocarditis may cause FUO, it is diagnosed chiefly from positive blood cultures in the presence of other suggestive findings (splenomegaly, microscopic hematuria, anemia, elevated sedimentation rate, and embolic phenomenon), not on the basis of echocardiographic findings. Echocardiographic findings are supportive, not diagnostic, of endocarditis and *cannot* exclude the possibility of endocarditis. Almost all children who develop endocarditis have some underlying cardiac anatomic abnormality that predisposes them to the development of endovascular infection. Gram-negative organisms rarely cause endocarditis, whereas gram-positive organisms such as staphylococci and streptococci are the most common causes of endovascular infection.

8. True or false: Children with FUO should have whole-body CT scans to diagnose occult neoplasm.

False. Although this approach may be necessary in some cases, the work-up is directed at subtle abnormalities in physical exam, such as regional adenopathy, splenomegaly, or musculoskeletal abnormalities. Suggestive history is important, such as travel to foreign countries, family history of autoimmune disorders, inflammatory bowel disease, or exposure to unusual environmental sources of infection or animals.

9. Describe the three-tiered hierarchy of evaluation for children with FUO.

The most broadly based, highest-yield, and most cost-effective testing is done first, and the lowest-yield, most esoteric testing is done last if no diagnosis is made despite persistence of symptoms. A template for evaluation is below.

Level I. CBC, comprehensive metabolic profile, chest x-ray (when indicated), sinus films (when indicated), blood cultures, sedimentation rate and C-reactive protein, stool and urine cultures, and purified protein derivative (PPD) test. Directed viral serologic tests may be indicated, based on history (e.g., cytomegalovirus and Epstein-Barr virus, not Monospot). In the absence of positive findings, level II studies are indicated.

Level II. Antinuclear antibody (ANA) and anti–double-stranded DNA titers, angiotensin-converting enzyme level (ACE), antistreptolysin O (ASO) titer, directed serologic tests (based on travel and exposure history), directed radiologic procedures (bone scan, CT of sinuses/mastoids or magnetic resonance imaging [MRI] or CT of region of complaint or abnormal physical findings), human immunodeficiency virus (HIV) test, and rapid plasmin reagin (RPR) test for syphilis (if indicated). Usually by the time level II testing is completed, the fever has resolved or a diagnosis is made. If fever persists, proceed to level III.

Level III. This level, which is uncommon in children but more common in adults, is reached after nearly 2 weeks of evaluation for FUO. Whole-body gallium scan for infection or adenopathy usually directs biopsy efforts. Bone marrow exam should be done with cultures for acid-fast bacillus (AFB) and fungus as well as routine bacterial cultures. Granulomas or other findings may further direct appropriate serologic testing. Liver biopsy is performed in rare cases for further evaluation of granulomatous hepatitis in the absence of other positive findings.

10. Ten days ago a boy returned from a 3-week stay in India with fevers, chills, crampy abdominal pain, and diarrhea that tested negative for occult blood. He took mefloquine weekly while in India and for 1 week after his return. Which of the following is the likely diagnosis: malaria due to *Plasmodium falciparum*, brucellosis, typhoid fever, or intestinal tuberculosis?

His stool and urine cultures were positive for *Salmonella typhi*, and he was treated with intravenous cefotaxime for 4 days until afebrile, then continued on oral trimethoprim-sulfa for 2 weeks. Malaria is common in India, but the history of ongoing mefloquine prophylaxis makes malaria unlikely.

11. Another patient presents with fevers 3½ weeks after returning from 2 months in India. The physical exam is negative with the exception of a large cervical lymph node. What should be done to make a diagnosis?

Tuberculosis (TB) should be considered in this setting. The PPD test was positive. Chest x-ray revealed no evidence of active pulmonary TB, but this does not exclude extrapulmonic infection such as cervical adenitis due to TB. Throat culture yielded *Staphylococcus aureus*, and cervical node biopsy was negative for AFB and granulomas and positive on bacterial culture for *S. aureus*. The patient responded well to oral antistaphylococcal medications. He was also treated with isoniazid for 6 months for tuberculosis prophylaxis. Common illnesses remain common, even in returning travelers!

12. A 14-day-old infant has fevers as high as 104°F. Septic evaluation revealed no cerebrospinal fluid abnormalities, and blood culture was positive for *S. aureus*. White blood cell count was 30,000, and the sedimentation rate was 85 mm/hr. The infant did not move his right leg on presentation, maintaining a frog-leg position at rest, and cried when his diaper was changed with painful range of motion of the hip. Erythema at the umbilical stump site is minimal. The practice at the hospital where he was born was to wash the umbilical stump with soap and water (no gentian violet, no alcohol). What is the diagnosis?

S. aureus may be a skin contaminant in blood cultures, but in the setting of pain with motion of the right hip, umbilical erythema, and poor umbilical stump care, concern for a deep-seated staphylococcal infection in the region of the hip is high. Plain films of the leg revealed no osteomyelitis, and ultrasound revealed no sign of septic joint. CT scan of the pelvis revealed a large psoas muscle abscess. The abscess was not drained but resolved with prolonged intravenous antibiotic therapy. Because of the lack of umbilical-related infections and the purple stain of gentian violet, many hospitals have changed umbilical care policies to use of alcohol alone. This hospital, in fact, had changed its policy to use of soap and water alone! After an increase in umbilical stump infections, the hospital mandated alcohol use. The author's preference is gentian violet, because it is highly effective against staphylococci and, unlike alcohol, you can tell that it has been used!

13. True or false: Patients with Kawasaki disease are easily diagnosed by the presence of fever, rash, swelling and tenderness of hands and feet, hypertrophic tongue papillae, elevated sedimentation rate, and elevated C-reactive protein.

False. Kawasaki's disease may present without any of the characteristic physical findings except the one hallmark symptom of fever. Other physical findings, including rash and hand/feet swelling, may be totally absent. Sedimentation rate and C-reactive protein are reliably elevated, but not always in the "astoundingly high" range. In toxic-appearing children with FUO, Kawasaki's disease should be included in the differential diagnosis. An echocardiogram should be considered; treatment includes intravenous immune globulin and aspirin within 7 days of the onset of fever. Side effects of therapy are minimal compared with the potentially devastating outcome if the disease is not treated appropriately.

14. A 5-year-old boy presents with fevers up to 104.5°F for 6 days and a flushed, slapped-cheek appearance to his face. The mother, who is 24 weeks pregnant, reports that these symptoms have been "going around the school" and asks what can be done to stop the fevers. Your partner prescribes ibuprofen and acetaminophen. The mother calls back on Friday night in a panic because a friend told her that exposure to the boy's illness may cause her to lose the pregnancy. What do you do?

In most settings parvovirus B19 infection can be diagnosed on the basis of history and physical examination alone. In this setting, with an expectant mother at risk, serologic tests must be obtained, and the obstetric physician should be notified of possible exposure. If serologic tests are positive for acute infection, the mother should be tested to determine whether she is immune. The unborn child is at risk only if mother has an acute infection. Parvovirus may cause a persistent infection with fevers lasting for weeks in patients with dys- or hypogammaglobulinemia or HIV infection. Diagnosis involves findings of high levels of parvovirus IgM in the absence or presence of high levels of parvovirus IgG. HIV serology should be checked in all patients with this persistent infection. Treatment is intravenous immune globulin.

15. A 9-year-old boy presents with a chronic cough, recurrent asthma attacks refractory to oral and aerosolized steroids and beta agonists, and low-grade fevers up to 100°F for months. A previous doctor had treated him with many courses of antibiotics but had avoided macrolides because of an erythromycin allergy with hives. What is your diagnosis?

The diagnosis is chronic chlamydial pneumonia with hyperreactive airways secondary to infection. Because the boy's 16-month-old cousin recently succumbed to neuroblastoma, the parents were naturally anxious. PPD was nonreactive, and CT scan of the chest revealed no anatomic pulmonary or vascular findings. Sedimentation rate was 50, and the serologic test for *Chlamydia pneumoniae* was positive (> 1:512). The boy was treated with doxycycline for 28 days, and the fevers and poor asthma control resolved. Sedimentation rate normalized. The boy avoided the normal rotation of antibiotics because of his uncommon macrolide allergy. Because doxycycline is far less active as a calcium chelator than tetracycline, it may be used in children under age 8.

16. A 7-year-old girl presents with daily fevers up to 102–103°F for 2½ weeks. Her mother is a nurse, her father a general surgeon. Initially they were not worried, but now their daughter refuses to walk and needs to be carried to the bathroom. You find an enlarged spleen, peripheral nonblanching petechial rash, and no erythema or swelling of any joints. Despite this profile, the patient refuses to bear weight. What tests should you order?

CBC revealed normal white cell count, low hemoglobin at 8.6, and platelet count of 36 k. Ferritin was elevated at 1200 and LDH at 936. The sedimentation rate was 56, and C-RP level was 25; AST and ALT were elevated at twice normal. Chest-ray showed no abnormality. This unfortunate child has signs of chronic illness with low hemoglobin and decreased bone marrow function with low platelets. Although juvenile rheumatoid arthritis is of concern, the significant hematologic findings are worrisome for acute hematologic malignancy.

The second battery of tests should include CT scan of the chest, MRI of the spleen and liver, blood cultures, and bone marrow exam and biopsy. Bone marrow exam revealed acute lymphoblastic leukemia.

17. The 19-year-old daughter of a local pediatrician complains of fevers up to 100.5°F nearly every day for 2 months. She also complains of tender swollen erythematous plaques in the anterior tibial regions, just proximal to the ankles. She denies diarrhea or crampy abdominal pain. She is anxious to return to school in southern Arizona because her legs are less tender in the warm weather. Which of the following is the likely diagnosis: Crohn's disease with erythema nodosum, psoriatic arthritis, cryoglobulinemia, or coccidiomycosis?

The association of college in southern Arizona should suggest coccidiomycosis, which was confirmed by positive serologic tests and is a common cause of erythema nodosum. The chest x ray was unremarkable. The patient improved with oral fluconazole, which was given for 4 weeks. Antibody titers decreased, and she remains asymptomatic.

18. Four weeks ago a 19-year-old Hispanic male returned from a 1-month stay at his family's home in rural Mexico. He has been running fevers up to 103°F every day for 10 days. He works as a landscaper. His chest x-ray shows no abnormality, and he has chills with each spiking fever (daily at sundown). Laboratory abnormalities include sedimentation rate of 125 mm/hr, ferritin > 3000, CRP of 25, and liver enzymes elevated at 3 times normal. Blood and urine cultures are negative, and surface echocardiogram reveals no abnormality. Bone marrow exam reveals normal cellular elements with noncaseating granulomas. PPD is positive. Which of the following is the likely diagnosis: brucellosis, sarcoidosis, Q fever, extrapulmonic tuberculosis, or disseminated fungal infection?

Markedly elevated titers of *Coxiella burnetii* established a diagnosis of Q fever. Bone marrow cultures eventually yielded *C. burnetii,* which is a hazard to laboratory workers. The patient was treated with doxycycline, and his fever abated. Q fever endocarditis, which has a mortality rate of 40%, is a concern in chronic infections, but the lack of findings on echocardiogram and lack of relapse after 4 weeks of oral doxycycline therapy support a low probability of this condition. Because Q fever is an agent that can be used for bioterrorism, it is immediately reportable to the state health department.

Noncaseating granulomas commonly are found with fungal infections and sarcoidosis. Tuberculosis (TB) is classically associated with caseating granulomas. Bone marrow was cultured for AFB and fungus, but a positive culture may require 4–6 weeks. Levels of angiotensin-converting enzyme (ACE), which is associated with sarcoidosis, were minimally elevated. Serologic tests for histoplasmosis (risk factors include exposure to bat droppings and adobe construction dust) were negative. Histoplasmosis and TB are unlikely because of the negative findings on chest X ray. Histoplasmosis frequently reveals pneumonic changes in acute illness and small calcified granulomas with old or chronic disease. Serologic tests for histoplasmosis, blastomycosis, and coccidiomycosis have good predictive value when positive but poor predictive value when negative. In all situations, paired sera-reflective acute and convalescent titers are important to establish a diagnosis. Brucellosis, which is not uncommon in rural Mexico, was unlikely because of negative serologies.

19. A 14-year-old girl presents with daily fevers up to 101.5°F for 3 weeks. She also has severe low-level back pain that comes and goes. She denies postural improvements of back pain. She is unable to sleep more than 1 or 2 hours because of back pain. Before developing the fevers, she had a sore throat that was positive on culture for beta-hemolytic streptococci. She has shaking chills each day after the febrile spike. She has no history of travel or heart murmur. Laboratory tests reveal normal white blood cell count; borderline anemia with hypochromic, microcytic indices; elevated sedimentation rate at 39 mm/hr; C-RP of 17; and normal serum chemistries and liver enzyme studies. Plain films of the back revealed no bony spinal abnormalities. MRIs of the lumbar and thoracic spine revealed no evidence of spinal canal tumor, abscess, or bone infection or destruction. Bone scan revealed increased uptake in the lumbar spine articular facets, which did not correlate with MRI findings. What should be done next?

Blood work, including CBC; cultures (multiple sets); and repeat sedimentation rate, CRP, and ferritin liver functions. CRP level and sedimentation rate were similar to the previous values. Ferritin (an acute-phase reactant that is markedly elevated in neuroblastoma) was normal. LDH (commonly elevated in lymphoma) and alkaline phosphatase were normal for age. Blood cultures were negative, as was the test for HLA-B27, which is closely associated with postinfectious inflammatory syndromes (e.g., Reiter's syndrome, ankylosing spondyloarthritis). Antinuclear antibody, ACE level, and Lyme western blot tests were negative. Serologic tests for *Brucella* spp., which can cause severe sacroiliac pain in chronic infections, were negative. Gallium scan, which is sensitive for regional adenopathy or infection, revealed no focal increased uptake through 72 hours after injection. Fevers and back pain continued despite treatment with indomethacin, and repeat MRI 5 weeks after onset of fever revealed increased T2-weighted signal in the L2–L3 disc space and adjacent vertebral bodies consistent with discitis. The patient was placed on intravenous ceftriaxone for 6 weeks, and back pain gradually improved over the first 10 days on therapy.

This case teaches several lessons. Tests such as gallium scan cannot reliably rule out diagnoses, and high-yield tests, such as MRI of the region of pain, may need to be repeated if symptoms do not improve or fevers do not resolve. A negative initial work-up is nothing more than a negative initial work-up. The pursuit of a diagnosis must be dogged and dedicated. Involvement of other specialists (e.g., rheumatologist, hematologist) may be crucial.

20. A 13-year old girl has been running fevers up to 103°F since her return from a soccer tournament 1 week ago. She has no upper respiratory tract symptoms and no signs of pneumonia. Her father, who accompanied her on the trip, was just hospitalized for a case of pneumonia that is progressing despite therapy. Two other teammates have similar fevers, and one other adult chaperone is hospitalized on a ventilator for pneumonia. Liver function studies are minimally elevated. Her father, who is a smoker, had abdominal pain and diarrhea before the onset of pneumonia. He has markedly elevated liver enzymes and

hyponatremia with serum sodium level of 124. Of interest, the patient's heart rate remains normal (in the 70s) during the febrile spikes. The patient's mother thinks that all of these cases are connected. What is the likely diagnosis?

The key is the father's hyponatremia with elevated liver enzymes and temperature-pulse discordance, which are classic findings of *Legionella* infection. This infection is acquired through a common environmental source, such as evaporative water coolers, hot tubs, or contaminated hot water supplies. All of the soccer families stayed in the same hotel, which had old water heaters caked with lime. The water temperature was warm enough to encourage growth of *Legionella* organisms but not hot enough to kill them. Pneumonia can follow a prodrome of abdominal pain and diarrhea but usually occurs only in persons with impaired lung function, such as patients with chronic obstructive pulmonary disease or underlying immune deficits. It can occur in normal persons as well.

Pontiac fever can be seen in persons infected with Legionella species who do not develop pneumonia. It usually resolves even without therapy in 2-3 weeks. Temperature-pulse discordance is common in *Legionella* infection, as it is in rheumatic fever and typhoid infection. It can also be observed with higher-than-expected heart rates in thyroiditis and thyroid disease. Heart rate is expected to rise 10 beats per minute for every degree centigrade over 37°. Calcium channel blockers, beta blockers, and amiodarone can block this response. Although a urine sample that tests positive for *Legionella* antigen is diagnostic, a negative result does not exclude infection. The urinalysis tests for the one serotype that causes two-thirds of human *Legionella* infections but does not test for the serotypes that cause the other one-third of infections. Antibiotics used to treat *Legionella* infection include erythromycin, doxycycline, and azithromycin. Although quinolones have been reported to have activity against *Legionella* spp., treatment failures have been observed.

21. True or false: The most important aspects of an FUO work-up are a detailed, expansive history and a detailed physical examination.

True. Many cases can be diagnosed by a thorough history that reveals some long-forgotten exposure or important detail of illness. Secondly, physical exam with directed evaluation of any abnormal findings is important. Lastly, diligence in pursuing the diagnosis is important. FUO is the most difficult and exhausting work-up for any adult or child (except for chronic fatigue, of course).

XII. Special Infectious Disease Problems

37. HUMAN IMMUONDEFICIENCY VIRUS INFECTION IN CHILDREN

David P. Regis, M.D., and Linda L. Lewis, M.D.

1. When do most perinatal transmissions of HIV occur?

The most common mode of pediatric HIV transmission is perinatal transmission. It is estimated that approximately 65% of vertical transmissions occur during the intrapartum period.

2. List common risk factors for perinatal HIV transmission.

- High maternal viral load
- Advanced maternal disease/immunosuppression
- Rupture of membranes > 4 hours
- Prematurity
- Low birth weight
- Breastfeeding
- Micronutrient deficiency (vitamin A)
- Smoking
- Chorioamnionitis
- Intercurrent sexually transmitted diseases
- Invasive procedures (e.g., amniocentesis, chorionic villous sampling, fetal blood sampling)
- High risk behaviors

3. What is the rate of maternal-fetal transmission of HIV?

Based on data from the Pediatric AIDS Clinical Trials Group Protocol 076 (PACTG 076) and international antiretroviral prophylaxis clinical trials, the rate of transmission to infants whose mothers received no prophylaxis ranges from 17% to 45%. Prophylaxis reduced this rate by up to 70%, with documentation of perinatal transmission rates as low as 3-4% in developed countries and 5–10% in developing countries, even in woman with advanced disease. For women receiving antiretroviral therapy who have undetectable viral burdens and avoid breastfeeding the rate can be < 2%.

4. What are the recommended prophylactic regimens for pregnant women with HIV?

The most experience involves the ACTG 076 study regimen with oral zidovudine (ZDV) given to the mother during pregnancy, intravenous ZDV given intrapartum to the mother, and and oral ZDV started in the infant within 6–12 hours of birth. Other regimens use combinations of oral ZDV, nevirapine, and 3TC or nevirapine alone for both mother and infant. The table below summarizes several possible regimens for women who have not received prior therapy. The current recommendation in the U.S. is to treat all pregnant women with HIV therapy that is appropriate for their stage of disease, using at least the PACTG 076 regimen if they otherwise are not candidates for therapy and additional drugs as suggested by current adult treatment guidelines. However, little is known about the pharmacokinetics and safety of antiretrovirals other than ZDV during pregnancy.

Prophylactic Regimens for HIV-Infected Women with No Prior Antiretroviral Therapy

DRUG(S)	MATERNAL REGIMEN	INFANT REGIMEN	STUDIED IN
ZDV	Oral ZDV during pregnancy, then 2 mg/kg IV bolus followed by continuous infusion of 1 mg/kg/hr until delivery	2 mg/kg orally every 6 hr for 6 wk	ACTG 076; data from U.S. compared with placebo

Continued on following page

Prophylactic Regimens for HIV-Infected Women with No Prior Antiretroviral Therapy (Cont.)

DRUG(S)	MATERNAL REGIMEN	INFANT REGIMEN	STUDIED IN
ZDV + 3TC	ZDV: 600 mg orally at onset of labor followed by 300 mg orally every 3 hr until delivery *and* 3TC: 150 mg orally at onset of labor followed by 150 mg orally every 12 hr until delivery	ZDV: 4 mg/kg orally every 12 hr *and* 3TC: 2 mg/kg orally every 12 hr for 1 wk	PETRA: data from clinical trial in Africa compared with placebo
Nevirapine	One 200-mg dose orally at onset of labor	One 2-mg/kg dose orally at 48–72 hr*	HIVNET 012; data from clinical trial in Africa compared with oral ZDV to mother and 1 wk of ZDV to infant
ZDV + nevirapine	ZDV: 2-mg/kg bolus IV, followed by continuous infusion of 1 mg/kg/hr until delivery *and* Nevirapine: single dose of 200mg orally at onset of labor	ZDV: 2-mg/kg bolus orally every 6 hr for 6 wk *and* Nevirapine: single dose of 2 mg/kg orally at age 48–72 hr	Not studied

*If the mother received nevirapine < 1 hour before delivery, the infant was given 2 doses, one as soon as possible and the other at 48–72 hours.
Adapted from: Public Health Service Task Force Recommendations for Use of Antiretroviral Drugs in Pregnant HIV-1-Infected Women for Maternal Health and Interventions to Reduce Perinatal HIV-1 Transmission in the United States, February 4, 2002.

5. What is the primary complication of ZDV therapy in neonates?

The primary complication of the 6-week course of ZDV is anemia. Therefore, the newborn should have a baseline complete blood count with differential at birth before starting ZDV and a repeat hematologic evaluation at the end of therapy and at 12 weeks of age when any toxic effects attributed to ZDV should be resolved. More intensive monitoring is recommended for infants with anemia at birth or prematurity as well as infants who are given combination antiretroviral therapy or whose mothers received combination antiretroviral therapy.

6. What is the most appropriate screening test for infants born to mothers with HIV?

Because the HIV enzyme-linked immunosorbent assay (ELISA) tests only for the presence of antibodies, it almost assuredly will be positive in the newborn period because of transfer of maternal antibodies across the placenta. Therefore, the ELISA gives many false-positive results. The earliest age at which an ELISA is considered reliable for the diagnosis of HIV is 18 months. Therefore, the diagnostic test of choice is the qualitative HIV DNA polymerase chain reaction (PCR), which tests for the presence of viral DNA in the blood. This test is preferred over the quantitative HIV RNA PCR, which may give a false-negative result in the neonate who is infected but has little or no active viral replication at the time of sampling.

7. How sensitive is DNA PCR for HIV testing in the newborn?

HIV DNA PCR is positive in approximately 38% of infected infants tested in the first 48 hours of life. It is not until the second week of life, when most infections are already established, that the sensitivity rises to 93% by 14 days of life and as high as 95% after the first month of life.

8. True or false: Cord blood is an acceptable specimen for HIV testing of the neonate born to a mother with HIV.

False. There is a significant risk of contamination with maternal blood.

9. How is the diagnosis of HIV infection confirmed in the newborn whose mother has HIV?

To confirm the diagnosis, two separate specimens from the infant must test positive on virologic assays (DNA or RNA PCR). A presumptive diagnosis can be based on either one positive result (not from the cord blood) or presentation with an AIDS-defining illness. In either case, however, confirmatory testing is recommended. Currently, the American Academy of Pediatrics recommends that the infant be tested in the first 48 hours of life, at 1–2 months, and at 3–6 months of age, with confirmatory testing repeated at any time a positive result is obtained. HIV infection can be reasonably excluded by documenting two or more negative virologic tests at or after 1 month of age with at least one of the tests done at or after 4 months of age.

10. Will the use of ZDV in neonates delay the diagnosis of those who are actually infected with the virus?

Current data do not suggest any delay in the diagnosis of HIV in the neonate who has received the prophylactic ZDV regimen. However, it is currently unknown whether more highly potent combination antiretroviral therapy has any effect on virologic testing.

11. True or false: It is safe for an HIV-infected mother to breastfeed her infant.

False. The vertical transmission of HIV from mother to infant via breastmilk is well established and is estimated to increase the risk of transmission by as much as 50%. In the U.S., where alternatives to breastfeeding are available, new mothers infected with HIV should be counseled not to breastfeed their newborn to reduce the chance of transmission.

12. Should pregnancy preclude a woman infected with HIV from taking combination antiretroviral therapy?

No—although data about combination antiretroviral therapy during pregnancy are limited. Early studies appeared to show an elevated risk of preterm delivery among infants whose mothers received combination antiretroviral therapy (with or without protease inhibitors); however, preliminary data from more recent studies do not support this finding. Likewise, there is concern for exacerbation of pregnancy-induced hyperglycemia by the use of protease inhibitors as well as the potential for mitochondrial toxicity from the nucleoside analogs in both mother and infant. At this time, however, it is unclear whether these conditions are induced or exacerbated by their respective agents. Their occurrence appears to be rare and should be compared with the benefits of reducing the transmission of a fatal infection by 70% and the reconstitution and maintenance of the mother's immune system. The decision ultimately lies with the mother and her health care provider after careful consideration of the effects of the particular therapy on both mother and fetus/newborn. with close monitoring during pregnancy and after delivery for adverse events.

13. Are there any particular antiretroviral drug combinations that a pregnant woman should avoid?

Because of reports of several maternal deaths due to lactic acidosis with prolonged use of the combination of d4T (stavudine) and ddI (didanosine) in HIV-infected pregnant women, this combination should be prescribed with caution and only when other combinations have failed or caused intolerable toxicity or side effects. Likewise, efavirenz should not be used during pregnancy because of the potential for teratogenicity identified in animal toxicology studies.

14. How does viral RNA load affect perinatal HIV transmission?

Viral RNA load, expressed as copies/ml, is an indication of the level of viral replication within the patient and is used as a measure of disease burden as well as efficacy of therapy. High viral load is a risk factor for transmission. Conversely, women on combination therapy with undetectable viral loads (defined by the lower limits of detection for a particular assay, usually < 50 or < 400 copies/ml) have < 2% chance of transmitting HIV to their child. Two points must be emphasized: there is no absolute cut-off for viral load and perinatal transmission, and transmission has been documented even with undetectable RNA levels.

15. What role do cesarean sections play in the management of perinatal HIV transmission?

In women who have received no antiretroviral therapy and present for care late in pregnancy, a scheduled cesarean section can reduce transmission by up to 50%, depending on maternal viral load. The HIV/AIDS Treatment Information Service and the American College of Obstetricians and Gynecologists have chosen 1,000 copies/ml as the cut-off for recommending a scheduled cesarean section; this is the point at which the potential risks of such a procedure begin to be overshadowed by the benefits of reducing the risk of transmission. For woman who are on therapy and have viral RNA loads < 1,000 copies/ml, a cesarean section is unlikely to provide added benefit. Currently, no data are available about performing a cesarean section on women who are at higher risk of transmission and who are already in labor or have ruptured membranes. Some data suggest little effect on the reduction of transmission, especially with membranes that have been ruptured > 4–6 hours.

16. For an HIV-infected mother who is pregnant with twins, which twin is at higher risk for transmission of the virus?

The first twin delivered has the higher risk of being infected (35% vs. 15%) for reasons not completely understood but most likely due to longer exposure to vaginal secretions in late pregnancy and during labor.

17. What is the current recommendation for antiretroviral therapy in infants, children, and adolescents infected with HIV?

Currently the most strongly recommended regimen in infected infants, children, and adolescents (who are not pregnant) consists of a combination of two nucleoside reverse transcriptase inhibitors (NRTIs) and a protease inhibitor (PI). Another strongly recommended regimen for children who can swallow capsules includes efavirenz, a non-nucleoside reverse transcriptase inhibitor (NNRTI), plus two NRTIs or efavirenz in combination with the PI nelfinavir and one NRTI. Compared with monotherapy, combination therapy has been shown to slow disease progression, improve survival rates, provide greater and more sustained virologic and immunologic response, and delay the emergence of resistant mutants.

18. Explain the acronym HAART.

Highly **a**ctive **a**ntiretroviral **t**herapy is a common term to denote combination antiretroviral regimens shown to be highly effective in clinical trials.

19. What are the major differences between pediatric/perinatal HIV infection and adult HIV infection?

Perinatal HIV infection occurs during a child's growth and development, thus affecting the immune system before it can mature. Consequently, virologic parameters differ from those seen in adults, as do manifestations of disease. Close monitoring of growth and development is essential because deterioration may be an early indication of disease and corrective measures can affect immune function, drug activity, and quality of life.

20. True or false: A detectable HIV RNA level within the first 48 hours of life (early/in utero HIV infection) is a prognostic indicator for more rapid disease progression.

False. Although some investigators have proposed that infants with early HIV infection may be at risk for rapid disease progression, more recent prospective studies have suggested that HIV RNA levels at 1 month of age are more predictive for progression of HIV infection than those measured at the time of initial positive status. However, the overall predictive value is only moderate, and a better predictor may be how the combination of the CD4+ T-cell counts/percentage and RNA levels trend over time.

21. Which is a better marker of identifying disease progression in children, CD4+ T-cell number or percentage?

Although both absolute CD4+ T-cell count and CD4+ T-cell percentage indicate the level of immune suppression for a given age, the absolute CD4+ T-cell count changes with age, whereas

CD4+ T-cell percentage does not. Therefore a change in CD4+ T-cell percentage may be a better marker for disease progression.

22. At what levels of CD4+ T-cell percentage are children considered immune suppressed? How are HIV-infected children classified clinically?

The Centers for Disease Control and Prevention (CDC) published the following classification scheme to identify levels of immune suppression based on CD4+ T-cell measurements. A similar scheme categorizes clinical severity based on indicator signs/symptoms and secondary diseases.

CDC 1994 Revised Classification of HIV Infection in Children < 13 Years of Age

IMMUNOLOGIC CATEGORY	CD4+ T-CELL %
Category 1: no suppression	≥ 25%
Category 2: moderate suppression	15–24%
Category 3: severe suppression	< 15%

CLINICAL CATEGORY	DEFINITION
Category N: no symptoms	No signs or symptoms attributed to HIV infection or only one of the symptoms listed in category A.
Category A: mild symptoms	≥ 2 of the following symptoms but none of the symptoms from categories B or C: lymphadenopathy > 0.5 cm at 2 sites; hepatomegaly; splenomegaly; dermatitis, parotitis; recurrent or persistent upper respiratory infection, sinusitis, or otitis media.
Category B: moderate symptoms	Symptoms other than those in categories A or C, including anemia, neutropenia, or thrombocytopenia lasting ≥ 30 days; single episode of bacterial meningitis, pneumonia, or sepsis; oropharyngeal candidiasis lasting > 2 months in a child > 6 months old; cardiomyopathy; cytomegalovirus (CMV) infection before 1 month of age; chronic or recurrent diarrhea; hepatitis; > 2 episodes per year of herpes simplex virus (HSV) stomatitis; HSV bronchitis, pneumonitis. or esophagitis before 1 month of age; two episodes of herpes zoster or episode involving more than one dermatome; leiomyosarcoma; lymphoid intersitial pneumonitis/pulmonary lymphoid hyperplasia (LIP/PLH); nephropathy; nocardiosis; fever > 1 month; toxoplasmosis before 1 month of age; disseminated varicella infection.
Category C: severe symptoms	Any condition listed in the 1987 surveillance case definition of AIDS with the exception of LIP (e.g., *Pneumocystis carinii* pneumonia, CMV retinitis, extrapulmonary cryptococcal infection, mycobacterial infections).

Adapted from: CDC: 1994 revised classification system for human immunodeficiency virus infection in children less than 13 years of age. MMWR 43:1-17, 1994.

23. When should therapeutic changes be considered in a pediatric patient with HIV?

Changes in therapy are based on changes in HIV RNA copy number, but in the setting of an otherwise clinically stable infection there can be considerable interpatient variation in RNA levels. Over the course of a few days, copy numbers can range up to threefold ($0.5 \log_{10}$) in adults and probably higher in infants. Therefore, only changes greater than fivefold ($0.7 \log_{10}$) for children < 2 years old, and changes greater than threefold ($0.5 \log_{10}$) for children ≥ 2 years, on two different measurements, should be considered significant. Immunologic criteria that warrant a change in therapy include a change in immune classification, a persistent decline in CD4+ T-cell percentage of five or more percentiles for those with CD4+ T-cell percentages < 15%, or a > 30% decline in absolute CD4+ T-cell count in < 6 months. Clinical events that may warrant therapeutic changes include progressive neurodevelopmental deterioration, unexplained growth failure despite adequate nutrition, or other signs of disease progression in conjunction with any of the above changes in virologic or immunologic status.

24. What extrinsic factors may cause a transient elevation in HIV RNA levels?

The two major extrinsic causes of transient elevations in RNA levels are recent immunizations and concurrent illness.

25. Are there any advantages of using one HIV RNA quantitation assay over another?

No. It is important, however, that the same assay be used to monitor each patient, if possible, because variation among assay methods can be considerable.

26. At what age should children receiving HIV medications be dosed as adults?

Children with Tanner stage V should be dosed according to adult schedules. Children who are Tanner stage III or IV should be dosed according to pediatric recommendations but should be monitored closely for efficacy and toxicity during this stage of relatively rapid development.

27. Should all HIV-infected children receive antiretroviral treatment?

Most experts agree that treatment should be offered to all infected children meeting the following criteria: (1) those who are < 1 year old; (2) those who are symptomatic. regardless of age; and (3) those demonstrating significant increases in HIV RNA levels or decreases in CD4+ T-cell percentages (< 25%). Few data are available for asymptomatic children with stable, low RNA levels and relatively normal immunologic status. Ultimately, the decision to treat such children should be based on input from provider, patient, and parent. Careful consideration should be given to the family's ability to adhere to a proposed regimen. The provider may wish to postpone therapy if adequate adherence is unlikely, because lack of adherence has been associated with rapid selection of resistant mutants, especially to the protease inhibitors.

28. Should the initial antiretroviral therapy for an infant with HIV be based on the mother's regimen?

Not necessarily. However, if antiretroviral resistance patterns are known for the mother, consideration should be given for testing of the infant's isolate to help direct therapy.

29. What are the goals of combination therapy?

The goals of therapy are to maximize suppression of viral replication while maintaining or reconstituting immune function and to minimize the emergence of resistant HIV. Ideally, HIV RNA levels should be below the limits of detection of the assay, although this goal is not always possible.

30. When should one expect to see a maximal response once antiretroviral therapy has been initiated?

In infants, who tend to have higher HIV RNA levels, it may take 8–12 weeks before the maximal response is noted. When RNA levels are closer to those seen in adults (< 100,000 copies/ml), 4 weeks is a reasonable time to judge the extent of efficacy for a given regimen.

31. What is the most effective way of preventing opportunistic infections in children with HIV?

Administration of a potent HAART regimen is the most effective way of preventing opportunistic infections by reconstituting and maintaining adequate immunity.

32. True or false: Children with HIV who are moderately immunosuppressed (CD4+ T cells between 15% and 24%) should not receive the measles/mumps/rubella (MMR) vaccine.

False. Only children who are severely immunosuppressed (CD4+ T cell < 15%) should avoid vaccination with the live MMR vaccine. In fact, it is recommended that children with HIV receive the MMR vaccine as soon as possible after their first birthday with consideration for a booster as soon as 1 month after. This recommendation contrasts to that for the varicella vaccine, which should be given only to asymptomatic, nonimmunosuppressed (CDC Category N1) HIV-infected children.

33. True or false: Infants born to HIV-infected mothers should be placed on prophylaxis for *Pneumocyctis carinii* pneumonia (PCP).

True. Beginning at 4-6 weeks of age, infants born to mothers infected with HIV or suspected of having HIV should receive appropriate PCP prophylaxis. Therapy should be continued until the child is considered not infected with HIV (by testing as outlined in question 9) or until 12 months of age. If the child's immune status is adequate (CD4+ T cells > 15%) and the child has not had PCP, consideration should be given to stopping prophylaxis at that time.

34. What is the first-choice agent for PCP prophylaxis?

The first choice for PCP prophylaxis is trimethoprim-sulfamethoxazole (TMP-SMZ) at 150 mg/m^2 TMP and 750 mg/m^2 SMZ, divided into two doses per day and given 3 days per week. This regimen carries the extra benefit of simultaneous prophylaxis against *Toxoplasma gondii* infections. Alternative schedules and regimens are available for patients who are unable to adhere to the regimen or cannot tolerate TMP-SMX because of allergy or side effects.

35. Summarize guidelines for households of HIV-infected persons that have or want a pet.

To avoid exposure to *Cryptosporidium, Salmonella,* and *Campylobacter* spp., HIV-infected children and their household members should avoid purchasing dogs or cats younger than 6 months, adopting stray animals, or bringing animals with diarrhea into the household. In households with pets, the HIV-infected person should avoid contact with the feces of the animal to avoid exposure to *Cryptosporidium* as well as *Toxoplasma*. If a dog or cat brought into the home is younger than 6 months or is a stray, the owners should ask the veterinarian to test the animal's stool for *Cryptosporidium*, *Salmonella*, and *Campylobacter* spp. Contact with reptiles also should be avoided to reduce the risk of salmonellosis, and gloves should be worn during cleaning aquariums to avoid exposure to *Mycobacterium marinum*.

36. Should HIV–infected persons receive the influenza vaccine?

Yes. All people with HIV should receive the influenza vaccine annually. In addition, other people living in the same household with an immunocompromised person should consider immunization against influenza. During an outbreak of influenza A, consideration should be given to prophylaxis for children aged 1–9 years with rimantadine or amantadine at 5 mg/kg/day, divided into 2 doses; adult doses are used for for children > 10 years. Although the newer neuraminidase inhibitors, oseltamivir and zanamivir, are probably effective, there is little experience with their use in the pediatric population.

37. What are the most common diagnoses for an HIV-infected child found to have a focal brain lesion on head imaging for evaluation of headache?

The most common causes of a focal brain lesion in patients with HIV include toxoplasmosis, primary central nervous system lymphoma, and progressive multifocal leukoencephalopathy. Although some of these diseases have classic findings on radiologic imaging, no finding is pathognomonic, and there is considerable overlap among radiologic presentations and initial clinical manifestations. Current guidelines recommend empirical treatment for toxoplasmosis based on radiologic findings and serologic titers, with follow-up imaging after 2 weeks of therapy to identify a therapeutic response. If no response is noted, other diagnostic procedures should be considered.

38. A chest x-ray is performed on an HIV-infected child with signs and symptoms of cough, dyspnea and hypoxia. The study shows diffuse, multifocal lesions. What are some of the diagnostic considerations?

Radiographic findings of the chest in children infected with HIV are not always specific, and interpretation should take the patient's immune status into consideration. Tuberculosis and other bacterial infections should be carefully investigated, and consideration also should be given to PCP, fungal infections, and lymphoid interstitial pneumonitis/pulmonary lymphoid hyperplasia, an insidious and slowly progressive disease that also includes generalized lymphadenopathy, hepatosplenomegaly, and digital clubbing. Viral pneumonia, including CMV, may present with similar findings.

39. What are the most common AIDS-defining conditions in children?

The most common AIDS-defining infection in children is PCP. Other common AIDS-defining conditions include lymphoid interstitial pneumonitis, recurrent bacterial infections, HIV wasting syndrome, HIV encephalopathy, esophageal candidiasis, cytomegalovirus disease, and *Mycobacterium avium-intracellulare* complex infection.

40. In an otherwise previously healthy child, are there any particular illnesses that should make a practitioner consider testing for HIV infection?

In general, the identification of any infection or recurrence of infection that would be considered unusual in an otherwise normal host should prompt HIV testing. Some of the more common HIV-related opportunistic pathogens are listed above. If you think that HIV is a possibility, perform the test.

41. What are the different classes of antiretroviral drugs? How do they work?

The first class of antiretroviral drugs discovered was the nucleoside reverse transcriptase inhibitors (NRTIs). These drugs mimic the natural nucleosides of human DNA and exert their antiviral effect by being incorporated into the growing chain of viral DNA and functioning as DNA chain terminators. The non-nucleoside reverse transcriptase inhibitors (NNRTIs) act in a similar way. Protease inhibitors (PIs) block cleavage of viral protein precursors into proteins that form the virus core or yield functional viral enzymes. Other classes of drugs under investigation include inhibitors of HIV integrase and drugs that block entry of HIV into cells.

42. Metronidazole (Flagyl) should not be given in conjunction with either ritonavir (Norvir) or lopinavir/ritonavir (Kaletra) oral solution formulations. Why?

Because both Norvir and Kaletra oral solutions are formulated with a large amount of ethanol (about 40% by volume), administration with Flagyl may result in a disulfiram (Antabuse) reaction.

43. Why should Agenerase (amprenavir) oral solution not be given to children less than 4 years of age?

Agenerase is highly insoluble in water and requires propylene glycol to maintain it in solution. Younger children may not have the liver enzyme (alcohol dehydrogenase) required to metabolize propylene glycol effectively.

BIBLIOGRAPHY

1. Centers for Disease Control and Prevention: Guidelines for the use of antiretroviral agents in adults and adolescents. MMWR 47 (RR-5):1–82 (1998).
2. Centers for Disease Control and Prevention: Pediatric HIV/AIDS surveillance L262 slide series through 2000 (www.cdc.gov/hiv/graphics/pediatri.htm).
3. Centers for Disease Control and Prevention: Revised classification system for human immunodeficiency virus infection in children less than 13 years of age. MMWR 43 (No. RR-12):1–10, 1994.
4. Kline MW: Infectious complications of HIV infection. In Long SS, Pickering LK, Prober CG (eds): Principles and Practice of Pediatric Infectious Diseases. New York, Churchill Livingstone 1997, pp 755–761.
5. Penn ZJ, Ahmed S: Human immunodeficiency virus in pregnancy. Curr Obstet Gynaecol 10:190–195, 2000.
6. Public Health Service Task Force: Recommendations for use of antiretroviral drugs in pregnant HIV-1-infected women for maternal health and interventions to reduce perinatal HIV-1 transmission in the United States, February 4, 2002 (http://www.hivatis.org).
7. Report of the Committee on Infectious Diseases: Red Book 2000, 25th ed. American Academy of Pediatrics, 2000, pp 325–350.
8. Shearer WT, et al: Viral load and disease progression in infants infected with human immunodeficiency virus type 1. N Engl J Med 336:1337–1342, 1997.
9. U.S. Public Health Service/Infectious Diseases Society of America: Prevention of Opportunistic Infections Working Group: 1999 USPHS/IDSA guidelines for the prevention of opportunistic infections in persons infected with human immunodeficiency virus. Clin Infect Dis 30: S29–S65, 2000.
10. Working Group on Antiretroviral Therapy and Medical Management of HIV-Infected Children: Guidelines for the use of antiretroviral agents in pediatric HIV infection. December 14, 2001 pp 1-68. (http://www.hivatis.org).

38. INFECTIONS IN THE IMMUNOCOMPROMISED CHILD

Jeffrey M. Bergelson, M.D.

1. Should immunocompromised patients receive routine immunizations?

The major safety concern is the use of live attenuated virus (measles, mumps, rubella [MMR], oral polio vaccine, varicella, rotavirus, vaccinia) or live attenuated bacterial vaccines (bacille Calmette-Guérin [BCG], oral typhoid Ty21a) in patients with cellular or humoral immune deficiency. Fatal vaccine-associated poliovirus, vaccinia, BCG, and measles infections have occurred in patients with severe immunodeficiency. These vaccines are generally contraindicated, but there are a few exceptions.

2. What are the specific issues related to varicella vaccine?

Varicella vaccine has been given safely to children with acute lymphocytic leukemia whose disease has been in remission for at least 1 year but who still receive maintenance chemotherapy; the decision to immunize should be made in consultation with the child's oncologist. Varicella vaccine can also be given safely to HIV-infected children with normal CD4 lymphocyte counts, and its safety is now being studied in HIV patients with mild immunosuppression.

3. Can MMR be given to children with HIV infection?

Because of the severity of wild-type measles infection in children with HIV (40% mortality rate), immunization with MMR is recommended for HIV-infected children who are not severely immunocompromised. Two doses should be given: the first at age 12 months, the second 1 month later. MMR should not be given be given to HIV patients with severe immunosuppression.

4. True or false: Immunizations should not be given to patients receiving corticosteroid therapy.

False. In patients receiving corticosteroids, decisions about immunization should be made after considering both the steroid dose and the duration of treatment. Live vaccines can be given safely to children receiving physiologic or low therapeutic doses (< 2mg/kg/day of prednisone or < 20 mg in children weighing more than 10 kg). In patients receiving higher doses, administration of live vaccines should be delayed until steroids have been discontinued for at least 1 month.

5. True or false: Inactivated virus vaccines can be given safely to any immunocompromised child.

True. Inactivated virus vaccines (inactivated polio vaccine; hepatitis B; diphtheria, pertussis, tetanus [DPT]; Pneumovax; Prevnar, hepatitis A; rabies) can be given safely to any immunocompromised patient. However, some immunodeficient patients may not generate appropriate immune responses in response to vaccination. If at all possible, patients should receive routine immunizations before undergoing medical procedures that involve long-term immunosuppression (e.g., splenectomy or solid organ transplant).

6. Should siblings of immunocompromised children receive live virus vaccines?

Children vaccinated with MMR do not transmit virus to close contacts, and it is safe (and desirable) to immunize the siblings even of patients with severe immunodeficiency. Varicella vaccine can be transmitted only by vaccinees (5%) who develop a rash, and it is extremely rare for contacts of healthy vaccinees to develop even mild vaccine-associated illness. Given the much greater risks associated with transmission of wild-type virus within a family, it is recommended that siblings of immunocompromised children receive varicella vaccine; if a rash develops, direct contact with the susceptible child should be avoided.

7. What infections are associated with asplenia?

Asplenic children are at high risk of overwhelming infection caused by encapsulated bacteria (pneumococci, *Haemophilus influenzae*, and meningococci). After dog bites, they may suffer sepsis caused by capnocytophaga, an unusual gram-negative organism. In addition, babesiosis (and possibly malaria) may be particularly severe in asplenic patients.

8. In which patients has antibiotic prophylaxis been shown to be effective after splenectomy?

In young children (< 5 years old) with sickle cell disease, penicillin prophylaxis significantly reduces the incidence of pneumococcal sepsis. The efficacy of chemoprophylaxis has not been well studied in adults or in patients with asplenia or splenic dysfunction due to other causes. The risk of overwhelming infection is much greater in patients whose spleens were removed because of malignancy than in those splenectomized after trauma. Young children are at higher risk than adults.

9. How long should antibiotic prophylaxis be continued?

Some authorities recommend lifelong chemoprophylaxis, although compliance with prolonged regimens is imperfect and pneumococci resistant to penicillin are increasingly common. In sickle cell patients who have received pneumococcal vaccine, who have no history of severe pneumococcal infection, and who have not undergone surgical splenectomy, it appears safe to discontinue antibiotic prophylaxis after age 5 years.

Whether or not chemoprophylaxis is administered, immunization with 7-valent pneumococcal vaccine (for children < 5 years old) and or 23-valent polysaccharide vaccine (children > 2 years old) is essential for management for all asplenic children, along with immunization against *H. influenzae* and meningococci. Despite immunization and chemoprophylaxis overwhelming infection can still occur. Asplenic children with fever should be evaluated thoroughly, and if sepsis is suspected, empirical antibiotic therapy (cefotaxime + vancomycin) should be administered.

10. What effect do steroids have on the immune system?

Steroids have multiple effects on the immune system and impair both neutrophil and lymphocyte function. The immunosuppressive effects depend on both dose and duration of steroid therapy: patients receiving 2 mg/kg/day of prednisone (2 mg in adults) have significant impairment of cell-mediated immunity; the immune deficit is less severe in those receiving lower doses (or inhaled steroids). The risk of infection is greater with steroid courses longer than 3 weeks than it is with short courses, but even short pulses of high-dose steroids are immunosuppressive. After prolonged steroid treatment, immunosuppression may persist for 1–3 months.

11. What infections should cause concern in a patient taking steroids?

Perhaps the most tragic (and preventable) complication of steroid therapy is fatal varicella infection. Vaccination against varicella is especially important in children who are likely to be treated with steroids in the future. Seronegative patients treated with steroids should be specifically instructed to report immediately any exposure to chickenpox. Varicella immune globulin should be administered within 48 hours of exposure (and may be effective even at 96 hours), and patients who develop infection should be treated with acyclovir.

Steroid therapy predisposes patients to reactivation of mycobacterial infection and herpesvirus infection and to endemic fungal infections such as coccidioidomycosis and cryptococcosis. Systemic *Aspergillus* infections may occur. Reactivation of *Strongyloides stercoralis* may cause pulmonary infiltrates, fever, and sepsis in patients who were initially infected in endemic areas.

12. All patients taking high dose steroids for 1 month or more should receive prophylaxis with trimethoprim-sulfa. What infections are you trying to prevent?

Pneumocystis carinii pneumonia (PCP), toxoplasmosis, and nocardial infections.

13. What infections are associated with cancer chemotherapy?

Patients with cancer who become severely neutropenic (absolute neutrophil counts < 200) have a high risk of bacterial and fungal infection. Neutropenia due to chemotherapy is a particular danger because it is often associated with damage to the mucosal lining of the gastrointestinal tract. Because bacteremia due to gram-negative enteric bacteria (including *Pseudomonas* species) can be quickly lethal, it is standard practice to treat neutropenic cancer patients with broad-spectrum anti-pseudomonal antibiotics (e.g., ceftazidime or piperacillin plus tobramycin) as soon as they develop fever. Many neutropenic patients who remain febrile despite antibiotics have undetected fungal infections; empirical antifungal therapy (typically amphotericin B) is added if fever persists for 5–7 days. After neutropenia resolves, patients with acute lymphoblastic leukemia and some other leukemias may develop *P. carinii* pneumonia; prophylaxis is indicated.

14. What antibiotics can be used for a patient with fever and neutropenia who is severely allergic to penicillin?

Therapy should include an antibiotic with broad activity against gram-negative organisms as well as activity against common gram-positive organisms. Combinations of vancomycin plus aztreonam or vancomycin plus ciprofloxacin are usually tolerated by patients with penicillin allergy.

15. Do all patients with fever and neutropenia need broad-spectrum IV antibiotics?

Patients with moderate neutropenia (absolute neutrophil count of 500–1000) and neutropenia not related to chemotherapy (e.g., transient neutropenia due to drug toxicity or viral infection) may be at much lower risk of infection than cancer patients with no neutrophils. The decision to administer empirical antibiotics to such patients should be based on clinical evaluation.

16. What infections are associated with solid organ transplantation?

In the first month after transplantation, patients develop bacterial infections related to the surgical procedure, often involving the transplanted organ. Renal transplant patients have urinary tract infections, lung transplant patients develop bacterial pneumonia, liver transplant patients have infections of the biliary tree. Wound infections, catheter-related infections, pneumonia, and urinary tract infections can occur in any of these patients. Infections caused by *Candida* species also occur in the early period, often related to antibiotic treatment, intravascular or urinary catheters, and abdominal surgery. Herpes simplex virus may reactivate during this early period

Infections after the first month are most often related to immunosuppressive therapy and are caused by opportunistic pathogens, including *P. carinii* pneumonia, cytomegalovirus (mononucleosis, marrow suppression, pneumonia, hepatitis), varicella zoster, and meningitis caused by *Listeria monocytogenes*. Posttransplant lymphoproliferative disorder, related to Epstein-Barr virus, occurs at this stage and is best controlled by reduction in immunosuppression. Primary toxoplasmosis (affecting the lung, brain, or other organs) occurs most often in heart transplant recipients.

Patients receiving continued immunosuppression may develop infections caused by *Nocardia, Mycobacteria, Cryptococcus,* or *Histoplasma* species or by *Coccidioides immitis. Aspergillus* infections are common. Reactivation of *Strongyloides* infection is uncommon in the United States but should be considered in patients who have traveled to endemic countries or who have eosinophilia.

17. What infections are associated with bone marrow transplantation?

Recipients of bone marrow transplants (BMT) may be at increased risk of infection because of the underlying disease (e.g., leukemia, aplastic anemia). At the time of transplantation they undergo ablative chemotherapy, resulting in severe neutropenia and mucositis, and are at risk for bacterial infections and fungal infections

Once neutropenia has resolved, allogeneic BMT patients continue to have marked cellular and humoral immunodeficiency for at least 6–12 months, a period during which they are subject to opportunistic infections caused by pathogens—such as *P. carinii*, cytomegalovirus (CMV), and cryptococci—similar to those affecting solid organ transplant patients. Because of impaired humoral immunity, they are also at risk for infections caused by pneumococci and other encapsulated bacteria.

In patients suffering from graft-vs.-host disease and receiving steroids or other immunosuppression, immune deficits are particularly prolonged and severe. *Aspergillus* species and CMV are important problems in these patients.

18. True or false: Respiratory syncytial virus (RSV) can cause life-threatening infection in a bone marrow transplant.

True. Pneumonia caused by RSV is particularly severe if acquired in the early posttransplant period.

19. Are there any activities that should be avoided by a child who recently received a bone marrow transplant?

Individual transplant centers give specific instructions to their patients about such things as hobbies, diet, and pets to limit their exposure to opportunistic infections. The greatest risk of infection is in the first few months after transplant; significant immune reconstitution occurs in most patients by 9 months. Some risks are greater than others, and patients may receive conflicting advice about whether swimming is permissible and whether Fluffy must be exiled or autoclaved.

Transplant patients often die from fungal and viral infections, and they are uniquely susceptible to infections caused by intracellular pathogens such as *Listeria* and *Salmonella* species and *Toxoplasma gondii*. All transplant recipients should receive prophylaxis for *P. carinii*. They should avoid heavy exposure to fungi and spores released by gardening, digging, or building reconstruction. They should avoid contact with people who have respiratory infections and exposure to chickenpox or zoster. Such exposures should be reported immediately.

Transplant recipients should eat only fully cooked meat and poultry and avoid undercooked eggs as well as unpasteurized milk or cheeses. Petting healthy cats and dogs may be acceptable (hands should be washed afterward), but contact with reptiles is best avoided. The transplant patient should not clean the cat litter box, fish tank, or birdcage. Weasels have no place in the home.

20. Summarize the important facts about infections in the immunocompromised child.

IMMUNE DEFICIT	CLINICAL SITUATION	TYPE OF INFECTION	EXAMPLES
Neutrophil dysfunction	Chronic granulomatous disease Leukocyte adhesion deficiency Cancer chemotherapy	Bacteria	Gram-positive, Gram-negative, *Aspergillus, Candida* spp.
Antibody deficiency	Agammaglobulinemia	Encapsulated bacteria	Pneumonia and sinusitis due to pneumococci, *H. influenzae*
		Picornaviruses	Chronic echovirus meningo-encephalitis
Lymphocyte dysfunction	HIV Bone marrow transplant Solid organ transplant Corticosteroid therapy Severe combined immunodeficiency	Latent viruses	Herpes simplex Cytomegalovirus Epstein-Barr virus
		Intracellular bacteria	*Listeria monocytogenes Mycobacterium* spp. *Nocardia* spp. *Legionella* spp.
		Intracellular fungi	*Histoplasma* spp. *Cryptococcus* spp. *P. carinii*
		Parasites	*Toxoplasma* spp. *Strongyloides* spp.

Table continued on following page

IMMUNE DEFICIT	CLINICAL SITUATION	TYPE OF INFECTION	EXAMPLES
Splenic dysfunction	Sickle cell disease Hodgkin's disease Splenectomy	Encapsulated bacteria	Bacteremia due to pneumo-cocci, *Neisseria menin-gitidis*, *H. influenzae*
		Babesia Capnocytophaga	
Complement deficiency	Congenital disorder	*N. meningitidis*	

BIBLIOGRAPHY:

1. Cunha B (ed): Infections in the Immunocompromised Host. Infectious Disease Clinics of North America. Philadelphia, W.B. Saunders, 2001.
2. Centers for Disease Control and Prevention: Guidelines for preventing opportunistic infections among hematopoietic stem cell transplant recipients. MMWR 49(RR-10):1–125, 2000.
3. Hughes WT, et al: Guidelines for the use of antimicrobial agents in neutropenic patients with unexplained fever. Clin Infect Dis 25:551–573, 1997.
4. Molrine DC, Hibberd PL: Vaccines for transplant recipients.Infect Dis Clin North Am1 5:273–305, 2001.

39. RECURRENT INFECTIONS

Elena Elizabeth Perez, M.D., Ph.D., and Kathleen E. Sullivan, M.D., Ph.D.

1. What patterns of infection suggest an underlying immunodeficiency?

Immunodeficiency should be suspected when any of the following factors are present in the clinical history:

- Significant infections at more than one site
- Infections with normally nonpathogenic organisms
- Failure to thrive
- Persistent candida
- Unusually persistent viral or bacterial infections
- Paucity of secondary lymphoid tissue
- Recurrent infections with autoimmune disease

2. Are multiple infections always a sign of immunodeficiency?

Healthy children can have an average of 6–8 uncomplicated upper respiratory infections per year. Frequent or persistent infections may be a sign of underlying immunodeficiency, but there is no absolute number of infections that should prompt a further evaluation. The clinical history (including severity, site, and cause of infection and age at presentation) is more important in determining whether to pursue an immunologic evaluation.

3. The immune system is complex. How do I approach this problem?

Usually immunodeficiencies involving cell-mediated immunity present earlier in life with failure to thrive, severe viral infections, or chronic diarrhea. Defects in humoral immunity often present later in infancy when protection from maternal antibody wanes and often involve recurrent sinopulmonary infections. Disorders of the innate immune system, such as those involving macrophages, neutrophils, or complement, can present at any time.

4. What are possible causes of delayed separation of the umbilical cord?

The umbilical stump usually falls off within 1–2 weeks after birth. Neutrophils are recruited to areas of inflammation or wound healing, where they help to mediate tissue remodeling among other functions. When the umbilical stump remains attached longer than the first 1–2 weeks of life, there are three main causes:

1. Aggressive cleaning of the umbilical stump reduces neutrophil migration into the area and impairs separation.

2. Agranulocytosis can be associated with delayed separation of the umbilical cord because of absent neutrophils.

3. The classic immunodeficiency associated with delayed separation of the umbilical cord is leukocyte adhesion deficiency (LAD).

5. What is LAD?

LAD is a rare autosomal recessive disorder that can be life threatening. Only about 200 patients have been diagnosed with LAD to date. It is often associated with recurrent bacterial and fungal infections (skin, gut, gingiva, lung) and delayed wound healing. The most severe form involves a total absence of CD11/CD18 and presents with neutrophilia and severe recurrent bacterial infections due to inability of neutrophils to migrate to sites of inflammation. A variant of the disease, named LAD-2, involves an error in fructose metabolism. LAD-2 is characterized by increased neutrophil counts, recurrent infections, and mental retardation. When immunodeficiency is suspected as a cause for delayed separation of the umbilical cord, a complete blood count and differential should be obtained along with a flow cytometric analysis of CD11b and CD18 expression on neutrophils.

6. A 4-month-old boy admitted for a 6-week history of progressive wheezing poorly responsive to outpatient management has an absolute lymphocyte count of 800 cells/mm³. What is the most likely immunodeficiency?

The diagnosis of severe combined immunodeficiency (SCID) should be considered in any infant with severe or persistent infections during the first year of life. Clinical recognition of SCID is crucial to the survival of the infant and constitutes a medical emergency. Typical infections with SCID include viral pneumonitis, candidal infection, and chronic diarrhea. Absence of palpable lymph nodes, lack of tonsils, absence of thymic shadow on chest radiograph, and a complete blood count with a lymphocyte count < 2800 cells/mm³ are suggestive of SCID. Approximately 95% of all patients with SCID have an absolute lymphocyte count < 2800 cells/mm³. SCID is fatal within the first year of life without a bone marrow transplant.

Infants suspected of having SCID should receive only irradiated blood products, including red cells, platelets, white cells, and plasma, to prevent graft vs. host disease. They must not receive any live viral vaccines. Protective isolation should be instituted and known infections treated aggressively. Bone marrow transplantation is curative for SCID, and HLA typing of the child and all available first-degree relatives should be undertaken as soon as possible. IVIG should be begun once the diagnosis is established as well as prophylaxis for *Pneumocystis carinii*.

7. Who was the most famous fictional patient with SCID?

The boy in the plastic bubble, played by John Travolta.

8. A 14-year-old girl with a minor injury to her neck after lacrosse presents to the emergency department with airway compromise. What is the probable underlying cause?

Hereditary angioedema or C1 esterase inhibitor deficiency is characterized by attacks of intermittent angioedema of the submucosa or skin. The episodes are often associated with stress or trauma. Attacks in the intestines are associated with abdominal pain, vomiting, and diarrhea. Attacks involving the airway can result in potentially life-threatening obstruction. Long-term prophylaxis is usually undertaken with tranexamic acid for prepubertal patients or attenuated androgens for postpubertal patients. Plasma transfusions before surgical procedures have been used to prevent iatrogenic angioedema. Treatment of acute episodes is controversial, although there is universal agreement that antihistamines and epinephrine are ineffective. Fresh frozen plasma and attenuated androgens have been advocated in the acute setting, although paradoxical increases in angioedema have been seen with fresh frozen plasma. The best option is a concentrated C1-inhibitor, currently under study for approval by the Food and Drug Administration (FDA). Infusions are extremely effective in the treatment of acute episodes. This agent has an excellent track record in Europe. Initial management in this case should include airway stabilization and attenuated androgen administration.

9. Is neutropenia commonly associated with other immunodeficiencies?

Neutropenia is typically an isolated finding as a consequence of intercurrent illness, inherited neutrophil defects, or an autoimmune process. Mild neutropenia is defined by an absolute neutrophil count (ANC) between 1000 and 1500/mm³; moderate neutropenia is defined as an ANC between 500 and 1000/mm³; and severe neutropenia is defined as an ANC < 500/mm³. Patients with severe neutropenia have an increased susceptibility to severe and fatal infections. The most common infections are cellulitis, abscesses, pneumonia, and septicemia. Organisms most commonly found with neutropenia are *Staphylococcus aureus*, *Streptococcus* sp., *Nocardia* sp., *Escherichia coli*, *Klebsiella pneumoniae*, *Pseudomonas aeruginosa*, *Enterobacteriaciae* sp., *Candida* sp., and *Aspergillus* sp.

Chronic neutropenia is characterized by an ANC < 500 cells/mm3 for more than 6 months and may have many different causes. Drug-induced neutropenia, congenital neutropenia, cyclic neutropenia, myelodysplastic syndromes, and hypersplenism should be considered. Schwachman-Diamond syndrome, vitamin deficiency (transcobalamin, vitamin B12, folate), and inborn errors of metabolism (Gaucher's disease, glycogen storage disease type 1B) are rare causes of chronic neutropenia. Neutropenia is associated with a few uncommon inherited immunodeficiencies: X-linked agammaglobulinemia, hyper-IgM syndrome, Chediak-Higashi syndrome, cartilage-hair hypoplasia, reticular dysgenesis, and dyskeratosis congenita. HIV also has been associated with neutropenia.

10. When is intravenous immunoglobulin (IVIG) helpful for immunodeficiency?

Therapy with IVIG has had a significant effect on mortality and quality of life for patients with primary antibody deficiencies. Patients with immunologic diseases such as X-linked agammaglobulinemia, common variable immunodeficiency, SCID, hyper-IgM syndrome, hyper-IgE syndrome, and Wiskott-Aldrich syndrome receive clinical benefit from therapy with IVIG. Use of IVIG in patients with primary antibody deficiencies is clinically indicated in the presence of markedly diminished immunoglobulin levels or a demonstrated inability to form functional antibody. IVIG is not indicated for selective IgA deficiency, nor is it useful for congenital neutrophil defects. In measuring serum immunoglobulin concentrations, it is important to use age-matched normative data because of significant developmental variation.

The success of IVIG therapy depends greatly on patient adherence. The initial dose is 400 mg/kg every 4 weeks. All currently available IVIG preparations are equivalent and interchangeable. However, they do vary in IgA content, which may be an important factor for patients who have antibodies to IgA. Nonanaphylactic reactions, which occur in 5–10% of patients, include back pain, abdominal pain, headache, nausea, vomiting, chills, fever, and rash. These symptoms often respond to slowing the rate of infusion or changing products. Anaphylactic reactions are rare and occur mainly as a response to IgA in the infusion.

11. What known infectious agents are transmitted by IVIG?

None. Transmission of infectious agents such as hepatitis C occurred in the past, but there have been no reports of transmission with currently available products. To date, there have been no documented cases of HIV transmission, Creutzfeldt-Jakob disease, or transmissible spongiform encephalopathy disease in patients receiving IVIG. However, because IVIG is considered a blood product, the theoretical risk of transmission of infectious agents does exist. Patients should be counseled about this risk before consenting to IVIG therapy.

12. A toddler with recurrent otitis media and two episodes of pneumonia recently stopped growing. Suggest a reasonable approach to screening for immunodeficiency.

A basic screening for immunodeficiency before referral may include the following: complete blood count with differential, noting absolute lymphocyte count and ANC; quantitative levels of IgG, IgA, IgM, and IgE; and titers to prior vaccines, including tetanus, *Haemophilus influenzae*, diphtheria, and *S. pneumoniae*. This strategy rules out all of the congenital defects in antibody formation and detects eight of the 10 most common inherited immunodeficiencies. HIV testing should be pursued if risk factors are present.

13. A few infections are characteristic of a specific underlying medical condition. Match the infections below with the specific condition.

a. 1-week-old baby with poor growth,   1. Terminal complement component
    lethargy, jaundice, and E. coli sepsis   deficiencies
b. 3-year-old child with *Burkholderia*   2. Severe combined immunodeficiency
    cepacia osteomyelitis
c. 5-month-old child with disseminated   3. Chronic granulomatous disease
    parainfluenza disease
d. Recurrent meningococcal meningitis   4. Galactosemia
Answers: a, 4; b, 3; c, 2; d, 1.

14. List the cutaneous manifestations of specific immunodeficiencies, which often serve as important diagnostic clues.

Ataxia telangiectasia: ocular and cutaneous telangiectasias
Wiskott-Aldrich syndrome: petechiae and eczema
Leukocyte adhesion deficiency: aggressive bacterial cutaneous ulcers
C1, C2, C4 complement deficiencies: cutaneous lupus
Chronic mucocutaneous candidiasis: candidal infection and nail dysplasia
Chediak-Higashi syndrome: pigmentary dilution

Omenn syndrome: erythematous dermatitis

Hyper-IgE syndrome: eczema and cold abscesses

C1 inhibitor deficiency: angioedema

Chronic granulomatous disease: cutaneous abscesses

NEMO (X-linked recessive anhidrotic ectodermal dysplasia with immunodeficiency: anhidrotic ectodermal dysplasia

Dyskeratosis congenita: reticular hyperpigmentation

Griscelli syndrome: pigmentary dilution

Cartilage hair hypoplasia: thin, fine hair

15. What is the most common inherited immunodeficiency?

Mannose-binding lectin deficiency is the most common immunodeficiency (approximately 4% of the United States population); however, it has a very limited phenotype. The second most common is IgA deficiency, which occurs in 1:500 Caucasians; it is much less frequent in other ethnicities. IgA deficiency is often asymptomatic; in symptomatic patients, the most common manifestation is recurrent infections of the mucosal surfaces. IgA deficiency is also associated with a predisposition to allergic and autoimmune diseases.

16. Most serious immunodeficiencies present in childhood. Name the immunodeficiencies that present in adolescence or adulthood.

Mild variants of any of the congenital immunodeficiencies may present later than usual, but this occurrence is unusual. The most common immunodeficiency to present in adolescence is common variable immunodeficiency, in which attrition of immunoglobulin production and function occurs. Hypogammaglobulinemia may occur months to years after the onset of symptoms. Other immunodeficiencies that present in adolescence or adulthood are secondary to lymphomas, thymomas, or HIV..

17. Which components of the human immune system are developmentally regulated?

T-cell function is nearly normal at birth, as are T-cell numbers. There is little established memory at birth, but proliferation of T cells is normal. Cytokine production is diminished, but this finding reflects the fact that nearly all of the T cells are naive. Immunoglobulin production is the most strongly developmentally regulated component. IgG, IgA, and IgM are not produced in utero. IgG production begins to become apparent after 3 months of age, when maternal antibody has diminished. IgM is produced shortly after birth, and IgA is produced in significant quantities beginning at 6 months to 1 year of age. Antibody responses to protein antigens are intact, but responses to polysaccharide antigens are diminished. Complement components are also produced in increasing quantities during the first year of life. Neutrophil function is relatively deficient at birth and improves in the first year of life.

BIBLIOGRAPHY

1. Gaspar HB, Gilmour KC, Jones AM: Severe combined immunodeficiency-molecular pathogenesis and diagnosis. Arch Dis Child 84:169–173, 2001.
2. Mallory SB, Paller AS: Congenital immunodeficiency syndromes with cutaneous manifestations. Part I. J Am Acad Dermatol 23:1153–1158, 1990.
3. Mallory SB, Paller AS: Congenital immunodeficiency syndromes with cutaneous manifestations. Part II. J Am Acad Dermatol 24:107–111, 1991.
4. Rich RR, Fleisher TA, Shearer WT, et al (eds): Clinical Immunology: Principles and Practice, 2nd ed. St. Louis, Mosby, 2001.
5. Stiehm ER (ed): Immunologic Disorders in Infants and Children, 4th ed. Philadelphia, W.B. Saunders, 1996.
6. Stiehm ER: Human intravenous immunoglobulin in primary and secondary antibody deficiencies. Pediatr Infect Dis J. 16:696–707, 1997.
7. Ugochukwu N, Frigas E, Tremaine WJ: Hereditary angioedema: A broad review for the clinician. Arch Intern Med 161:2417–2429, 2001.

40. INFECTIOUS DISEASES IN TRAVELERS

M. Cecilia Di Pentima, M.D., M.P.H., FAAP

1. Characterize travelers' diarrhea (TD) in children.

Although there are different definitions of TD, the best definition for pediatric patients is a syndrome characterized by a twofold increase in the frequency of unformed bowel movements, commonly associated with abdominal cramps, nausea, bloating, urgency, fever, and/or malaise. It usually starts abruptly during travel or soon after returning home. Each episode is generally self-limited with a median duration of 3–4 days. Persistent diarrhea for longer than 4 weeks is unusual.

2. Is antibiotic prophylaxis recommended for children travelling abroad?

The Centers for Disease Control and Prevention (CDC) currently does not recommend antibiotic prophylaxis for children. Concerns that justify this approach include potential side effects and lack of scientific data to support the use of antimicrobial prophylaxis in children with TD. Ciprofloxacin, the drug of choice for prophylaxis of TD in adults, is not approved for routine use in children. A second alternative, doxycycline, is not recommended for children under 8 years of age. A third alternative, trimethoprim-sulfamethoxazole, has fallen out of favor because increasing numbers of resistant strains of *Escherichia coli*, *Shigella*, and *Salmonella* spp. have been isolated in developing countries. The use of antibiotic prophylaxis should be considered in immunocompromised children, who are at higher risk for severe TD.

3. Which travel-related vaccines are contraindicated for children under 1 year of age?

Yellow fever vaccine is contraindicated in infants younger than 4 months of age and Japanese encephalitis vaccine in children under 1 year of age.

4. Which vaccines are required for travelers visiting Mecca during the hajj season?

Meningococcal and yellow fever vaccines.

5. What are the advantages of pre-exposure rabies vaccine?

Pre-exposure vaccination against rabies eliminates the need for rabies immunoglobulin after exposure and reduces the number of postexposure injections. Children traveling to rural areas in developing countries are at highest risk for rabies exposure.

6. Which acute febrile illness affected almost 50% of American athletes participating in the Eco-Challenge-Sabah 2000 multiexpedition race in Borneo, Malaysia?

The responsible pathogen is *Leptospira* sp., which contaminates the Segama River. Athletes participating in water sports are at higher risk for acquiring leptospirosis.

7. Where is the Puente de Verrugas (Verruga) Bridge? What outbreak occurred during its construction?

The Puente de Verrugas is part of the world's highest railroad, built by American engineer Henry Meiggs in Peru. The railroad travels through the Peruvian Andes from Lima to Oroya. Between August and September 1871, the local hospitals reported an outbreak of an unknown disease associated with intermittent high fever, anemia, and hepatitis among immigrant workers from Asia, Chile. and England. During the construction of the railroad, thousands of workers died of bartonellosis, also known as Verruga peruana or Oroya fever. The causative agent is *Bartonella bacilliformis*. The construction of the bridge took the highest toll.

8. A missionary family with three children (2 weeks, 24 months, and 4 years of age) is moving to Zimbabwe in 4 months. How would you advise them about immunizations?

The parents should complete as many doses of the primary series as possible before departure. Different considerations apply to the children; the pediatrician should bear in mind the need for:

- Earlier immunization
- Shorter intervals between doses
- Repeat vaccines at later dates

When infants are travelling abroad, an accelerated schedule is recommended for the following vaccines: diphtheria-tetanus-pertussis (DTaP), hepatitis B, *Haemophilus influenzae* type b (Hib), and polio (inactivated polio vaccine [IPV]).

Accelerated Schedule for Routine Immunization Before International Travel

VACCINE	ROUTINE VACCINATION	ACCELERATED SCHEDULE
DTaP or DT	2, 4, and 6 mo	6, 10, and 14 wk
Hib	2, 4, and 6 mo	6, 10, and 14 wk
IPV	2, 4, and 6 mo	6, 10, and 14 wk
Hepatitis B	Birth, 1–2 mo, and 6 mo	0, 1, and 4 mo
Pneumococcal conjugate vaccine	2, 4, and 6 mo	6, 10, and 14 wk
Measles		6 mo, 12–15 mo
MMR	12–15 mo, 4–6 or 11–12 yr	12 and 13 mo
Varicella	12–18 mo	

DTaP = diphtheria, tetanus, and pertussis; Hib = Haemophilus influenzae type B; IPV = inactivated polio vaccine; MMR = measles, mumps, and rubella.

For older children, it is important to document a complete vaccination schedule. For updated information on routine and travel immunizations review the CDC web-site at www.cdc.gov and the World Health Organization (WHO) website at www.who.int.

9. What is the most important toxicity associated with repellents containing N,N-diethyl-metatoluamide (DEET)?

Neurotoxin reactions can be seen with high DEET concentrations or when excessive volumes are used. Reactions described include toxic encephalopathy, seizure, and acute manic psychosis.

10. What is the most common cause of fever in return travelers?

Malaria is the most common cause of fever in travelers returning from tropical regions.

11. True or false: When counseling families about the risk of acquiring infections abroad, you should reassure them that if they follow your advice, they will return home without any unusual concerns.

False (see figure on following page).

12. Which drugs are available for malaria chemoprophylaxis in children?

Mefloquine, doxycycline and atovaquone/proguanil (Malarone) are the current drugs recommended for children traveling to areas at high risk for malaria: South America, Africa, the Indian subcontinent, Asia, and the South Pacific. However, contraindications may apply based on the child's weight and/or underlying conditions. Chloroquine is indicated only for selected regions in which chloroquine-sensitive *Plasmodium falciparum* is common and can be safely given to children. Always review the CDC website for updated information.

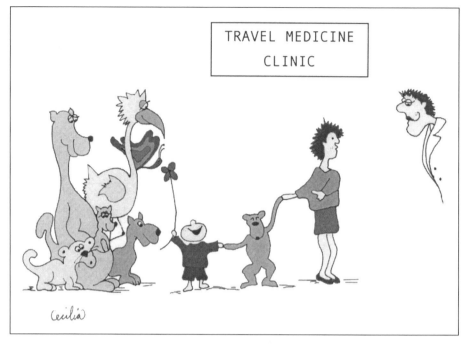

After the Wilsons returned from an exciting trip to Australia, Mrs. Wilson shows up at Dr. Wise's office: "Doc, didn't you say that if we follow all your instructions carefully, Junior would not catch anything weird!"

13. How is ciguatera poisoning acquired?

Ciguatera poisoning is acquired by eating fish, especially large carnivorous coral reef fish, such as sea bass, snapper, and barracuda.

14. How many American children under the age of 16 travel abroad every year?

Approximately 1,500,000 children travel abroad every year from the United States.

15. What is the "economy class" syndrome"?

Also known in England as the bomb shelter syndrome during World War II, the economy class syndrome or traveler's thrombosis is massive pulmonary embolus after the patient arises from a prolonged sitting position.

16. Influenza is clearly associated with winter seasons in temperate climates. How should you advise travelers to the tropics about the risk of exposure to influenza?

In the tropics, transmission of influenza virus occurs throughout the year, and vaccination should be considered for high-risk children and adults.

17. Travelers returning from tropical countries in Africa, Central and South-America, and Asia may bring with them more than souvenirs. Tungiasis is closely related to which of the following: (a) leishmaniasis, (b) African trypanosomiasis, (c) American trypanosomiasis, (d) myasis, or (e) gnathostomiasis?

(d). Tungiasis, like myasis, is an ectoparasitosis caused by the female of *Tunga penetrans*, a small flea that burrows into the skin, where it lays it eggs. Leishmaniasis and trypanosomiasis are caused by protozoan parasites, and gnathostomiasis is a helminthic infection.

18. **Match the following illnesses reported by the WHO during the first quarter of 2002 with the country of outbreak.**

a. Ebola virus	1. India
b. Plague	2. Kosovo
c. Tularemia	3. Gabon
d. *Neisseria meningitidis*, serogroup A	4. Afghan refugee camps in Pakistan
e. Cholera	5. Ethiopia
f. Leishmaniasis	6. Democratic Republic of Congo

Answers: a, 3; b, 1; c, 2; d, 5; e-6, f, 4.
World Health Organization web-site at www.who.int.

19. **You strongly recommend that patients camping with their children in Arizona should stay away from pit vipers with which of the following characteristics:**
   a. Triangular head, round eyes, small teeth, and double row of ventral scales
   b. Triangular head, elliptical eyes, single row of ventral scales, and a musical rattle
   c. Round head, elliptical eyes, double row of ventral scales, and a long tail
   d. Round head and eyes, small teeth, single row of ventral scales, and a short tail

Approximately 7,000 people are bitten by poisonous snakes in the United States, resulting in 9–14 deaths every year. Close to half of the poisonous snakebites involve children. Venomous pit vipers have a triangular head, elliptical eyes, heat-sensing pits between the eyes and the mouth, a single row of ventral scales, and rattles on the tail. The exception is baby rattlesnakes, which have only "buttons" that are quite venomous. They are cute and dangerous!

20. **True or false: The number of cases of imported malaria in nonendemic areas doubled in the past 10 years.**

True—mainly because travelers are taking more adventurous trips. A second factor is more worrisome, the development of multi-drug resistance among *P. falciparum* strains.

21. **What is the risk of acquiring tuberculosis during an airplane flight?**

The risk of acquiring tuberculosis during a short flight is negligible. Nevertheless, it is estimated that the prevalence of transmissible tuberculosis in the air travel population is approximately 50–100 cases per 100,000 passengers. In other words, there may be one encounter per 3–60 flights; the risk is higher in routes that involve high endemic countries or areas. Based on the ventilation system of modern airplanes, if an encounter occurs, the time of exposure required for the transmission of *Mycobacterium tuberculosis* is approximately 10 hours.

22. **Name the three syndromes described in association with high altitude.**

Acute mountain sickness (AMS), high-altitude pulmonary edema (HAPE), and high altitude cerebral edema (HACE). With rapid ascent to high altitude (> 2500 meters above sea level), AMS may develop, depending on the severity of acute hypoxia. If descendence does not occur promptly, AMS can progress to HAPE or HACE, with progressive clinical deterioration, cyanosis, and potentially coma.

23. **Should acetazolamide prophylaxis be prescribed in children?**

Slow ascent is the most effective preventive measure against altitude illness, and the use of acetazolamide should be avoided unless rapid ascent is unavoidable or the child has a previous history of altitude illness. Paresthesias, skin rash and dehydration are common side effects of acetazolamide. Allergy to sulfa is a contraindication to acetazolamide use.

24. **Chikungunya is an "exotic" (a) Brazilian meal, (b) town in Nigeria, (c) virus, (d) African snake, or (e) reef fish.**

(c). Chikungunya virus, a member of the family Togaviridae and the genus Alphavirus, is transmitted by *Aedes aegypti* mosquitoes. In Swahili *chikungunya* means "that which bends up."

25. Match the following antimalarial agents with the corresponding characteristic(s).

a. Chloroquine	1. Active against liver stages of *Plasmodium* spp.
b. Mefloquine	2. Recommended for travelers to Southeast Asia
c. Primaquine	3. Not recommended in patients with epilepsy.
d. Doxycycline	4. Contraindicated in infants weighing < 11 kg
e. Atovaquone/Proguanil	5. Bitter taste
1, c and e.	

2, d and e. Resistance to mefloquine and chloroquine has been reported in Southeast Asia.

3, b. Mefloquine also is not recommended for patients with severe psychiatric disorder or cardiac conduction abnormalities.

4, e.

5, a, b, and e. Parents will be grateful if you advise them to break open the gelatin capsule and mix the drug with applesauce, chocolate syrup, or jelly.

For updated information about travel prophylaxis, review the CDC and WHO websites.

26. True or false: Ten percent of all helicopter evacuations from the Nepalese Himalayas are secondary to diarrheal diseases.

True.

Travel scenario: A freelance photographer and his family returned from Peru after a 2-week trip. They spent the first 3 days in Lima, then flew to Cuzco, where they spent 2 days adjusting to the high altitude before a 2-day trek on the Inca Trail. They spent 1 night in Machu Pichu, returned to Cuzco by train, and flew back to Lima on the following day. The original plan was to spend the rest of the week in Lima, but they decided to fly to Iquitos, where they took a 3-day boat trip down the Amazon River with an overnight stay at a "jungle hotel." Activities included hiking in the jungle, visiting regional Indian tribes, and participating in an evening tour by canoe for alligator spotting.

27. Three days after arrival to the United States, the 13-year-old son developed high fever, chills, retroocular pain, back-pain, and headaches for two days. Later that night an emergency physician diagnosed a viral syndrome. He defervesced within 48 hours and remained afebrile for the next two days. He presents at your office on the fourth day, with fever and a rash that began on his trunk and spread to his face and extremities. His physical examination reveals mild hepatosplenomegaly, subtle conjunctival injection, and a diffuse bright red maculopapular rash that blanches with pressure. How should the patient be managed?

By admission to the hospital for observation. The patient has dengue fever.

28. Three weeks after arrival the 9 year-old daughter develops intermittent episodes of high fever, chills, and headache followed by profuse diaphoresis. Episodes recur every 36–48 hours, and each episode last approximately 10 hours. Clinical assessment reveals mild splenomegaly and jaundice. What is your management strategy?

Chloroquine followed by primaquine. The patient has malaria due to *Plasmodium vivax*. In both cases, knowledge of risk factors, epidemiologic distribution of infectious diseases, and incubation periods helps to narrow the differential diagnosis and guide evaluation and management. If you review dengue fever, malaria, leptospirosis, and typhoid fever, diagnosis of the two children is simple. Approach the differential diagnosis based on fever patterns, incubation period, and physical findings. When travelers change itineraries, appropriate prophylaxis may have not been prescribed.

29. A 3-year-old boy with Down syndrome accompanied his parents on a short trip to Tibet. They arrived in Katmandu, Nepal the night before, and early the next morning they flew to Lhasa, which is located 3,749 meters above sea level. A few hours after arrival his parents noticed that he was unusually fussy, which they attributed to the cold weather and the long flight of the day before. As the day progressed, he developed emesis, respiratory distress, fever, and progressive lethargy. What is the most likely diagnosis?

Manifestations of altitude illness in nonverbal children, particularly those under 3 years of age or with learning or communication difficulties, may be confused with behavioral changes. Typical symptoms include increased fussiness, decreased appetite and playfulness, vomiting, and difficulty in sleeping, which usually begin 4–12 hours after ascent. Children with Down syndrome are more prone to develop pulmonary edema at lower altitudes. The Lake Louis Score has been modified to include nonspecific manifestations in young children to help parents recognize early signs of altitude illness.

Children's Lake Louise Score (CCLS)*

RATE	0	1	2	3	4	5	6	TOTAL
Appetite (A) How well has your child eaten today?	Normal	Slightly less than usual	Much less than normal	Vomiting or not eating				
Playful (P) How playful is your child today?	Normal	Slightly less than usual	Much less than normal	Not playing				
Sleep (S) How well has your child slept today?	Normal	Slightly less than	Much less than	Not able to sleep				
Fussiness (FS)	No fussiness		Intermittent fussiness			Constant		
Amount								
Intensity								

* AMS is diagnosed if the CLLS score is ≥ 7, with a fussiness score ≥ 4 and A + P + S ≥ 3.
Modified from Pollard AJ, Niermeyer S, Barry P, et al: Children at high altitude: An international consensus statement by an ad hoc committee of the International Society for Mountain Medicine, March 12, 2001. High Alt Mec Biol. 2001;2:389–403.

30. Match the following scenarios with the causative virus.

a. Abrupt onset of fever, chills, and headache, myalgia, and arthralgia during travel in the tropical rain forest and Pacific coastal plains of South America. Initial symptoms are followed by transient abdominal pain, backache, nausea, vomiting, photophobia, and dizziness. Most symptoms resolve within 5 days except the arthralgias, which last for 2 months.

b. Arrival in the United States 2 days ago after recent exposure to an unknown febrile illness in Nigeria. Acutely ill in your office, the patient reports headaches, dizziness, and diffuse myalgia. Positive findings on physical examination include temperature of 41°C, hemorrhagic mucous membranes, petechiae, and persistent oozing from a venopuncture site.

c. Febrile illness characterized by fever, hypotension, subconjunctival and gingival bleeding, epistaxis, petechiae, tremor, and dysarthria after exposure to a febrile illness in Bolivia.

    1. Marayo virus
    2. Machupo virus
    3. Lassa virus
    Answers: a, 1; b, 3; c, 2.

31. This summer you plan to spend 1 week in Jamaica with your family. List three safety tips that can help prevent TD.

The major causes of infection are ingestion of contaminated food or drinks and lack of sanitation standards to which families in the United States are accustomed. Although preventive measures may not be enough to eliminate completely the likelihood of acquiring TD, the following table lists tips to help families enjoy the trip without unpleasant interruptions.

Safety Hints to Reduce the Risk for Traveler's Diarrhea

FOR ALL FAMILIES	FOR COMPULSIVE FAMILIES
1. Use appropriate handwashing techniques.	1. Do not expect to find clean facilities. Bring alcohol gel or alcohol swabs.
2. Breastfeeding is safer than bottle feeding.	2. Check that all milk products have been pasteurized or boiled.
3. Eat only well-cooked or canned meals.	3. Meats and fish that are still hot when served are safer.
4. Avoid high-risk foods.	4. Examples include seafood and undercooked meat, raw vegetables, cream pastries, mayonnaise, custards, fruits that cannot be peeled, and food from street vendors.

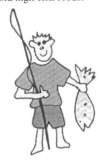

5. Avoid high-risk beverages.	5. Examples include tap water, ice cubes (unless boiled or purified), bottled noncarbonated water, and fruit juices that may be diluted with tap water.

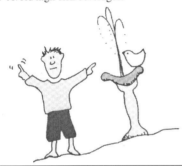

32. After returning from a hunting safari in South Africa, the patient presents with acute onset of blistering that began on the day before arrival and evolved within 24 hours to a painless, ulcerative lesion with marked edema but no fever or lymphadenopathy. What is the diagnosis?

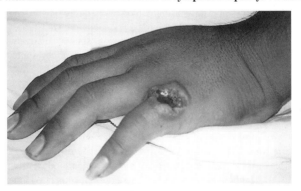

Cutaneous anthrax.

33. A patient returned 2 months ago from a 12-month missionary assignment in the Brazilian Amazon Jungle. Three months ago he noted a subcutaneous nodule on the back of his neck that progressed to an ulcerated lesion. Despite treatment with 1 week of oral ciprofloxacin and 3 weeks of topical steroids, the ulceration worsened. The lesion is painless and nonpruritic, and the patient has remained afebrile throughout the entire course of the illness. No lymphadenopathy is noted. What is your approach to management?

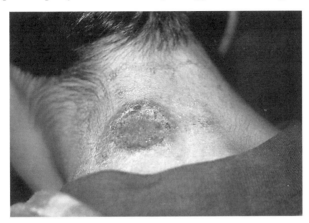

The patient has cutaneous leishmaniasis, which may resolve without treatment. Observation is recommended initially. If treatment is needed, sodium stibogluconate is the agent of choice.

34. During a hiking trip at Big Bend National Park in Texas, the patient developed acute onset of a painful, erythematous lesion with subsequent blistering and ecchymosis. Was the patient bitten by a tick, spider, snake, fire ant, flea, or rabid bat?

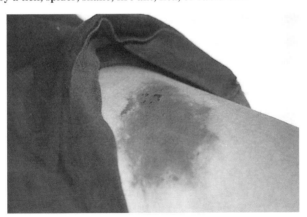

The patient was bitten by a brown recluse spider (*Loxosceles reclusa*).

35. A member of an archeologic expedition to Ica, Peru, presents with a 3-month history of a progressive nodular skin lesion that worsened with sun exposure. Associated symptoms include pruritus with intermittent burning sensation and pain and occasional headaches and abdominal pain. No fever is noted. Was the patient exposed to *Mycobacterium tuberculosis*, free-living amoebas, sandflies, rabbits, *Paracoccidioides brasiliensis*, or human immunodeficiency virus?

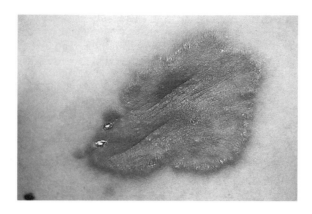

A free-living amoeba (*Balamuthia mandrilaris*).

BIBLIOGRAPHY

1. Centers for Disease Control and Prevention, U.S. Department of Health and Human Services: Health Information for International Travel 2001-2002. Bethesda, MD, CDC, DHHS, 2001.
2. Centers for Disease Control and Preventions: Travelers' Health. Available at www. cdc.org.
3. DuPont HL, Steffen R (eds): Textbook of Travel Medicine and Health, 2nd ed. Hamilton, Ontario, B. C. Decker, 2001.
4. Pollard AJ, Niermeyer S, Barry P, et al: Children at high altitude: an international consensus statement by an ad hoc committee of the International Society for Mountain Medicine, March 12, 2001. High Alt Med Biol 2:389–403, 2001.
5. Strickland TG (ed): Hunter's Tropical Medicine and Emerging Infectious Diseases, 8th ed. Philadelphia, W. B. Saunders, 2000.
6. World Health Organization: International Travel and Health. Available at www.who.int

41. IMMIGRANTS, REFUGEES, AND INTERNATIONAL ADOPTEES

M. *Cecilia Di Pentima*, M.D., M.P.H., FAAP

1. The 1990s witnessed an increased migratory movement worldwide. The United States is not an exception. Estimate the impact of immigrants and their children on population growth in the United States during the past decade: (a) 10%, (b) 20%, (c) 40%, (d) 50%, or (e) 70%.

(e) 70%.

2. Which immigrant group is the most vulnerable to infection: (a) internationally adopted children, (b) refugee children, (c) children of illegal immigrants, (d) children of legal immigrants, or (e) all share the similar risk factors.

(c). Children of illegal immigrants are at highest risk because parents may be frightened to seek medical attention, fearing deportation. In general, refugees receive a more comprehensive medical evaluation before immigration to the United States, and most of them are eligible for Medicaid or temporary health care subsidized by federal funds from the Office of Refugee Resettlement.

3. A 10-year-old Ecuadorian boy presents to the emergency department with a chin laceration. He recently arrived in the United States with his parents. True or false: His general health will improve in the next five years because he will have access to better medical care in the United States.

False. Recent reports from the Institute of Medicine have shown that the health condition of immigrant children deteriorates after arrival to the United States because of poor access to health care, language barriers, and cultural adaptation.

4. Which of the following is the most commonly diagnosed infectious disease among immigrant children: (a) tuberculosis, (b) hepatitis B, (c) hepatitis A, (d) hepatitis C, or (e) human immunodeficiency virus infection?

(a). The risk of tuberculosis in immigrant children is 100 times higher than for children born in the United States.

5. Name five infectious disease screening tests recommended by the American Academy of Pediatrics for all international adoptees.

1. Hepatitis B virus testing
2. Human immunodeficiency virus 1 serology
3. Syphilis serology
4. Stool examination for ova and parasites
5. Tuberculosis skin test

6. A 30-month-old Chinese girl recently was adopted by an American family. Immunization records from the Chinese orphanage include three doses of hepatitis B and four doses of DTaP (diphtheria, tetanus, pertussis) and polio vaccines. Her hepatitis B evaluation shows positive hepatitis B surface antigen (HBsAg) and negative antihepatitis B virus surface (HBV) antibody. You conclude that (a) her HBV vaccine records are accurate and no further doses are needed; (b) her records are inaccurate and she needs three doses of HBV vaccine; (c) she needs further evaluation for HBV infection; (d) the laboratory confused the specimens and you need to repeat the tests; or (e) none of the above.

(c). Children with a positive HBsAg require further evaluation to determine whether they have a transient acute or chronic HBV infection or whether they are HBV carriers.

7. **Describe the approach to DTaP and polio immunization in the above patient: (a) repeat all immunization series; (b) test antibody response to diphtheria and tetanus; (c) assume her immunizations are complete, (d) give DTaP and polio booster doses; or (e) refer the patient to an infectious diseases specialist.**

(b) Immunization records from international adoptees, particularly from orphanages in Eastern Europe, Russia, and China, do not always reflect appropriate protection. Evaluation of antibody titers is recommended, except when children are young and vaccination records are incomplete. In such cases, repeating the doses in question is an easier and acceptable approach.

8. **Which of the following statements about the prevalence of HBV infection among internationally adopted children is true: (a) the overall prevalence is < 1%; (b) prevalence is higher in children from Latin America; (c) the highest reported rates are among Rumanian children; (d) the overall prevalence > 20%; or (e) none of the above?**

(c). The overall prevalence of HBV infection is between 1% and 15%. The highest rates (up to 20%) have been reported in Rumanian children, followed by adoptees from China (3%) and Korea (6%).

9. **True or false: Because of the high incidence of hepatitis C virus infection in children from China, Russia, Eastern Europe, and Southeast Asia, routine screening for hepatitis C should be performed.**

True.

10. **Most infants in developing countries receive at least one dose of bacille Calmette-Guérin (BCG) vaccine. Is confirmation of BCG vaccination by immunization record or scar a contraindication for tuberculin skin testing in asymptomatic infants?**

No. A positive tuberculin skin test (10 mm in an asymptomatic infant) should prompt evaluation for latent tuberculosis infection.

11. **What is a complex humanitarian emergency?**

The end of the cold war marked the beginning of increasing frequency and worsening magnitude of mass population migrations, resulting in significantly increased mortality rates. The term *complex humanitarian emergencies* (CHEs) was introduced in the early nineties to define acute humanitarian crises affecting large populations, mainly involving political instability, civil war, food shortages, and population displacement, all of which are associated with collapsing public health infrastructures. Mortality rates may be 60 times higher than the baseline rates for the affected population.

12. **The proportion of deaths during CHE is significantly higher among children under 5 years of age. Most deaths among displaced children are due to (a) cholera, (b) measles, (c) malaria, (d) noncholera infectious diarrhea, or (e) all of the above.**

(e). Preventable infectious diseases are the major cause of morbidity and mortality for all age groups. However, children under 5 years of age are the most vulnerable and have the highest mortality rates.

13. **Which of the following people were refugees and recipients of a Nobel Prize: (a) Albert Einstein, (b) Madeline Albright, (c) Rabindranath Tagore, (d) Winston Churchill, or (e) none of the above?**

(a). Albert Einstein was a refugee and received the Nobel Prize in Physics in 1921. Madeline Albright was a refugee but did not receive a Nobel Prize. Rabindranath Tagore and Winston Churchill were awarded Nobel Prizes in Literature in 1913 and 1953, respectively.

14. **In the event of an outbreak of meningococcal meningitis in a refugee camp, you should consider vaccination if which of the following criteria are met: (a) laboratory tests confirm meningococcal disease; (b) an outbreak is confirmed to be due to serogroup A or C organisms;**

(c) *Neisseria meningitidis* group A is affecting children under 1 year of age, or group C is affecting children ≥ 2 years; (d) all of the above; or (e) none of the above?
Answer: (d).

15. True or false: You should strongly consider chemoprophylaxis to control an epidemic of meningococcal disease in a refugee camp.
False. Mass chemoprophylaxis is ineffective and is discouraged in a refugee setting.

16. Which vaccine should be considered a priority in CHEs?
During the 1980s, refugee camps in Somalia and Sudan had high measles-specific death rates. Since 1985, measles immunization is considered part of the initial emergency relief effort. It is recommended that all children between the ages of 6 months and 12 years of age receive measles vaccine and a dose of vitamin A soon after they arrive to a refugee camp. A complete expanded program on immunization (EPI) should be planned as part of the long-term health program.

BIBLIOGRAPHY

1. American Academy of Pediatrics. Refugees and immigrants: Medical evaluation of internationally adopted children for infectious diseases. In Pickering LK (ed) 2000 Red Book: Report of the Committee on Infectious Diseases. Elk Grove Village, IL, American Academy of Pediatrics, 2000.
2. Centers for Disease Control and Prevention.Disasters: Famine-affected, refugee and displaced populations. In: Friede A, O'Carroll PW, Nicola RM, et al (eds): A Guide to Action. Williams & Wilkins, Baltimore, 1997, pp 1104–1149.
3. Hernandez DJ, Charney E (eds): From Generation to Generation: the Health and Well-being of Children in Immigrant Families. Committee on the Health and Adjustment of Immigrant Children and Families, National Research Council and Institute of Medicine. Washington, DC, National Academy of Press; 1998. Available at www.nap.edu.
4. Toole MJ: Mass population displacement: A global public health challenge. Infect Dis Clin North Am 9:353–366, 1995.
5. Toole MJ, Malkki RM: Famine-affected, refugee and displaced populations: Recommendations for public health issues. MMWR 41:1-76 (No RR-13), 1992.

42. CONGENITAL AND PERINATAL INFECTIONS

Susan E. Coffin, M.D., M.P.H.

1. How are perinatal infections transmitted?

INFECTIOUS AGENT	COMMON ROUTES OF TRANSMISSION*		
	TRANSPLACENTAL	INTRAPARTUM	POSTNATAL
Viruses			
Cytomegalovirus	+++	++	+
Enteroviruses	+	+++	+++
Hepatitis B	+	+++	+
Hepatitis C	++	+++	—†
Human immunodeficiency virus	+	+++	+
Herpes simplex virus	+	+++	+
Parvovirus	+++	—	—†
Rubella	+++	—	—†
Varicella-zoster	+++	—	—†
Bacteria			
Group B streptococci	+++	+++	+++
Enteric bacilli (including *Escherichia coli*)	+++	+++	+
Listeria sp.	+	+++	+
Treponema pallidum	+++	—	—†
Other			
Chlamydia sp.	—	+++	—†
Toxoplasma gondii	+++	—	—†

+++ = most common route of transmission, ++ = occasional route of transmission, + = rare route of transmission.
* Common routes of transmission that lead to clinically significant disease.
† Postnatal transmission can occur but is unlikely to cause disease more severe than that seen in older infants.

2. For what does the acronym TORCH stand?
Toxoplasmosis, **r**ubella, **c**ytomegalovirus (CMV), and **h**erpes.

3. Which congenital infections are associated with intrauterine growth retardation (IUGR)?
Prenatal infection with rubella, CMV, syphilis, or toxoplasmosis may lead to IUGR. Congenital herpes simplex virus (HSV) infection, although rare, also may lead to IUGR.

4. Name the most common infectious causes of neonatal thrombocytopenia.
CMV, toxoplasmosis, rubella, enteroviruses, and severe bacterial infection.

5. Which common congenital or perinatal infections result in hepatomegaly?
Rubella, CMV, Toxoplasma gondii, disseminated HSV, human immunodeficiency virus (HIV), syphilis, or bacterial sepsis (e.g., Escherichia coli, group B streptococci [GBS]).

6. Which congenital or perinatal infections can cause pneumonitis?
Neonatal pneumonitis may be associated with infections caused by rubella, HSV, CMV, toxoplasma gondii, syphilis, enteroviruses, or bacterial pathogens (e.g., *E. coli*, GBS).

7. What are the infectious causes of neonatal heart disease?

Congenital rubella infection can cause peripheral pulmonary artery stenosis. Congenital parvovirus and neonatal enterovirus infections may induce myocarditis.

8. What congenital infections are associated with rashes?

Description of rash	Infectious agent
Petechiae or purpura	CMV, enteroviruses, rubella
Vesicles	HSV, syphilis, *Candida* sp.
Bullae	*S. aureus*
Maculopapular	Syphilis, enterovirus, HSV, toxoplasmosis

9. Which neonatal skin lesions may be confused with HSV?

Erythema toxicum neonatorum and milia.

10. Describe the diagnostic workup for an infant born with microcephaly.

Prenatal infections that can cause microcephaly include CMV and toxoplasmosis. Rubella has been reported to cause hydrocephalus or microcephaly. Therefore, a thorough evaluation of potential infectious causes of microcephaly should include the following:

- Urine for viral culture.
- Maternal and infant serum for toxoplasmosis IgM, IgA, and IgG.
- Review of maternal records for rubella antibody status.

TORCH antibodies are IgG and acquired transplacentally from the mother late in gestation. Proof of infection requires paired acute and convalescent sera.

11. Describe the association between the pattern of brain calcifications and the underlying cause of congenital microcephaly.

Infectious agent	Pattern of calcifications
CMV	Periventricular
Toxoplasmosis	Parenchymal > periventricular

12. Which congenital infections may be associated with hearing deficits?

CMV is now the most common infectious cause of neonatal hearing loss. Prenatal infection with toxoplasmosis or rubella also may cause congenital hearing loss.

13. Which eye abnormalities are associated with congenital infections?

Eye abnormality	Infectious agent
Cataract	Rubella, toxoplasmosis, HSV, varicella-zoster virus (VZV)
Chorioretinitis	Toxoplasmosis, rubella, CMV, HSV, syphilis, VZV
Microphthalmia	CMV, toxoplasmosis, rubella, HSV

14. What are the common clinical manifestations of perinatal group B streptococcal infections?

CLINICAL FEATURE	EARLY ONSET	LATE ONSET	LATE LATE ONSET
Time of onset	< 7 days	7–30 days	> 30 days
Typical features	Respiratory distress, pneumonia, shock, meningitis (5–10%)	Bacteremia, meningitis, septic arthritis	Bacteremia, osteomyelitis, septic arthritis

15. What are the risk factors for early-onset group B streptococcal (GBS) disease?

Maternal history of a previous infant with invasive GBS disease, maternal colonization with GBS at 35–37 weeks' gestation, documented GBS bacteriuria during pregnancy, and delivery before 37 weeks' gestation. In addition, maternal temperature > 38.0°C or rupture of membranes more than 18 hours before delivery are associated with an increased risk of neonatal GBS infection.

16. How should an infant born to a mother who is colonized with GBS be managed?

All women who are colonized with GBS and have other risk factors for invasive GBS disease should be given intrapartum penicillin. In the absence of risk factors, women should be offered intrapartum penicillin if GBS was isolated from maternal vaginal and rectal cultures at 35–37 weeks' gestation.

17. Describe the management of an infant born to a mother who did not undergo prenatal screening for GBS colonization.

Intrapartum penicillin should be given if any of the following risk factors are present:
• Maternal history of a previous infant with invasive GBS disease
• Documented GBS bacteriuria during pregnancy
• Delivery before 37 weeks' gestation
• Maternal temperature > 38.0°C
• Rupture of membranes more than 18 hours before delivery

18. Which viruses can be transmitted by breast milk?

Both CMV and HIV can be transmitted from mother to infant during breast-feeding. However, maternal CMV infection is *not* a contraindication to breast-feeding a healthy neonate because postnatal CMV infection is not associated with serious disease for most full-term infants. In contrast, maternal HIV infection is a contraindication to breast-feeding in developed countries. The benefits of breast-feeding may outweigh the risks of HIV transmission in certain underdeveloped countries.

19. What are the neonatal consequences of maternal varicella infection?

There is a low (< 5%) risk of congenital defects when a pregnant women develops primary varicella infection (chickenpox) before 20 weeks of gestation. Infants whose mother had onset of varicella infection within 5 days before delivery or within 48 hours after delivery are at high risk for severe disease and should receive varicella-zoster immunoglobulin.

20. Are infants born to women with active Lyme disease at risk of infection?

Although rare cases of transplacental transmission of *Borrelia burgdorferi* have been reported, no evidence indicates that maternal Lyme disease causes congenital abnormalities or complications during pregnancy. Maternal Lyme disease is not a contraindication to breast-feeding.

21. Which congenital infections may be asymptomatic at birth but cause serious disease later in life?

INFECTIOUS AGENT	LATE MANIFESTATIONS
CMV	Sensorineural hearing loss
Hepatitis B	Cirrhosis, hepatocellular carcinoma
Hepatitis C	Cirrhosis, hepatocellular carcinoma
Papillomavirus	Respiratory papillomatosis
Rubella	Sensorineural hearing loss
Syphilis*	Malformations of teeth and bone, deafness, keratitis
Toxoplasmosis*	Chorioretinitis, seizures, hypotonia

* Early treatment is believed to reduce the risk of sequelae.

22. What are the major risk factors for perinatal HSV infection?

Primary maternal infection, active genital lesions (cervix > labia > buttocks), invasive fetal monitoring (especially scalp electrodes), and prolonged rupture of membranes.

23. What are the common clinical manifestations of perinatal HSV infection?

	SITE OF INFECTION		
	SKIN, EYE, MUCOUS MEMBRANE	CNS	DISSEMINATED
Frequency	40%	35%	25%
Time of onset	7–14 days	14–21 days	5–10 days
Clinical features	Grouped vesicles on erythematous base; conjunctivitis	Fever, lethargy, seizures	Shock, respiratory distress, hepatomegaly

24. Which of the following tests is the most sensitive and specific for the diagnosis of herpetic disease of the central nervous system (CNS): MRI of the brain, viral culture of CNS, polymerase chain reaction (PCR) of cerebrospinal fluid, or fever?

PCR of cerebrospinal fluid.

25. What are the current treatment recommendations for neonatal HSV infection?

Intravenous acyclovir should be administered to infants with HSV infection for 14–21 days, depending on the site of infection. Skin, eye, and mouth disease can be treated for 14 days; CNS or disseminated disease is typically treated for 21 days.

26. What are the major risk factors for perinatal transmission of HIV infection?

Primary maternal infection, high viral load, and breast-feeding.

27. Describe the management of infants born to mother with active or untreated sexually transmitted diseases other than syphilis or HIV.

INFECTIOUS AGENT	POSSIBLE CLINICAL MANIFESTATIONS	MANAGEMENT
Chlamydial infection	Conjunctivitis, pneumonitis	Infants born to infected mothers are at high risk of chlamydial conjunctivitis or pneumonitis; however, prophylactic antibiotics are not recommended.
Gonorrhea	Conjunctivitis, bacteremia	Universal prophylaxis with erythromycin ophthalmic ointment reduces but does not eliminate the risk of neonatal gonococcal infection. Infants born to infected mothers should be treated with a single dose of ceftriaxone, 125 mg IM.
Hepatitis B	90% risk of chronic infection without intervention	Hepatitis B vaccine and HBIG at birth.
HSV	Perinatal HSV (see above)	Asymptomatic infants born to women with active genital lesions should have viral cultures of nasopharynx and rectum obtained at 24–48 hr of life. Some experts recommend empiric acyclovir for babies born to women with active primary genital lesions.
Papillomavirus	Laryngeal papillomatosis	Expectant management.
Trichomonal infection	Vaginal discharge or UTI	Metronidazole for symptomatic infants.

IM = intramuscularly, HBIG = hepatitis B immunoglobulin, HSV = herpes simplex virus, UTI = urinary tract infection.

28. Which newborns are at risk for congenital syphilis?

Newborn should be considered at risk for congenital syphilis if any of the following conditions are present:

- Untreated, inadequately treated, or undocumented treatment of maternal syphilis
- Treatment of syphilis in pregnancy with a nonpenicillin regimen
- Absence of a documented 4-fold fall in maternal titers on Venereal Disease Research Laboratory (VDRL) or rapid plasmin reagin (RPR) test despite appropriate therapy
- Infant's VDRL or RPR is 4-fold or greater than mother's titer
- Abnormal physical examination consistent with congenital syphilis

29. Describe the appropriate work-up for infants at risk for congenital syphilis.

- Physical examination
- Quantification of serum nontreponemal (VDRL or RPR) and treponemal (microhemagglutination-*Treponema pallidum* [MHA-TP] or fluorescent treponemal antibody, absorbed [FTA-ABS]) antibodies (not to be performed on cord blood sample)
- Radiographs of long bones
- Complete blood count

Examination of the cerebrospinal fluid for cell count, protein content, and VDRL titer should be performed for all at-risk infants who have a suspicious physical examination or a quantitative serum nontreponemal antibody titer that is 4-fold greater than the mother's titer.

30. How should syphilis serologies be interpreted?

NONTREPONEMAL TEST (e.g., VDRL, RPR)		TREPONEMAL TEST (e.g., MHA-TP, FTA)		
MOTHER	INFANT	MOTHER	INFANT	INTERPRETATION
–	–	–	–	No evidence of maternal syphilis, incubating syphilis, or prozone phenomenon.
+	+	–	–	No maternal syphilis infection (false-positive nontreponemal test with passive transfer of antibodies to infant).
+	+ or –	+	+	Maternal syphilis with possible infant infection; mother treated for syphilis during pregnancy; or mother with latent syphilis and possible infection of infant.
+	+	+	+	Recent or previous syphilis in the mother; infant at risk for syphilis.
–	–	+	+	Mother successfully treated for syphilis, or mother with false-positive serology.

Adapted from American Academy of Pediatrics: Report of the Committee on Infectious Diseases, 25th ed. Elk Grove Village, IL, American Academy of Pediatrics, 2000.

31. How should a neonate with congenital syphilis be treated?

1. Patients with suspected or proven disease should be treated for 10 days with parenteral penicillin.

2. Asymptomatic infants with a normal laboratory evaluation may be treated with either parenteral penicillin for 10–14 days or a single dose of benzathine penicillin.

BIBLIOGRAPHY

1. American Academy of Pediatrics: Report of the Committee on Infectious Diseases, 25th ed. Elk Grove Village, IL, American Academy of Pediatrics, 2000.
2. Duff P (ed): Perinatal infectious disease. Semin Perinatol 22:241–346, 1998.

3. Fowler MG, Simonds RJ, Roongpisuthipong A: Update on perinatal HIV transmission. Pediatr Clin North Am 47:21–38, 2000.
4. Moodley P, Sturm AW: Sexually transmitted infections, adverse pregnancy outcome and neonatal infection. Semin Neonatol 5:255–269, 2000.
5. Morita JY, O'Brien KL, Schuchat A: Prevention of perinatal group B streptococcal infections. Pediatr Infect Dis J 18:279–280, 1999.
6. Remington JS, Klein JO: Infectious Diseases of the Fetus and Newborn Infant. 5th ed. Philadelphia, W.B. Saunders, 2001.

43. LYME DISEASE

Stephen C. Eppes, M.D.

1. From where does the term *Lyme disease* derive?
a. Swollen joints have the shape of a Lyme.
b. The original description was by Dr. Lyme.
c. It was originally felt to be a form of scurvy, preventable by eating limes.
d. The condition was first recognized in Old Lyme, Connecticut.
Answer: (d). What was initially felt to be a clustering of cases of juvenile rheumatoid arthritis (JRA) in Old Lyme, Connecticut lead to an epidemiological investigation which suggested an infectious etiology. Note that the name of the town has no "s" or "z", so that the correct pronunciation is Lyme disease.

2. Name the etiologic agent that causes Lyme disease.
Borrelia burgdorferi is responsible for virtually all cases in North America. In Europe, *B. afzelli* and *B. garinii* also cause Lyme borreliosis. Like other spirochetes, these organisms share the ability to invade a variety of tissues and cause persistent infection, with both early and late manifestations.

3. Which is the reservoir of *B. burgdorferi*: (a) the deer tick, (b) the Lone Star tick, (c) the white footed mouse, or (d) the white tailed deer?
Answer: (c). The white-footed mouse, *Peromyscus leucopus*, is frequently spirochetemic, even though asymptomatic, and is the reservoir of infection. The deer tick, *Ixodes scapularis*, feeds on the mouse and acquires the spirochete, which can then be transmitted to humans. The deer is important in the life cycle of the tick; the second winter of the tick's 2-year life is most often spent on the white-tailed deer.

4. True or false: Humans are a dead-end host for *B. burgdorferi*.
True. When ticks are attached for a minimum of 24–48 hours, *B. burgdorferi* can be deposited in the dermis, after which the disease manifestations may begin. Unlike syphilis, for example, there is no transmission from person to person, and humans do not act as a reservoir.

5. What geographic areas of the United States are most affected by Lyme disease?
Most states have reported cases of Lyme disease, but the areas which are most highly endemic are the Northeast, Mid-Atlantic region, upper Midwest (parts of Minnesota and Wisconsin), and, less commonly, northern California.

6. At what time of year do most cases of Lyme disease occur?
Most cases present as early infection and tend to occur during the warmer months, corresponding to peak tick activity. However, Lyme arthritis is a late manifestation (occurring on average 6 months after tick bite) and may be seen at any time of year.

7. The characteristic skin lesion of early Lyme disease is (a) erythema annulare, (b) erythema migrans, (c) erythema marginatum, or (d) acrodermatitis chronicum atrophicans?
Answer: (b). Erythema migrans (EM) is the hallmark of early Lyme disease and is recognized in 60–90% of cases (see figure on following page). Other early manifestations (during the first several weeks after tick bite) include malaise, fever, headache, myalgias, and arthralgias.

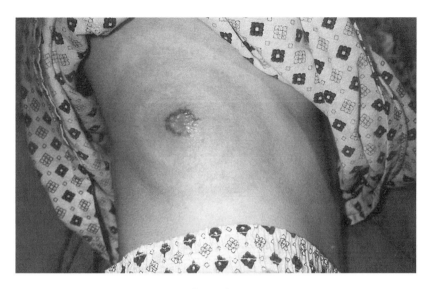

Erythema migrans.

8. Disseminated infection, usually occurring within 3 months after the tick bite, is accompanied by which of the following manifestations: (a) more pronounced fever and achiness, (b) meningeal signs, (c) facial palsy, (d) multiple EM, (e) all of the above, or (f) a, c, and d only?

The answer is (e), all of the above.

9. The facial palsy associated with Lyme disease is (a) central or (b) peripheral?

Answer: (b). Peripheral facial nerve palsy (PFNP) is the most common cranial neuropathy associated with Lyme disease (others occur, especially of cranial nerves III and VI). The lack of function of the upper face/forehead musculature distinguishes this from central lesions, in which these muscles are spared. Even though the neurologic injury is peripheral, concomitant meningitis (central nervous system [CNS] involvement) is present in more than half of cases.

10. Cardiac involvement in Lyme disease is most often (a) first-, second-, or third-degree heart block, (b) pericarditis, (c) myocarditis, or (d) all of the above?

Answer: (a). Fluctuating degrees of heart block are most frequently observed (in about 10% of cases). Electrocardiography should be considered in cases of early Lyme disease. While uncommon, third-degree heart block can lead to a fatal outcome.

11. Contrast the findings in Lyme meningitis and viral meningitis.

FINDING	LYME MENINGITIS	VIRAL MENINGITIS
Presentation	Subacute, days to weeks	Acute, one to a few days
Fever	Variable	Almost always
Erythema migrans	Common	Absent
Cranial neuropathy	Common	Rare
Papilledema	Common	Rare
CSF WBC count	Mean: 80/mm^3	Mean: 300/mm^3
CSF neutrophils	Absent or low	Frequent, especially early

CSF = cerebrospinal fluid, WBC = white blood cell.

12. Name four late manifestations of Lyme disease.

Arthritis, chronic neurologic disease, acrodermatitis chronicum atrophicans, and borrelial lymphocytoma. By far the most common is arthritis, which presents in a mean of 6 months after the tick bite. Ninety percent of arthritis occurs in the knees; the ankles are the second most common location. Small joint involvement is rare. The characteristic joint findings are moderate-to-large effusions and limitation of motion, usually without pronounced pain or tenderness, although a more "septic" appearance may be seen, mainly in young children. Synovial fluid white blood cell counts are high, often 30,000–100,000. Lyme arthritis should be considered in previously healthy children in a Lyme-endemic area who present with a swollen knee. Chronic CNS disease is reported more commonly in adults than children. Some experts question whether chronic CNS infection even occurs, but a subtle encephalopathy (memory loss, impaired cognition) in patients who have had Lyme disease has been reported in the literature. The other two late conditions involve the skin and are seen primarily in Europe.

13. True or false: A patient from a Lyme-endemic area with an annular erythematous skin lesion of at least 5-cm diameter with central clearing (bulls-eye appearance) can be accurately diagnosed with Lyme disease on clinical grounds alone.

True. If the finding is this characteristic, it is diagnostic; the diagnosis can be reported to health departments without laboratory documentation. Laboratory testing should be reserved for patients with atypical skin lesions or other disease manifestations that are not accompanied by recognizable EM.

14. Which of the following laboratory tests are useful in identifying infection with *B. burgdorferi*: (a) culture, (b) polymerase chain reaction (PCR), (c) antibody testing (serology), or (d) rapid antigen detection?

Answers: (a), (b), and (c). The most commonly used tests in clinical practice are designed to detect the presence of antibody to *B. burgdorferi*. IgM antibody becomes detectable about 2 weeks after infection and disappears within a few months, whereas IgG antibody appears somewhat later and may persist for years. Culture methods have been important research tools but are of limited clinical value. Likewise, PCR has been used mainly in research settings. PCR testing of cerebrospinal fluid (in the setting of neuroborreliosis) has low sensitivity but is occasionally helpful. PCR testing of synovial fluid has been useful in guiding decisions about managing chronic Lyme arthritis.

15. Match the diagnostic method with its description:

a. Older serologic test used less today because of more challenging methodology

b. Measures IgG, IgM or total antibody to *B. burgdorferi*

c. Uses electrophoretically separated *B. burgdorferi* proteins to measure IgM or IgG antibody response to individual antigens (more specific)

1. Enzyme linked0immunosorbent assay (ELISA))
2. Western blot
3. Immunoflourescent assay (IFA)

Answers: a, 3; b, 1; c, 2..

16. Although a generally sensitive test, ELISA may be falsely positive in which of the following conditions: (a) syphilis, (b) pregnancy, (c) autoimmune diseases, or (d) viral infections?

Answers: (a), (c), and (d). Other spirochetal infections may cause falsely positive ELISA for *B. burgdorferi;* however, Lyme disease is not associated with nontreponemal tests for syphilis (e.g., rapid plasma reagin or Venereal Disease Research Laboratory test). Autoimmune diseases (e.g., lupus erythematosus) and certain viral infections (e.g., Epstein-Barr virus, parvovirus B19) also may cause false positive ELISA results. The western blot is recommended for confirmation of ELISA results and is especially useful in identifying false positives (which are often low or borderline by ELISA).

17. Which statement about *B. burgdorferi* antibody testing is false?

a. Early antibiotic therapy can reduce the antibody response after infection.

b. Over the years, there has generally been good standardization of these tests, leading to good intra- and interlaboratory agreement.

c. Because some patients continue to have detectable antibody long after adequate antibiotic treatment and apparent cure, it is of little value to perform follow-up serologic testing.

d. Standard criteria are used for interpreting western blots, including the number of "bands" and their molecular weights.

Answer: (b). The other three statements are true.

18. Which of the following oral antibiotics have been shown to be efficacious in treating Lyme disease: (a) doxycycline, (b), amoxicillin, (c) cefuroxime axetil, (d) levofloxacin, (e) all of the above, or (f) a, b, and c only?

Answer: (f).

19. Penicillin G, cefotaxime, and ceftriaxone have been effective in treating Lyme disease. Ceftriaxone has favorable pharmacokinetics, allowing once-daily dosing and also attains effective CSF concentrations. In which of the following situations is ceftriaxone recommended?

a. Lyme meningitis

b. Third-degree heart block associated with early Lyme disease

c. Arthritis refractory to oral antibiotics

d. Abducens palsy associated with early Lyme disease

e. All of the above

Answer: (e).

20. What are the advantages and disadvantages of doxycycline?

Doxycycline is generally the agent of choice for early Lyme disease for the following reasons (1) good tissue penetration (including CNS), (2) demonstrated efficacy (both in vitro and in vivo), and (3) activity in human granulocytic ehrlichiosis (which may be simultaneously transmitted with *B. burgdorferi* during deer tick attachment). **Disadvantages** include photosensitivity reactions, esophageal ulcerations, and potential dental toxicity for the fetus and young child (although short courses of doxycycline can be safely given, even in children younger than 8 years).

21. Match the antibiotic choice to the clinical situation (numbered answers can be used more than once).

a. 6-year-old boy with swollen knee and high positive ELISA	1. Amoxicillin for 30 days
b. 9-year-old girl with peripheral facial palsy whose parents refuse lumbar puncture	2. Cefuroxime axetil for 21 days
c. 15-year-old boy with papilledema and multiple EM	3. No antibiotic
d. 12-year-old girl with arthritis of hands and knees with positive ELISA but negative western blots	4. Amoxicillin for 21 days
e. 4-year-old boy with EM, fever, and PR interval of 0.24 seconds	5. Ceftriaxone for 14 days
f. 5-year-old girl with EM and documented rash with penicillin in the past	6. Doxycycline for 21 days
g. 8-year-old boy with lymphocytic CSF pleocytosis and low positive ELISA	
h. 13-year-old boy with history of Lyme arthritis adequately treated 3 years ago, weakly reactive serology, and mother under treatment for chronic Lyme's disease	

Answers: a, 1; b, 6; c, 5; d, 3; e, 4; f, 2; g, 5; h, 3.

22. Which of the following is a useful measure for tick attachments?
a. **Pulling straight out by mouthparts using forceps or tweezers**
b. **Painting with fingernail polish or Vaseline**
c. **Burning tick's posterior with a hot match or cigarette**
d. **Rubbing with salt**
e. **Twisting counter-clockwise until the tick releases**
Answer: (a).

23. True or false: Prophylactic antibiotic treatment has been shown to reduce the likelihood of developing Lyme disease after deertick bites.

True. One study showed that a single dose of doxycycline, 200 mg, after a documented *Ixodes* tick bite reduced the frequency of Lyme disease in older adolescent and adult patients. This approach is not accepted in younger children. Several dozen patients would need to be treated in this way to prevent one case of Lyme disease.

24. Which of the following measures is recommended to prevent Lyme disease?
a. **"Tick checks" after outside exposure in an endemic area**
b. **Wearing light colored clothing when outside during tick season**
c. **Tucking pants legs into socks when outside during tick season**
d. **All of the above**
Answer: (d), although most children will not do (a), (b), and (c).

BIBLIOGRAPHY

1. Steere AC: Lyme disease. N Engl J Med 345:115–124, 2001.
2. Centers for Disease Control and Prevention: Surveillance for Lyme disease–United States, 1992–1998. MMWR 49 (No. SS-3):1–11, 2000.
3. Klein JD, Eppes SC, Hunt PC: Environmental and lifestyle risk factors for Lyme disease in children. Clin Pediatr 35:359–363, 1996.
4. Belman AL, Reynolds L, Preston T, et al: Cerebrospinal fluid findings in children with Lyme disease-associated facial nerve palsy. Arch Pediatr Adolesc Med 151:1224–1228, 1997.
5. Wormser GP, Nadelman RB, Dattwyler DK, et al: Practice guidelines for the treatment of Lyme disease. Clin Infect Dis 31(Suppl 1):S1–S14, 2000.

44. EMERGING INFECTIONS

Sharon A. Nachman, M.D.

1. What are *Leptospira?*

Leptospira are motile microorganisms, 6–20 µm in length and 0.1–0.2 µm in diameter. They are obligate aerobes with unique nutritional requirements for long-chain fatty acids. All *Leptospira* organisms are included in one of two different species: *L. interrogans*, which is pathogenic to humans and animals, and *L. biflexa*, which is free-living. *L. interrogans* is divided into more than 210 serovars and 23 serogroups. Virulence does not correlate with specific serovars, although serovar classifications can be used epidemiologically to identify common-source outbreaks.

2. What are some of the other names for leptospirosis?

Weil's disease, Swineherd's disease, rice-field fever, cane-cutter fever, swamp fever;, and hemorrhagic jaundice.

3. Discuss the epidemiology of leptospirosis.

Leptospirosis is a widespread infection transmitted among animals and occasionally from animals to humans. Asymptomatically infected wild or domestic mammals can harbor *Leptospira* for months in the proximal convoluted tubules of the kidney. After excretion in urine, the microorganism can survive for weeks or months in the environment under favorable conditions, such as temperatures of 28–32°C and a neutral or slightly alkaline pH.

4. What is a common source of exposure to leptospirosis?

Direct exposure to urine of infected animals or urine-contaminated water or soil, often through recreational or occupational hazards, represents the main source of infection for humans. The main source of exposure in developed countries is the dog or other household pets, followed by livestock, rodents, and other wild animals.

5. Describe the geographic distribution of leptospirosis.

Although the distribution is worldwide, tropical regions bear the brunt of impact. In developing countries, large percentages of the population often live in close contact with animals; thus, the spread of infection is much larger. Moreover, environmental conditions in tropical and subtropical American, including abundant rainfalls, nonacidic soil, and high temperatures, along with numerous natural water courses, are particularly favorable for the transmission of *Leptospira* infections.

6. How does infection with *Leptospira* occur?

Among the most common places of exposure is stagnant water, which is used by stray dogs for excreting urine. In some countries, 55–82% of domestic or stray dogs show serologic evidence of exposure to *Leptospira* as opposed to only 12.5% of cats. Other mechanisms of transmission of *Leptospira* are through abraded skin and intact mucous membranes, such as conjunctiva or nasopharyngeal and genital epithelium, allowing quick access to blood and lymphatic circulation. Of interest, inhaled aerosol spray also may carry the microorganism directly to the lung. Transplacental maternal-fetal transmission is also known to occur. Pathogenic *Leptospira* organisms are resistant to bactericidal activity of normal serum. Thus, in the absence of specific antibodies they undergo neither phagocytosis nor destruction by polymorphonuclear cells or macrophages. These pathogenic spirochetes adhere to epithelial cells but do not cause direct injury during penetration.

7. What is the incubation period of leptospirosis?

The incubation period ranges between 2 and 30 days, although most patients become ill after 5–14 days.

8. What are the common presenting signs?

None of the presenting features of leptospirosis are specific. In addition, it is not possible to tell clinically whether an attack will be mild or severe or what the outcome of the illness will be. Common signs include sudden onset of generalized headache, retroocular pain, muscle pain and tenderness, high fever, nausea with or without vomiting, conjunctivitis, a transient skin and mucosal rash, and photophobia. These signs and symptoms must be differentiated from those of influenza, hepatitis, and other viral illnesses, including aseptic meningitis. Depending on the location where the patient is living, other illnesses including rickettsiosis, borreliosis, brucellosis, toxoplasmosis, malaria, and dengue fever also must be considered.

9. What other signs and symptoms may be seen in leptospirosis?

Myalgia may be excruciating. In anicteric leptospirosis, spirochetes circulate hematogenously and can be recovered in cultures of blood, urine, and cerebrospinal fluid (CSF). Impairment of kidney and liver function is often reflected by a transient albuminuria and nitrogen retention. After 4–7 days, the patient may improve, the temperature subsides, and recovery is usually complete after 3–6 weeks of onset. In more severe forms, the course of illness may be prolonged and biphasic. After subsiding for 4–7 days, the fever suddenly recurs, rising to 40°C or higher. Headaches, rigors, and chills are more severe. Myositis occurs and occasionally tenderness of the abdominal wall may be so intense to mimic an acute surgical abdomen. Extremely elevated levels of creatine phosphokinase (CPK) are common and indicate active skeletal muscle inflammatory involvement. Occasional cases of monoarthritis or migratory polyarthritis have been reported.

10. Summarize the frequency of each symptom.
- Abrupt onset of fevers, rigors, myalgias and headache in 75–100% of patients
- Dry cough in 25–35% patients
- Nausea, vomiting and diarrhea in 50% of patients
- Muscle tenderness, enlarged liver or spleen, and enlarged lymph nodes in 7–40% patients

11. What is the most common symptom in patients with leptospirosis?

The most common finding seen in all patients with leptospirosis is a sudden, throbbing severe headache. Occasionally serous meningitis is seen in the second phase and recognized by rigidity and neck stiffness, photophobia, and severe headache and vomiting. Occasionally serous meningitis is the presenting form of leptospirosis in patients seeking hospitalization following an ill-defined fever. CSF labs are usually within normal limits except for an elevated pressure. Late in the disease CSF protein may increase, and moderate pleocytosis is seen. It may take up to 3 weeks for these symptoms and CSF levels to return to normal.

12. What is the most characteristic lesion of leptospirosis?

Vasculitis, mainly of small vessels, leading to fluid and cell leakage and eventually to frank hemorrhage, is considered the most characteristic lesion. Tissue lesions in leptospirosis are characterized by major cellular damage in the presence of few microorganisms, suggesting the involvement of toxic factors from the spirochete, or host, or both.

13. Describe the characteristic rash seen in leptospirosis.

Often a transient petechial red palatal enanthem occurs within the first day or two. Early in the illness, the skin is often suffused, exhibiting a pink tinge. Exanthematous rashes, usually morbilliform but not confluent and sometimes itchy, are recorded in 10–30% of patients during the first week and may last 1 to 2 days. Occasionally the rash may be purpuric and confluent. In the more severe form of leptospirosis, purpuric rashes may occur as part of a general hemorrhagic tendency. Capillary fragility is increased during that phase.

14. Describe the conjunctivitis seen in leptospirosis.
Conjunctival suffusion is probably the most characteristic and diagnostically helpful physical finding. Unlike bacterial or viral conjunctivitis, pus and serous secretions are absent. There is no matting of the eyelashes or eyelids. In a child, one should consider Kawasaki disease with this conjunctivitis.

15. Describe the kidney lesions observed in severe leptospirosis.
Abnormalities can be detected on urinalysis in 80–90% of patients. Often red cells, leukocytes, or granular casts are found in the urine. Hemoglobinuria and hyaline casts also are seen. Proteinuria and myoglobinuria are frequent findings. Renal failure may occur within 3 days of onset of disease. Blood urea nitrogen (BUN) and creatinine levels rise rapidly with corresponding increases in serum potassium, uric acid, and phosphate levels. It appears that the most severe lesions occur in the proximal tubules. Occasionally a hemolytic uremic syndrome has been observed, which is thought to result from the action of leptospiral toxins.

16. What laboratory tests are abnormal?
- Elevated erythrocyte sedimentation rate (ESR)
- Slight increase in neutrophil count
- Thrombocytopenia
- Elevated serum amylase
- Decreased serum C3

17. What other laboratory alterations are common in leptospirosis?
Other abnormalities include abnormal bleeding and coagulation times, prolonged prothrombin time, decreased levels of factor V, and shortening or prolongation of thrombin time.

18. Do these alterations mean that the patient has disseminated intravascular coagulation (DIC)?
These alterations are not related to DIC.

19. Infection with leptospira can result in acute renal failure and electrolyte abnormalities. What is the mechanism?
Bacterial glycolipoprotein inhibits the activity of the sodium-potassium-adenosine triphosphatase cycle of renal tubule epithelial cells. Thus, it is responsible for the electrolyte alterations seen in patients with leptospirosis who develop acute renal failure.

20. What mortality rate is associated with leptospirosis?
The mortality rate in severe leptospirosis usually ranges from 5% to 40%.

21. What unusual manifestations may be seen with leptospirosis?
Obstructive cerebral vascular disease, localized neuritis or polyneuritis, and cardiomyopathy. There is a high incidence of various ocular manifestations, such as conjunctival hyperemia, increased retinal vein caliber, optic disc redness or edema, subconjunctival hemorrhage, retinal vasculitis and hemorrhage. However, all of these are seen in the acute phase of leptospirosis; despite the systemic severity and high incidence of ocular disorders in the acute phase, the short-term visual outcome is good.

22. How does leptospirosis affect fetuses?
In the first and second trimester, death may result from hemorrhage, nephritis, or placentitis. However when the fetus and mother recover, sequelae are rare. On the other hand, infection of the mother during the third trimester may result in an apparently healthy fetus affected with congenital leptospirosis.

23. What is the prognosis in children vs. adults?

Leptospirosis has a better prognosis in children than in adults.

24. What is Weil's syndrome?

Originally described in 1886, Weil's syndrome is a severe form of leptospirosis associated with severe hepatic malfunction, jaundice, hemorrhages, and hemodynamic, pulmonary, and neurologic alterations. It has a high mortality rate (up to 82% of hospitalized patients). In this form of disease, the symptoms ascribed to anicteric patients, are more intense and prolonged. In addition, severe intense jaundice occurs about 3–7 days after the beginning of the illness. Frequently, serum bilirubin level are above 15 mg–100 cm^3. Although urine is dark, acholic feces are not usually observed. In addition, renal involvement is more frequent and severe in Weil's disease than in the anicteric form. Approximately 71% of patients with Weil's disease have concurrent renal failure. Hemorrhagic phenomena are relatively common in Weil's syndrome and may occur in the skin, mucosae, or internal organs. Thirty percent of patients in some series present with some kind of mucosal or cutaneous bleeding.

25. How is leptospirosis diagnosed?

Cases are considered confirmed when *Leptospira* organisms are isolated from any clinical specimen or when suggestive clinical symptoms are associated with seroconversion (a fourfold increase in the initial titer by serum-agglutination or presence of specific IgM class antibodies detected by enzyme-linked immunosorbent assay [ELISA]). The microscopic serum-agglutination and the ELISA are the most commonly used diagnostic techniques in clinical practice. Of interest, early use of antibiotics or steroids may delay or even completely prevent the appearance of specific antibodies during convalescence.

26. What is the recommended therapy for leptospirosis?

Recent double-blind, placebo-controlled studies have demonstrated that doxycycline, at a dose of 100 mg orally 2 times/day for 1 week, is beneficial in shortening the course of early leptospirosis. In addition, intravenous penicillin at the dose of 1.5 million units 4 times daily for 7 days, decreased the duration of fever and renal impairment in severe, late illness. Complications of therapy may include the Jarisch-Herxheimer reaction after penicillin.

27. What prophylaxis should be used in patients with presumed leptospirosis?

Prophylaxis should be individualized. For people exposed to single events with high risk of infections and people visiting endemic areas for a short time, single or weekly 200-mg prophylactic doses of doxycycline have proved efficacious.

28. How can leptospirosis be prevented?

Avoid areas of stagnant water, especially in tropical climates.

29. For the following cat- and dog-related zoonoses, match the disease with the mode of transmission.

Bacteria	Transmission
a. *Salmonella* species	1. Fecal-oral
b. *Campylobacter jejuni*	2. Environmental contamination
c. *Cryptosporidium parvum*	3. Direct contact
d. Giardiasis	4. Ingestion of dog and cat fleas
e. *Dipylidium caninum*	5. Skin penetration
f. *Toxocara canis*	
g. *Sarcoptes scabiei* var. *canis*	
h. *Ancylostoma caninum*	

Answers: a–d, 1; e, 1, 4; f, 1, 2; g, 3; h, 2, 5.

30. For the following dog-related zoonoses, match the disease with mode of transmission

Organism	Transmission
1. *Bordetella bronchiseptica*	a. Unknown
2. *Brucella canis*	b. Aerosol
3. *Leptospira* species	c. Indirect contact
4. *Malassezia pachydermatis*	d. Contact with urine or contaminated water

Answers: 1, b; 2, a; 3, d; 4, c.

31. For the following cat-related zoonoses, match the disease with mode of transmission.

Organism	Transmission
1. *Toxoplasma* sp.	a. Fecal-oral
2. *Bartonella* sp.	b. Transplacental
3. *Yersinia* sp.	c. Scratch, bite
	d. Direct contact with animal, flea bites

Answers: 1, a and b; 2, c; 3, d.

32. For the following bird-related zoonoses, match the disease with mode of transmission

Organism	Transmission
1. *Chlamydia psittaci*	a. Aerosol
2. *Salmonella* sp.	b. Direct contact
3. Paramyxovirus	c. Fecal-oral
4. Influenza virus	
5. *Aspergillus* sp.	
6. *Dermanyssus gallinae*	

Answers: 1, a; 2, c; 3–5, a; 6, b.

33. For the following rabbit-related zoonoses, match the disease with mode of transmission.

Organisms	Transmission
1. *Francisella tularensis*	a. Direct contact
2. *Trichophyton* sp.	b. Bites

Answers: 1, a and b; 2, b.

34. What emerging infection is related to reptiles and amphibians?
Salmonella species.

35. What emerging infection is associated with ferrets?
Influenza virus.

36. What is hantavirus?
Hantavirus belongs to the Bunyaviridae family. The organisms are lipid-enveloped, spheric viruses of 80–100 nm in diameter and consist of a trisegmented RNA genome. A prototype for this virus is Hantaan virus. This virus and closely related agents include Seoul, Dobrava-Belgrado, Cano Delgadito, and Puumala virus.

37. Where was hantavirus first described in the United States: (a) Washington, DC, (b) the three corners region, (c) the four corners region, or (d) Memphis, TN?
Answers: (c), the four corners region (including the states of New Mexico, Arizona, Utah and Colorado).

38. Hantavirus infections have been seen in other parts of the country. Name two.
New York and Pennsylvania.

39. How is hantavirus transmitted?

As with arenaviruses, hantavirus is transmitted from rodents to humans, mainly through inhalation of excreta from the infected host. There has been only one case of documented human-to-human transmission. The natural host of hantavirus is Murid rodents, which include Old World rats and mice, New World rats and mice, and voles.

40. What is the incubation period of hantavirus?

One to 6 weeks, followed by a prodromal phase for 3–5 days.

41. What are the symptoms of the prodromal phase?

Fever, headache, and myalgias. Other symptoms may include vomiting, diarrhea, abdominal pain, and dizziness. Cough and tachypnea, which are generally absent during the first days, appear at the end of the prodromal phase.

42. What are the findings on physical exam?

Tachypnea, tachycardia, hypotension, and rales on respiratory examination. Some South American cases also may present with conjunctival congestion, head and neck suffusion, and hemorrhagic and renal compromise. The different hantaviruses have different amounts of renal involvement, which may be due to the different viral genotypes.

43. What are common laboratory findings in hantavirus infection?

Laboratory evaluation shows leukocytosis with a left shift, atypical lymphocytes, thrombocytopenia, elevation of hepatic transaminases, marked increase in serum lactate dehydrogenase (LDH), and moderate prolongation of partial thromboplastin time (PTT).

44. What are the findings on chest x-ray?

Minimal initial changes of interstitial pulmonary edema, which rapidly progress to severe alveolar bilateral edema.

45. What is the unique pulmonary feature of hantavirus infection?

Hantavirus pulmonary syndrome (HPS). There is an absence of significant inflammatory response in the lung, in contrast with many other infectious pneumonias.

46. What is the differential diagnosis of HPS?

- Leptospirosis
- Psittacosis
- Rickettsial infections
- Arenaviral hemorrhagic fevers
- Influenza, histoplasmosis
- Atypical bacterial and viral community-acquired pneumonias

47. What are the definitive laboratory tests?

Serology showing the presence of IgM specific antibodies or seroconversion by IgG; a positive reverse-transcriptase polymerase chain reaction (PCR) for hantavirus RNA; or demonstration of viral antigens in tissues by immunohistochemistry.

48. What therapy is available for hantavirus infections?

There is currently no effective therapy for New World hantavirus infection.

49. What are the precautions for housestaff?

Universal precaution with barrier methods should be followed in all hospitalized cases. Patients should be placed in a private room, and any procedure associated with aerosol generation should have additional protection with gloves and HEPA filter mask.

50. What prevention methods could be used for hantavirus infection?

It is not possible to control the wild rodent populations at this time. There are no human vaccines against New World Hantavirus, and strategies for disease prevention are limited to minimizing contact with rodents and their excreta.

51. What is another name for variant Creutzfeldt-Jacob disease (vCJD)?

Transmissible spongiform encephalopathy (TSE). The members of this group include CJD, bovine spongiform encephalopathy (mad cow disease), and scrapie of sheep.

52. What is the nature of the TSE agent?

It is currently referred to as a self-replicating protein (prion). It is virus-like and possesses some nucleic acids, which carry genetic information. There have been no reported cases of vCJD in Australia, Canada or the United States. However, there are reports in France as well as the United Kingdom. Prion diseases are characterized by long incubation periods ranging from months to years. They are invariably fatal once classic symptoms have appeared. vCJD (a recently identified human prion disease) appears to arise from exposure to bovine spongiform encephalopathy agent.

53. How are vCJD and traditional forms of CJD different?

Traditional CJD was recognized to exist in only three forms: Sporadic cases, which have an unknown cause and occur throughout the world at a rate of 1 per 1,000,000 people (accounting for 85–90% of CJD cases; familial cases, which are associated with a gene mutation and make up an additional 5–10% of cases; and iatrogenic cases, resulting from the accidental transmission of the causative agent via contaminated surgical equipment as a result of cornea or dura mater transplants, or during the administration of human-derived pituitary growth hormone. Less than 5% of CJD cases were iatrogenic. CJD variant is strongly linked to exposure, probably through food, to a TSE of cattle called bovine spongiform encephalopathy.

54. What age group does vCJD affect?

Unlike traditional forms of CJD, vCJD affects younger patients (average age: 29 years), and has a relatively shorter duration of illness (median of 4.5 months as opposed 14 months). As of June 2001, the CJD surveillance unit has reported 95 cases of vCJD, including 88 confirmed and 7 probable. In addition, there are 6 cases in which vCJD is suspected, but diagnosis has not yet been confirmed.

55. Can vCJD be transmitted through blood?

The answer is unknown.

56. Describe the clinical features of vCJD.

Early in the illness, patients usually experience psychiatric symptoms, which most commonly take the form of depression or schizophrenia-like psychosis. Unusual sensory symptoms have been experienced by half of patients, including "stickiness" of the skin."

57. How is vCJD diagnosed?

There are no completely reliable tests for use before the onset of clinical symptoms. However, magnetic resonance imaging, tonsillar biopsy and CSF test may be useful diagnostic tests to eliminate or confirm other diagnoses. Currently, the only way to make a diagnosis or to confirm the diagnosis of vCJD is after pathologic examination of the brain. Characteristically multiple microscopic and abnormal aggregates encircled by holes are seen, resulting in a daisy-like appearance described by the term *florid plaques.*

58. What are some of the other human TSEs?

Kuru in Papua New Guinea and Gerstmann-Sträussler-Schenker syndrome.

59. How do you prevent the transmission of vCJD?

Currently, there is a statutory ban on the feeding of protein derived from cattle, sheep, and goats to any other ruminant. This ban has been in existence since 1999. The World Health Organization recommends the following: no part or product of any animal that has shown signs of TSE should enter any human or animal food chain; countries should not permit tissues that are likely to contain the BSE agent to enter any human or animal food chain; all countries should ban the use of ruminant tissues in ruminant feed; and pharmaceutical companies should avoid the use of bovine materials and materials from other animal species in which TSE occur in the preparation of vaccines.

60. Where did West Nile virus (WNV) originate?

It was first isolated in the West Nile district of Uganda in 1937. It has been commonly found in humans and birds and other vertebrates in Africa, Eastern Europe, West Asia, and the Middle East but was not documented in the Western Hemisphere until 1999.

61. How is the virus transmitted?

The basic transmission cycle involves mosquitoes feeding on birds infected with the West Nile virus. Infected mosquitoes transmit West Nile virus to humans and animals.

62. What are the clinical manifestations of WNV infection ?

The clinical description ranges from asymptomatic infection to a dengue-like illness with fever, lymphadenopathy, headache, abdominal pain, vomiting, rash, and conjunctivitis. CNS involvement and death occur in a minority of cases.

63. What is the incubation period?

Usually is 5–15 days.

64. To what viral family does WNV belong?

Flaviviridae virus (single-stranded RNA viruses).

65. Name some viruses related to WNV.

- Japanese encephalitis (Asia)
- St. Louis encephalitis (North and South America)
- Kunjin
- Murray Valley encephalitis (Australia)

66. Name two virulence factors of WNV?

E proteins and membrane fusion proteins.

67. What is the typical appearance of the rash in WNV infection?

The rash can be a roseola or macular papular rash in about half of patients; it lasts approximately 1 week and resolves without scaling.

68. Where does WNV replicate?

WNV replicates in local tissue in lymph nodes and is transported via the lymphatics to the blood. Virus can be isolated from the blood from 2 days before the onset of illness through the fourth day of illness.

69. How does CNS infection occur?

Although the exact mechanism is unknown, CNS infection probably occurs when virus crosses the blood-brain barrier by endothelial replication or axonal transport through olfactory neurons. Factors that enhance progression of CNS infections include hypertension and duration and level of viremia (presence of immune suppression).

70. Is lumbar puncture helpful?

CSF analyses include a normal glucose level, elevated protein, and lymphocytic pleocytosis with counts of 10–100 cell/mm^3. Although most patients' symptoms resolve completely, experimental infection in monkeys has shown a chronic progressive CNS infection, suggesting the possibility of viral persistence in the CNS.

71. What are the nonneurologic complications?
Myocarditis, pancreatitis, and fulminant hepatitis.

72. What laboratory diagnostic tests are useful in WNV encephalitis?
The most commonly used method is the IgM capture ELISA, which measures WNV-specific IgM antibody and has a sensitivity approaching 100%. IgM antibody may be detectable for several months after infection. Presence of intrathecal IgM strongly suggests a central nervous system infection.

73. How is WNV treated?
At this time there is no known treatment.

BIBLIOGRAPHY

1. Enria DA, Pinheiro F. Rodent-borne emerging viral zoonoses. Infect Dis Clin North Am 14:167–184, 2000.
2. Glaser C, Lewis P, Wong S: Pet-, animal-, and vector-borne infections. Pediatr Rev 21(7), 2000.
3. Hoots WK: The impact of Creutzfeldt-Jakob disease and variant Creutzfeldt-Jakob disease on plasma safety. Transfus Med Rev 15(2 Suppl 1):45–59, 2001.
4. Horga MA, Fine A: West Nile virus. Pediatr Infect Dis J 20:799–802, 2001.
5. Jackson GS: The molecular pathology of CJD: Old and new variants. Mol Pathol 54(5):393–399, 2001.
6. Lomar AV, Diament D, Torres JR: Leptospirosis in Latin America. Infect Dis Clin North Am 14:23–39, 2000.
7. Marfin AA, Gubler DJ: West Nile Encephalitis: An emerging disease in the United States. Clin Infect Dis 33:1713–1719, 2001.
8. Pickering LK (ed): 2000 Red Book: Report of the Committee of Infectious Diseases, 25th ed. Elk Grove Village, IL: American Academy of Pediatrics, 2000.

45. ZOONOSES

Robert N. Tiballi, D.O.

1. Define zoonoses.

Zoonoses are a wide and complex group of infectious diseases that commonly have their reservoir of infection in animal populations (usually vertebrates) and can infect humans. They can be transferred easily or inadvertently to humans via direct contact, inhalation, ingestion, animal bites, or arthropod intermediates. They can infect humans commonly or uncommonly and sometimes can be spread from human to human.

2. My son was bitten by a possum that ran off into the woods. Does he need rabies shots?

Possums are marsupials and do not carry rabies. No postexposure vaccination is needed.

3. My daughter was asleep in her room when a bat flew through the window. She was not bitten. Does she need rabies shots?

The most common exposure leading to human rabies in the United States in the past five years has been bat aerosol. The infected bat does not need to bite or scratch the human. Close contact allows sharing of respiratory aerosols between the bat and its victim. If the bat in the scenario above tests positive for rabies or cannot be located, the girl should receive postexposure rabies vaccination. Bats are the leading vector for human rabies in the United States. Worldwide, unvaccinated dogs are the major vector. Rabid bats can be found in most areas of the United States at any given time, whereas regional raccoon and skunk populations vary in rabies status.

4. My son was bitten by a strangely acting skunk. Can skunks carry rabies?

Yes. The offending animal should be captured, if possible, and tested for rabies. If capture is not possible, postexposure vaccination is indicated as a conservative measure.

5. We keep pet rabbits outside in a pen. Should they be vaccinated for rabies?

Rabbits can become infected with rabies. They should be vaccinated for rabies if kept outdoors.

6. My son was bitten by a squirrel. Does he need rabies shots?

Rodents, squirrels, mice, and rats do not carry rabies. Exposure to these animals carries no risk of contracting rabies.

7. A raccoon bit our dog. I shot the raccoon, and the animal control expert said that it was rabid. My children play with the dog all of the time. Do they need rabies vaccine?

If the dog was adequately vaccinated against rabies, there is no risk to children who play with the dog. If the dog's vaccination status has not been kept current, repeat vaccination is needed and the dog should be kept under quarantine for 2 weeks. If symptoms of rabies occur, the children also require vaccination, although their exposure is minimal if the dog was quarantined immediately after the bite.

8. My son was taunting the neighbor's dog, and it bit him. We washed out the wounds. Does he need antibiotics?

Dog and cat bites commonly involve exposure to *Pasturella multocida*. This extremely virulent organism can lead to dramatically progressive cellulitis and sepsis without aggressive treatment. Bites into tendon sheaths or bones carry a high (~90%) risk of tendon sheath abscesses or osteomyelitis. Such injuries should be aggressively treated with debridement, irrigation, and appropriate antibiotics. *P. multocida* is resistant to cephalexin and cefadroxil. Penicillinase-producing strains are becoming more common. Treatment should include high-dose amoxicillin/clavulanate or doxycycline.

9. Our daughter's horse has pneumonia. Now she is sick. The doctor in the emergency department said that she has pneumonia. She is not improving with a cephalosporin. What should we do?

Rhodococcus equi is a common cause of pneumonia in horses. It uncommonly causes infections in humans, but it may be an underrecognized cause of pneumonia in people with close contact with horses. It is not considered to be contagious from human to human. Active antibiotics include azithromycin, clarithromycin, erythromycin, clindamycin and vancomycin. Cephalosporins are not effective against this organism.

10. The local pharmacist tells you that her dog is sick with hepatitis and renal failure. She thinks that the dog has leptospirosis, the same infection that killed her other dog 4 weeks ago. She asks whether leptospirosis is contagious and whether she and her children should be given prophylactic antibiotics.

Leptospirosis is very uncommon in the United States. Americans usually are infected while traveling abroad. In humans leptospirosis most commonly causes hepatitis with jaundice and renal failure. The pharmacist and her children should be treated prophylactically because of the highly infectious nature of leptospirosis. Treatment is achieved with penicillin or doxycycline.

11. True or false: The most common cause of eosinophilia in toddlers and children is a dog parasite.

True. *Toxocara canis* is acquired via the fecal-oral route from dog to child. Treatment with antihelminthics is controversial.

12. Little Johnny just returned from a trip to Belize with his mother and father. He has an unusual serpiginous, tracking red streak on the bottom of his foot. Neither parent has similar lesions. The mother recalls that Johnny liked to walk on the beach without his shoes. Which is your diagnosis: (a) erythema chronicum migrans, (b) porphyria cutanea tarda, (c) contact dermatitis, or (d) cutaneous larva migrans?

Tropical tourist areas do their best to keep dogs off the beach. Otherwise, many tourists are subject to infectious reminders of their romantic walks. When they step on fecal remnants from dogs, they can be exposed to larvae from *Ancyclostoma brasiliense*, which burrows into the dermis and traverses the skin, causing the serpiginous course of pruritic erythema and the "creeping eruption" of cutaneous larva migrans. This infection is also common in the southeastern United States. When the infection is successfully treated with albendazole or ivermectin, intense itching of the foot may follow.

13. My daughter had enlarged lymph nodes. Biopsy revealed toxoplasmosis, which she probably contracted from our cat. I am worried that she will not be able to have children or that they will be infected. What can we do?

In most situations, people with normal immune systems who are infected with toxoplasmosis require no treatment. Pyrimethamine and sulfadiazine, the treatments of choice, are difficult to tolerate. Trimethoprim/sulfamethoxazole also has been used to treat the infection in nonpregnant, immunocompetent hosts, but it is less effective. Problems arise when a pregnant woman develops initial infection. Intrauterine infection of the unborn child is common. The effects in such children, born without prenatal treatment, can be devastating.

14. My wife had pneumonia that kept getting worse. Lung biopsy showed cryptococcal infection, which, according to the doctor, she probably contracted from our pet bird. Do we need to get rid of the bird? What about the children?

Birds can be infected with cryptococci, which can be transmitted to humans via excrement. Cryptococcal pneumonia transmitted from birds is rare in humans but can occur in a normal host. Most cryptococcal infections occur in HIV-infected people. Infection can be diagnosed by a blood test for cryptococcal antigen, which is about 95% sensitive for infection. Infections can be treated with fluconazole. The family members should have serum cryptococcal antigens checked and, if positive, be treated with fluconazole.

15. My daughter was bitten by her hamster. Should she take any antibiotics?

On rare occasions, hamsters have transmitted viruses to humans through bites. Bacterial infections are usually associated with particularly severe bites and caused by normal skin flora. The same is true for ferrets. Owning a ferret is still illegal in New York City.

16. Our dog has distemper. Can our children catch this disease from the dog?

Distemper does not infect humans. The illness can be prevented in dogs by a vaccine.

17. Our dog has parvovirus infection. Can our children catch this disease from the dog?

Canine strains of parvovirus do not infect humans. The canine and human strains. are different. Parvovirus can be deadly to dogs, but an effective animal vaccine is available.

18. We are traveling to Peru to go on a jungle excursion. According to the Centers for Disease Control and Prevention (CDC), we should receive yellow fever vaccine. What do you think?

The CDC website at CDC.gov has a section of advice for travelers. Yellow fever is endemic to many countries in the southern hemisphere. This mosquito-borne illness can be prevented by vaccination. Yellow fever and malaria killed thousands of workers on the Panama Canal. Almost all of them would have happily received the vaccine, if they had the opportunity.

19. While vacationing at Martha's Vineyard, we were bitten by mosquitoes. My father and I received doxycycline from a local doctor because we were worried about Lyme disease. Our two children (ages 4 and 6 years) received no medication. Do we need to worry about Lyme disease?

No. Lyme disease is spread by tick bites, not mosquito bites.

20. The children have fevers and night sweats. Maybe they were bitten by ticks, too.

Babesia microti, an intracellular parasite, is transmitted by tick bites and infects red blood cells. In the United States, it is most commonly seen in the coastal and island areas of Massachusetts (Cape Cod and Martha's Vineyard) as well as Rhode Island, Long Island, and Shelter Island and Washington states. Treatment is clindamycin or azithromycin plus quinine. It is possible to become infected with both Lyme disease and babesiosis in these hyperendemic areas.

21. My son accompanied me to Arkansas for a golfing weekend. He went into the woods to find lost golf balls and was bitten by a bunch of ticks. The local doctor put him on amoxyl to treat for Lyme disease. We returned home two weeks ago, and he has had a fever since. What is wrong?

Erlichia chaffeensis and *E. phagocytophilia* can coinfect ticks that carry Lyme disease. These organisms more commonly cause infection in the central United States, from Arkansas through Minnesota. Diagnosis is made by visualizing the morulae in the cytoplasm of white blood cells on peripheral smear. Patients usually have high fevers with thrombocytopenia and may manifest a petechial rash. Diseases are named for the type of white blood cell that the organism infects: human granulocytic erlichiosis (HGE) (*E. phagocytophilia*) and human monocytic erlichiosis (HME) (*E. chaffeensis*). Serologic tests are available to assist diagnosis, but treatment with doxycycline should begin once the infection is suspected.

22. A kitten scratched our daughter. She has a fever and swelling in her armpit. What is the cause?

Cats under the age of 18 months commonly are colonized and frequently bacteremic with *Bartonella henselae*. They have high concentrations of the bacteria between their footpads, and scratches from colonized cats can cause serious infections. Humans infected with *B. henselae* most commonly develop enlarged lymph nodes in the axilla or neck. Treatment consists of oral azithromycin or clarithromycin. Intravenous aminoglycosides are also effective.

23. Our dog likes to lick our newborn baby. Is it safe to let him do so?

A species of *Capnocytophaga* (DF-2) can colonize the mouths of dogs. This highly aggressive organism has caused sepsis and death in newborns who acquired infection from pet dogs through such contact. Neutropenic and splenectomized adults have developed sepsis and disseminated intravascular coagulation. This practice should be strongly discouraged. In a similar fashion, household presence of iguanas has been associated with *Salmonella* sepsis in newborns. Care providers are the vector for transmission of *Salmonella* from the reptile to the infant. Newborns should not be cared for by day care centers or in homes with reptile pets.

24. During our vacation in Florida, our son caught his foot on a sea urchin and now has a streak running up his leg as well as fevers and chills. The doctor prescribed a steroid for the sea urchin sting. Does he need antibiotics?

Vibrio vulnificus can cause infections in people who have skin ulcers or are cut or bitten while swimming in salt water. The organism commonly causes sepsis in people who survive shark bites and may cause cellulitis and lymphangitis in people who are stung by sea urchins or jellyfish. These infections are common in people who swim in the Gulf of Mexico. Ciprofloxacin, ceftazadime, and doxycycline are the drugs of choice.

25. Can people can catch pneumonia from birds?

Yes. People can become infected with *Chlamydia psitacci*, which may be present in ornithine birds that bypass normal import controls and quarantine. The birds become very sick with foaming at the beak and frequently succumb to the pneumonia.

26. My son helped me clean a deer. Since cleaning the heart and cavity organs, he has had a rash on his hands that is getting worse. What is it?

Erysipelothrix species commonly causes infections in deer. It may cause endocarditis in deer. Handling infected body organs can cause cutaneous infection in humans. Treatment is penicillin, cephalosporin, or fluoroquinolone.

27. Can you catch cysticercosis from another person whose brain is infected with the parasite?

Yes—if the person is also infected with the adult form of the parasite, an intestinal tapeworm. Brain infection represents the inadvertent human hosting of the intermediate stage of infection. This is the parasite that makes pork infectious if it is not adequately cooked. To become infected, one must ingest fecal material from the tapeworm-infected person. Such exposure leads to solid organ infection with the intermediate stage of the *Taenia* parasite. Deposition of the cystercads may occur in any body organ. Chance and blood flow determine the location of the infection (brain, lung, liver, kidney, dermis). People also can get a tapeworm from the person with neurocysticercosis if they eat the infected brain without proper cooking!

28. One of my patients has nodular densities that developed in a linear fashion after he scraped his knuckles while cleaning his aquarium. It looks like sporotrichosis, but it does not respond to antifungals. What is it?

Mycobacterium marinum infection is seen after skin abrasions. Contact with home aquariums, swimming pools, and fish can lead to infection. Treatment is usually required for 3–6 months or more. *M. marinum* is resistant to isoniazid and pyrazinamide but usually sensitive to clarithromycin, ethambutol, rifampin, and doxycycline. In refractory cases, drug sensitivities must be obtained.

46. BIOTERRORISM

Joel D. Klein, M.D., FAAP, and Theoklis E. Zaoutis, M.D.

1. **Match the bioterrorism infection with the clinical finding.**

Infection	Clinical finding
1. Anthrax	a. Cutaneous lesion
2. Smallpox	b. Pneumonia
3. Tularemia	c. Paralysis
4. Botulism	d. Adenopathy
5. Plague	

   Answers: 1, a, b; 2, a; 3, a, b, d; 4, c; 5. b, d.

2. **How many cases of human plague occur in the U.S. each year: (a) none, (b) 100–150, (c) 10–20, or (d) > 500?**

   (c). 10–20 cases occur annually, mostly in rural, scattered areas. The highest incidence is in New Mexico and Arizona.

3. **Explain the derivation of the term *bubonic plague*.**

   The word *bubo* refers to a tender swollen lymph node, which is the hallmark of human plague.

4. **Who wrote the novel *The Plague:* (a) John Donne, (b) John Grisham, (c) Daniel Defoe, or (d) Albert Camus?**

   (d). Camus describes the result of a plague epidemic in the port of Oran, Morocco.

5. **What is the classic chest x-ray finding in inhalation anthrax: (a) pleural effusion, (b) widening of the mediastinum, (c) pulmonary calcification, or (d) cardiac tamponade?**

   (b). Widening of the mediastinum results from massive mediastinal lymphadenopathy.

6. **Match the manifestation of Anthrax infection with the condition with which it may be confused.**

Anthrax manifestation	Confusing clinical condition
1. Cutaneous lesion	a. Bacillary dysentery
2. Inhalation anthrax	b. Influenza
3. Prodnomal myalgias, fever	c. Spider bite
4. Gastrointestinal anthrax	d. Community-acquired pneumonia

   Answers: 1, c; 2, d; 3, b; 4, a.

7. **Viral hemorrhagic fevers are considered possible agents for bioterrorism. For which of the following VHF viruses are the viral reservoirs unknown (a) Marburg, (b) hantavirus, or (c) Ebola?**

   (a) and (c). Hantavirus has a rodent reservoir.

8. **Smallpox vaccination offered within how many days after exposure will lessen the severity of infection?**

   a. **Vaccination is ineffective after exposure.**   c. **4 hours**
   b. **4 days**   d. **1 week**

   (c). If given in this time frame, smallpox vaccination may even prevent infection.

9. **Smallpox is only one of a number of poxviruses. Which of the following are genuine poxviruses: (a) monkey pox, (b) buffalo pox, (c) sealpox, (d) canary pox, or (e) all of the above?**

(e). Can you think of a literary reference to the pox? Hint: think of the Bard of Avon.

10. **True or false: The smallpox vaccine does not contain smallpox virus.**

True. It contains vaccinia virus.

11. **In view of a potential bioterroism threat, it is critical to distinguish smallpox (variola) from chickenpox (varicella). How can they be distinguished?**

	Variola	Varicella
Incubation	7–17 days	14–21 days
Prodrome	2–4 days	Minimal/none
Distribution	Centrifugal	Centripetal
Progression	Synchronous	Asynchronous
Scab formation	10–14 days after the rash	4–7 days after rash
Scab separation	14–28 days after rash	< 14 days after rash

12. **Which of the following antibiotics is appropriate for initial treatment of cutaneous anthrax: (a) ciprofloxacin, (b) doxycycline, (c) erythromycin, or (d) neomycin?**

Answer: (a) and (b).

13. **An accidental release of anthrax spores enabled scientists to learn about their potential as a biologic weapon. In what city did the accident occur: (a) Emerald City, (b) Santiago, (c) Sverdlovsk, (d) Hilo, or (e) Los Alamos?**

(c). Seventy-nine cases of anthrax occurred in the city of the former Soviet Union in 1979. Sixty eight of the patients died.

14. **Although a candidate for bioterrorism, botulism is occasionally a naturally occurring disease. What two forms of botulism are seen in the U.S.? List their major characteristics.**

	Infantile botulism	Foodborne botulism
Agent	*Clostridium botulinum*	*Clostridium botulinum*
Incubation	3–30 days	12–36 hours
Source of toxin	Germinating pores in food	Germinating spores in infant intestine
Signs/symptoms	Constipation, lethargy	Symmetric descending flaccid paralysis

15. **_Francisella tularensis_ is the spore-forming bacteria that causes tularemia. What are the minimal numbers of spores (inoculated or inhaled) required to cause disease?**

a. **Trick question: these spores cannot be inhaled.**   d. **> 1000**
b. **As few as 10**   e. **Not known**
c. **3.6 × 10**

(b). Tularemia a likely candidate for bioterrorism because of its extreme infectivity, ease of dissemination, and substantial capacity to cause illness.

16. **A terrorist biologic attack occurred in Oregon in 1984. What biologic agent was involved?**

Salmonella spp.

17. **In the above attack, what food was used to disseminate the biologic agent: (a) sushi, (b) veal cutlets, (c) salad, (d) rare hamburger, or (e) carrot juice?**

Answer: (c), served in a salad bar. The outbreak occurred in Dalles, Oregon and was the result of intentional contamination of salad bars by members of a religious commune.

BIBLIOGRAPHY

1. American Academy of Pediatrics, Committee on Environmental Health and Committee on Infectious Diseases: Chemical-biological terrorism and its impact on children: A subject review. Pediatrics 105:662–670, 2000.
2. Breman JG, Henderson DA: Current concepts: Diagnosis and management of small pox. N Engl J Med 346:1300–1307, 2002.
3. Henderson DA,.Inglesby TV, Bartlett JG, et al: Smallpox as a biologial weapon: Medical and public health management. JAMA 281:2127–2137, 1999.
4. Inglesby TV, O'Toole Tara, Henderson DA, et al: Anthrax as a biological weapon, 2002: Updated recommendations for management. JAMA 287:2236–2252, 2002.
5. Patt HA, Feigin RD: Diagnosis and management of suspected cases of bioterrorism: A pediatric perspective. Pediatrics 109:685–692, 2002.

XIII. Immunizations

47. VACCINE FACTS AND MYTHS

Edwin L. Anderson, M.D.

1. Tetanus is prevented in newborns infants by which of the following: good sanitary conditions, vaccination of women with tetanus toxoid vaccine, availability of penicillin, or modern newborn care?

Neonatal tetanus is prevented in the United States by prenatal immunization of women, followed by booster doses with the diphtheria-tetanus (dT) vaccine during pregnancy if it has been 10 years or longer since the last tetanus immunization. The etiologic agent of tetanus, *Clostridium tetani*, is worldwide in distribution and contaminates wounds. Neonatal tetanus is a common cause of neonatal mortality in developing countries.

2. How soon can the second vaccination for measles, mumps, and rubella (MMR) given?
a. When the child starts kindergarten   c. One month after the first vaccination
b. During adolescence   d. All of the above

(c). The second dose of measles vaccine is intended to produce seroconversion among vaccinees who did not seroconvert after their first dose. When completion of measles immunizations is considered urgent (e.g., during outbreaks, before travel or beginning school), the second dose can be given 1 month after the first.

3. After a patient with Kawasaki disease has been treated with 2 gm/kg of intravenous immunoglobulin (IVIG), how soon can the child be immunized with MMR?
a. 6 months   c. 11 months
b. 2 month   d. No particular waiting period

(c). Immunoglobulin preparations interfere with the serologic response to measles immunization; the degree of interference varies with the dose. After the large dose given to children with Kawasaki disease, the recommended interval between IVIG and measles vaccine is 11 months.

4. An infant perinatally infected with hepatitis B virus has what chance of developing a chronic hepatitis B infection?

Approximately 90%. Infected infants are at risk of developing chronic liver disease or primary hepatocellular carcinoma later in life.

5. Lawsuits for failure to vaccinate properly occur most often with which vaccine: (a) oral polio vaccine, (b) diphtheria-tetanus-pertussis (DTP), (c) hepatitis B virus, or (d) MMR?

(c). The key point here is failure to vaccinate properly—not adverse reactions. Failure to vaccinate infants properly, either through error or lost records, allows infants born to mothers who are HbsAg-positive to go unvaccinated.

6. True or false: The incidence of shingles after vaccination with the varicella vaccine is similar to the incidence of shingles after natural varicella infection:

False. The incidence of shingles after varicella vaccination is 2.6 cases/100,000 doses vs. 68 cases/100,000 person years for people younger than 20 years. Additional studies are ongoing to determine the exact incidence of shingles among children after wild-type varicella and varicella vaccination. The evidence thus far indicates that shingles due to the vaccine virus is rare.

7. Children who are exposed to pregnant women (a) should not be given varicella vaccine; (b) can be given varicella vaccine, or (c) should not be vaccinated until the infant is delivered

(b). Transmission of varicella vaccine virus is rare. A pregnant household member is not a contraindication to vaccination. Nursing mothers can be given varicella vaccine.

8. True or false: An immunocompromised child in the household is a contraindication to a varicella vaccination of a healthy child in the same home.

False. An immunocompromised child who is at risk for severe complications if infected with wild-type varicella virus can be protected from household exposure to clinical varicella by ensuring that other household members are immune to varicella. All susceptible persons living in the same household should be vaccinated.

9. A 12-year-old child was exposed to chickenpox but did not develop clinical disease. Which of the following statements is true?
  a. The child should be tested for antibody to the varicella-zoster virus before vaccination.
  b. The child should be vaccinated with varicella vaccine.
  c. There is nothing to worry about.

(b). Children and adults with a reliable history of varicella do not need to be vaccinated. However, people without a reliable history should be vaccinated. Serologic testing before vaccination is not indicated. There is no evidence of complications among immune people who receive varicella vaccine. Adults without a history of varicella should be vaccinated. The rate of complications from chickenpox is higher among adults.

10. When should a 4-year-old child who is asplenic be reimmunized with pneumococcal polysaccharide vaccine?
  a. Never—unless other risk factors are present
  b. Every 10 years
  c. 3–5 years after the previous dose.

(c). Children younger than 10 years should be reimmunized 3-5 years after a previous dose of pneumococcal polysaccharide vaccine. Asplenic children should receive two doses of the pneumococcal conjugate vaccine as well as a second dose of the 23-valent pneumococcal vaccine, as already recommended.

11. An infant has not completed the *Haemophilus influenzae* type B (Hib) immunization series and the specific Hib vaccine used is not known. Which of the following statements is true?
  a. Any of the Hib vaccines approved for infants can be used to complete the series.
  b. The series must be completed with the same Hib vaccine.

(a). When possible, the same Hib vaccine product should be used to complete a series. However, when the vaccine manufacturer is not known, the Hib vaccine products are considered interchangeable for primary as well as booster immunizations.

12. If a vaccination series is interrupted, what should you do?
  a. Start the series over.
  b. Resume the vaccination series.
  c. Hotline the parents

(b). A lapse in immunizations is not a reason to start a series over. Immunizations should be started with the next dose.

13. The hepatitis B vaccine is produced (a) by a recombinant process, (b) with hepatitis B surface antigen obtained from hepatitis B-positive carriers, or (c) from live viruses?

(a). The hepatitis B vaccine is produced by recombinant technology. The original plasma-derived vaccine is no longer produced in the United States.

14. True or false: Primary care doctors are experts on immunizations.

True. Approximately 50% of the immunizations given in the United States are administered in the offices of primary care physicians. No other group of physicians has the same amount of practical, daily experience with vaccines.

15. In a 4-month-old infant the minimal interval between dose 2 and dose 3 of the hepatitis B vaccine is (a) 1 month, (b) 2 months, or (c) 6 months.

(b). The third dose of hepatitis B vaccine can be given 2 months after the second dose as long as the infant is at least 6 months old and at least 4 months have passed since the first dose. Physicians need to be aware that the hepatitis B vaccine series can easily be completed in the first 6 months of life.

16. The usual number of Hib vaccinations in a series is four. Which Hib vaccine product requires only three doses: (a) Merck (Pedvax HIB), (b) Praxis (HibTITER), or (c) Lederle (ActHIB)?

(a). The Merck PedvaxHIB vaccine is licensed for doses at 2, 4, and 12–15 months of age. A dose at 6 months is not required. The same schedule applies for the Merck combination vaccine, HBV/Hib (COMVAX).

17. A 5-year-old boy received a "burst" of steroids for treatment of an acute asthma attack. When can he receive a live virus vaccine?

    a. One month later

    b. Two months later

    c. Immediately after treatment is discontinued

(c). Children receiving prednisone for less than 14 days can be immunized immediately after finishing treatment. This is especially true for children receiving the five day dose of 2 mg/kg of prednisone for management of acute asthma attacks.

18. For which of the following groups is influenza vaccine recommended?

    a. Pregnant women (after 14 weeks' gestation)

    b. Children older than 6 months with chronic pulmonary disease

    c. Any adult who wants to avoid influenza

    d. All of the above

(d). Pregnant women, adults and children with chronic pulmonary conditions, personnel taking care of patients, and any adult who wants to avoid influenza should receive the influenza vaccine. Use of the influenza vaccine, which is the most effective method of preventing influenza, continues to lag among all groups who would benefit. Physicians should identify and emphasize the value of the influenza vaccine to all at-risk groups.

19. The most common vaccine-preventable illness acquired by Americans traveling outside the United States is (a) typhoid fever, (b) meningococcal meningitis, (c) hepatitis A, or (d) influenza.

(c). Hepatitis A is the most frequent vaccine-preventable infection acquired by returning U.S. travelers. Travelers can easily be protected from hepatitis A infection with either of the currently available hepatitis vaccines.

20. True or false: The meningococcal vaccine is now required for college entry.

False. The meningococcal vaccine is recommended for college freshmen planning to live in a dormitory who want to reduce their risk of acquiring meningococcal disease. Students and parents should be made aware of meningococcal disease and the benefits of vaccination. The risk for meningococcal disease among non-freshmen college students is similar to that of the general population. Because the meningococcal vaccine is safe and efficacious, non-freshmen undergraduates also should be offered the vaccine.

21. The group of college students at greatest risk of invasive meningococcal disease is (a) fraternity members living in a separate house, (b) first-time freshmen college students living in a dormitory, (c) college students in general, or (d) day students.

(b). The overall incidence of meningococcal infections in the United States is approximately 1 case per 100,000 population. The incidence among freshmen living in dormitories is 4.6 per 100,000.

22. True or false: In evaluating a refugee child with a purified protein derivative test result greater than 10 mm and a normal chest radiograph, the history of bacille Calmette-Guérin (BCG) vaccination during early childhood should not change your decision to recommend isoniazid treatment for latent *Mycobacterium tuberculosis* infection.

True. In making decisions about the need for treatment of latent *M. tuberculosis* infection in a child or adult, the history of BCG vaccine should be ignored.

23. In an otherwise healthy child who has not received the varicella vaccine and has had a household exposure to chickenpox, clinical disease may be prevented by which of the following?
   a. Immediate initiation of oral acyclovir
   b. Administration of the varicella vaccine within 14 days after exposure
   c. Administration of varicella-zoster immunoglobulin within 7 days
   d. Immunization with the varicella vaccine within 3–5 days after exposure

(d.) Immunization within 3–5 days after exposure to varicella may protect the child from disease or at least modify the disease. Acyclovir is not recommended in this setting. Susceptible persons at risk of developing severe varicella should be given varicella-zoster immunoglobulin within 96 hours of exposure.

24. For which of the following groups is the anthrax vaccine recommended?
   a. Small animal veterinarians
   b. Workers in the wool and animal-hide industry
   c. Agricultural workers.
   d. Laboratory personnel directly engaged with live *Bacillus anthracis*

(d). The only group for whom the anthrax vaccine is routinely recommended is laboratory personnel working with live *B. anthracis*. These recommendations may change with the new threat of bioterrorism.

25. True or false: An asymptomatic infant infected with the human immunodeficiency virus should be vaccinated against measles.

True. Asymptomatic infants with HIV infection should receive measles vaccine at the usual age of 12 months. Children who are severely immunocompromised should not receive the vaccine. Physicians should consider giving the second dose of MMR vaccine earlier than the usual age of 4–6 years.

26. The highest risk of acquiring rabies in the United States is after exposure to (a) dogs, (b) bats, (c) raccoons, or (d) rabbits.

(b). In recent years approximately one-third of the cases of rabies diagnosed in the U.S. were related to rabid animal exposure outside the US. Between 1980 and 1996 bat-associated rabies viruses have been identified in 17 of the 20 cases of human rabies acquired in the U.S.

27. Hepatitis A vaccine is indicated for (a) travelers to Mexico, (b) children living in areas of the United States with an incidence of hepatitis A > 20 cases/100,000 population, (c) members of the military, or (d) all of the above.

(d). People traveling outside the U.S. should receive hepatitis A vaccine. Travelers to developed countries for a short period may not be at increased risk for acquiring hepatitis A infection. Young children are the main reservoirs of hepatitis A in the U.S., and until universal vaccination occurs, high rates of hepatitis A transmission will continue in many U.S. communities.

28. True or false: A mother who is breast-feeding her infant should not receive either the MMR vaccine or the varicella vaccine.

False. Mothers who are breast-feeding can and, if susceptible, should receive either MMR or varicella vaccine. They also should receive a second dose of MMR if they have not already done so. The viruses in the MMR vaccine are not transmitted by vaccine recipients. Transmission of varicella vaccine virus is rare.

29. DTP vaccine is contraindicated in which of the following infants?
 a. **Infants with swelling and redness about the injection site that resolved within 48 hours after vaccination**
 b. **Infants who had a fever of 103°F for a few hours on the day after vaccination**
 c. **Infants who were irritable for 1–2 hours after vaccination**
 d. **Infants who had generalized seizures beginning within 6 hours after vaccination, were difficult to control, and have required daily anticonvulsant medications**

(d). Swelling about the injection site, fever less than 104°F, and irritability are not contraindications to further DTP immunizations.

30. Why should the varicella vaccine be given at the same time as the MMR vaccine or 30 days later?

Children vaccinated with varicella vaccine less than 30 days after the MMR vaccine have an increased incidence of breakthrough disease with varicella. Simultaneous vaccination is also safe.

31. For which groups is routine serologic testing for the anti-hepatitis B surface antigen (HbsAg) indicated after immunization?
 a. **Hemodialysis patients**   d. **Infants born to HBsAg-positive**
 b. **Persons with HIV infection**   **mothers**
 c. **Sexual contacts of HBsAg-positive persons**   e. **All of the above**

(e). Routine testing for anti-HBsAg after immunization is not indicated in otherwise healthy, low-risk people. Infants born to HBsAg-positive mothers should be followed to determine whether they develop antibody after hepatitis B immunization or whether they become HBsAg-positive. People at risk of infection because of lifestyle, medical conditions, or immunocompromise should be tested for anti-HBsAg.

32. Recent shortages in supplies of DTP, influenza vaccine, and pneumococcal conjugate vaccine have been caused by (a) fewer vaccine manufacturers, (b) shortages in manufacturing vaccines, (c) stricter control by the FDA, or (d) all of the above.

(d). Shortages in vaccine supplies in recent years have been caused by many problems and may continue to worsen, primarily because of fewer vaccine manufacturers.

33. True or false: A child recovering from acute otitis media in the sixth day of a 10-day course of amoxicillin can receive regularly scheduled immunizations.

True. An asymptomatic child who is convalescing from an acute infection and is still receiving antibiotics can be immunized. The frequency of upper respiratory infections in infants and young children may cause significant delays in completing immunizations if primary care physicians do not insist on completing vaccination series in infants.

34. A 2-month-old girl with a birth weight of 1200 gm (a) should receive the regularly scheduled immunizations; (b) should receive a reduced dose of vaccine; (c) should already have been given a dose of hepatitis B vaccine; (d) can be immunized after her weight has reached 2500 gm, or (e) both a and c.

(e). Infants with birth weights less than 2000 gm should receive regularly scheduled immunizations at 2 months of age. They should receive hepatitis B prophylaxis at birth as recommended for full-term infants, but they should not be given reduced doses of vaccines. The initial dose of hepatitis B vaccine given at birth should not be counted in the required 3-dose series.

35. Pneumococcal conjugate vaccine is highly effective in preventing invasive *Streptococcus pneumoniae* disease (a) among children of all ages, (b) among children less than 2 years old, or (c) contains antigens from 10 serotypes of *S. pneumoniae*.

(b). The pneumococcal conjugate vaccine contains antigens from seven serotypes of *S. pneumoniae* that produce over 90% of invasive disease in children under 2 years of age. As children become older, the serotypes of *S. pneumoniae* causing serious disease broaden. The efficacy of this vaccine among older age groups has not been studied.

36. A 3-year-old child with sickle cell disease who has already received the pneumococcal polysaccharide vaccine should be considered for (a) a second dose of the same vaccine within 6 months, (b) a single dose of pneumococcal conjugate vaccine, or (c) two doses of the pneumococcal conjugate vaccine given at least 2 months apart

(c). Children aged 24–59 months at high risk of pneumococcal disease can benefit from the immunologic priming of the pneumococcal conjugate vaccine. They also should receive a second dose of pneumococcal vaccine as previously recommended.

37. The highest incidence of invasive pneumococcal disease occurs among (a) adults 65–74 years of age, (b) children less than 2 years of age, or (c) adults older than 80 years.

(b). The peak incidence of invasive pneumococcal disease occurs among children less than 2 years of age (166 cases/100,000 population). The second peak is among adults older than 80 years (98 cases/100,000).

38. True or false: The first dose of hepatitis B vaccine should be given before the infant is discharged from the hospital.

True. In 2001 the Advisory Committee on Immunization Practices (ACIP) recommended that the first dose of hepatitis B vaccine be given before the infant is discharged home. In 1991 the ACIP first recommended routine vaccination of all infants before discharge but allowed physicians the flexibility of vaccinating infants born to HbsAg-negative mothers at anytime up to 2 months of age.

39. True or false: Several immunizations have been linked to diseases such as autism, inflammatory bowel disease and multiple sclerosis.

False. Studies have disproved all of these associations. You must fight these myths in your practice.

BIBLIOGRAPHY

1. Centers for Disease Control and Prevention: Meningococcal disease and college students: Recommendations of the Advisory Committee on Immunization Practices (ACIP). MMWR 49(RR-7):13–20, 2000.
2. Centers for Disease Control and Prevention: Preventing pneumococcal disease among infants and young children: Recommendations of the Advisory Committee on Immunization Practices (ACIP). MMWR 49(RR-9):1–35, 2000.
3. Centers for Disease Control and Prevention: Use of anthrax vaccine in the United States: Recommendations of the Advisory Committee on Immunization Practices (ACIP). MMWR 49(RR-15):1–20, 2000.
4. Centers for Disease Control and Prevention: Prevention and control of influenza: Recommendations of the Advisory Committee on Immunization Practices (ACIP). MMWR 50(RR-4):1–44, 2001.
5. Centers for Disease Control and Prevention: Simultaneous administration of varicella vaccine and other recommended childhood vaccines, U.S., 1995-1999. MMWR 50(47):1308–1341, 2001.
6. Chin J: Control of Communicable Diseases Manual, 17th ed. Washington, DC, American Public Health Association, 2000.
7. Moran GJ, Talan DA, Mower W, et al: Appropriateness of rabies postexposure prophylaxis treatment for animal exposures. JAMA 284:1001–1007, 2000.
8. Pickering LK (ed): Report of the Committee on Infectious Diseases (2000 Red Book), 25th ed. Elk Grove Village, IL, American Academy of Pediatrics, 2000.
9. Plotkin SA, Orenstein WA (eds): Vaccines, 3rd ed. Philadelphia, W.B. Saunders, 1999.
10. Robinson KA, Baughman W, Rothrock G, et al: Epidemiology of invasive Streptococcus pneumoniae infections in the United States, 1995–1998. JAMA 285:1729–1735, 2001.

XIV. Fingertip Facts

48. EMERGENCY DEPARTMENT PERSPECTIVE

Fred Fow, M.D., and Amanda Pratt, M.D.

1. Name the four modes of acquisition for botulism.

1. Foodborne botulism
2. Inhalational botulism
3. Wound botulism
4. Infant botulism

2. What are the common risk factors for infant botulism?

Age less than 12 months, breast feeding, and consumption of honey.

3. Describe the management of infant botulism.

Management is strictly supportive. Patients need to be hospitalized to observe for potential respiratory compromise. Botulinum antitoxin is available and is most effective in preventing progression of disease and shortening the duration of respiratory failure if given early in the course of the illness.

4. In which states do you most commonly find Rocky Mountain spotted fever (RMSF)?

Despite its name, most cases are found along the East Coast from Maryland to Georgia and west to Oklahoma.

5. Describe the rash of RMSF.

The rash usually erupts after 3–5 days of fever. It starts as a blanching maculopapular exanthem on the wrist and ankles and spreads centrally over the next 2–3 days, usually sparing the face. Classically, the palms and soles are involved, and the rash usually becomes petechial or purpuric.

6. How is RMSF treated?

Tetracycline, doxycycline, and chloramphenicol are rickettsiostatic and the mainstays of therapy. Doxycycline is the drug of choice in children of all ages. Early treatment with specific antibiotics significantly decreases the mortality rate of RMSF.

7. What laboratory abnormalities are commonly seen with RMSF?

Hyponatremia, thrombocytopenia, and a white blood cell count that may be high, low, or normal but frequently shows a left shift.

8. What are the two human diseases caused by *Ehrlichia* spp. in North America?

Human monocytic ehrlichiosis (HME) and human granulocytic ehrlichiosis (HGE) are two distinct diseases with similar clinical manifestations.

9. Describe the similarities and differences between ehrlichiosis and RMSF.

Symptoms common to both ehrlichiosis and RMSF include fever, headache, myalgia, malaise, anorexia, nausea, and vomiting. They differ in that patients with ehrlichiosis have more frequent occurrence of leukopenia, anemia, and hepatitis and less frequently develop rash. When patients with ehrlichiosis develop a rash, less than 10% of cases involve the palms and soles.

10. What clinical symptoms are required for the diagnosis of Stevens-Johnson syndrome?

In addition to the cutaneous lesions of erythema multiforme minor, two or more mucosal surfaces must be involved.

11. Name the most common causes of Stevens-Johnson syndrome.

Mycoplasma pneumoniae is the most common infectious cause. Drugs, such as nonsteroidal anti-inflammatory agents, sulfonamides, and anticonvulsants (particularly phenytoin) are the most common precipitating factor. However, approximately 50% of cases have no known cause.

12. What is Nikolsky's sign?

Nikolsky's sign is the separation of the superficial layer of skin with gentle rubbing. This sign is commonly seen in patient's with staphylococcal scalded skin syndrome (SSSS), but it is not pathognomonic for the disease.

13. Who should be admitted to hospital with SSSS?

A good rule of thumb is to treat patients with SSSS as if they had burns.

14. What are the diagnostic criteria for staphylococcal toxic shock syndrome?

Three major criteria must be met:
1. Acute fever > 38.9°C.
2. Orthostatic hypotension or shock
3. Rash, starting as macular erythroderma that later leads to desquamation.

Any three of seven minor criteria must be met:
1. Mucous membrane inflammation
2. Gastrointestinal tract abnormalities
3. Muscle abnormalities
4. Central nervous system abnormalities
5. Hepatic abnormalities
6. Renal abnormalities
7. Decreased platelet count.

Two exclusionary criteria must be met:
1. Absence of another explanation for the symptoms
2. Negative blood cultures except for *Staphylococcus aureus*

15. How are staphylococcal and streptococcal toxic shock syndrome different?

Patients with staphylococcal toxic shock syndrome (TSS) usually have sudden onset of high fever with profuse watery diarrhea, erythroderma and hypotensive symptoms. Patients with streptococcal TSS usually have a less acute onset with a site of infection on the skin and complain of severe pain and hyperesthesia at the affected site that is out of proportion to objective findings. In staphylococcal TSS, multiorgan failure is a consequence of hypotension. In streptococcal TSS, multiorgan failure occurs regardless of hypotension and thus has a much worse prognosis.

16. Describe the initial management of patients with TSS.

Fluid replacement along with an antistaphylococcal/antistreptococcal antibiotic is the important initial management. Clindamycin should be started as well because it inhibits toxin production (Eagle effect). If a focal site of suppurative infection is identified, it should be drained. Initial laboratory tests include complete blood count (CBC), prothrombin time, partial thromboplastin time, fibrinogen, fibrin split products, electrolytes, blood urea nitrogen, creatinine, aspartate aminotransferase, alanine aminotransferase, and creatinine phosphokinase. Appropriate cultures should be obtained as well.

17. What is quinsy?

Another name for a peritonsillar abscess.

18. Describe the classic presentation of a patient with a peritonsillar abscess.

Patients have a muffled, or "hot potato," voice, trismus, drooling, fetid breath, and uvula deviation to the unaffected side. The trismus and muffled voice differentiate peritonsillar abscess from the more common simple pharyngitis.

19. Which age group is most commonly affected by peritonsillar abscess?

Peritonsillar abscess generally occurs in the adolescent population. In contrast, retropharyngeal abscesses tend to affect young children more commonly.

20. Describe the radiologic findings in a patient with a retropharyngeal abscess.

A lateral neck x-ray should be performed in patients suspected of having a retropharyngeal abscess if they are clinically stable. This radiograph shows an increase in the width of the prevertebral soft tissue, which normally should be less than half that of the adjacent vertebral body. Remember that exhalation and flexion can cause falsely thickened prevertebral soft tissue.

21. What are the clinical manifestations of a retropharyngeal abscess?

Affected children typically present with drooling, dysphagia, neck stiffness, and occasionally stridor secondary to airway edema.

22. What are the potential complications of a lateral pharyngeal abscess?

The lateral pharyngeal space contains the carotid sheath with the carotid artery and internal jugular vein, cranial nerves IX–XII, and the cervical sympathetic chain in the posterior portion. The anterior portion is close to the tonsillar fossa and internal pterygoid muscle. The complications of this abscess are potentially quite serious and depend on the extent of involvement of these various structures.

23. Name the organisms most commonly isolated from deep neck abscesses.

Group A streptococci, *Staphylococcus aureus*, and various oral anaerobic bacteria.

24. What are the criteria for the diagnosis of Kawasaki disease?

A child should have fever for a least 5 days and at least 4 of the 5 following findings:
1. Bulbar conjunctival hyperemia without exudate
2. Oropharyngeal erythema, strawberry tongue, and red cracked lips
3. Rash, which may be more morbilliform, maculopapular, scarlatiniform, or erythema multiforme-like
4. Hand and feet swelling with erythematous palms and soles
5. Cervical lymph node enlargement (> 1.5 cm in diameter), usually unilateral and single

The diagnosis also can be made if the child has fever, 3 of the above features, and evidence of coronary abnormalities. The diagnosis of atypical Kawasaki disease can be made without these criteria in a child (often an infant) with fever and coronary abnormalities. Other manifestations of Kawasaki's disease include urethritis, hepatitis, arthritis or arthralgia, aseptic meningitis, pericardial effusion, gallbladder hydrops, and congestive heart failure due to myocarditis.

25. What are the common laboratory features of Kawasaki disease?

The white blood cell (WBC) count in the blood is usually increased (> 20,000 cells/ml in 50% of cases) and shifted to the left.. Erythrocyte sedimentation rate (ESR) is high, often > 100. Platelets may be low, normal, or high initially but increase rapidly during the second week of the illness, eventually reaching levels as high as 1,000,000–2,000,000. Other lab indicators include sterile pyuria and mild proteinuria, elevated hepatic transaminases, mild anemia, hypoalbuminemia, hyponatremia, and hypophosphatemia.

26. How about EKG and echocardiogram findings?

During the acute phase of Kawasaki disease the EKG may show a prolonged PR interval, decreased QRS voltage, flattening of the T waves, and ST-wave changes. Ischemic changes may be seen later, in the subacute phase, from thrombosis of coronary aneurysms.

27. How is Kawasaki disease treated?

Intravenous immunoglobulin (IVIG), as a single dose, 2 gm/kg given over 10–12 hours, and aspirin, 80–100 mg/kg/day divided into 4 doses, are the initial treatment. Aspirin is continued at a lower dose, 3–5 mg/k/day, after several days of defervescence. Dipyridamole may be added in patients with coronary aneurysms. For patients without coronary abnormalities, aspirin is continued for 6–8 weeks or until the platelet count and ESR normalize. In patients with coronary abnormalities, low-dose therapy is continued indefinitely. A second dose of IVIG may be necessary in some children with persistent (> 48–72 hours) or recurrent fever or other persistent inflammatory signs (e.g., conjunctivitis and rash).

28. Which types of animals are high-risk and which types are low-risk for transmitting rabies to humans?

Low-risk animals include healthy vaccinated dogs, cats, and ferrets that can be observed for 10 days (incubation period of animals rabies) as well as squirrels, hamsters, guinea pigs, gerbils, chipmunks, rats, mice and other small rodents, rabbits, and hares. Rabies prophylaxis is unnecessary for exposure to these animals unless signs of animal rabies are noted.

Higher-risk animals include rabid, suspected rabid, or escaped dogs, cats, ferrets, skunks, raccoons, woodchucks, foxes, most other carnivores (e.g., coyotes), and bats (known or probable exposure).

29. What are the wound treatment and irrigation guidelines for postexposure rabies prophylaxis in a child not previously vaccinated against rabies?

Wash the wound immediately and thoroughly with soap, water, and a virucidal agent (e.g., providone-iodine solution). Do not forget tetanus prophylaxis and antibiotics (if indicated). Rabies immune globulin (RIG), 20 IU/kg, should be infiltrated into the wound. The full dose should go into the wound if possible. Otherwise, any remaining RIG should be given intramuscularly at a site far from the site where the rabies vaccine will be given. Human diploid cell vaccine (HDCV), rabies vaccine adsorbed (RVA), or purified chick embryo vaccine (PEC), 1.0 ml intramuscularly, is given at the same visit and on days 3,7, 14, and 28. The location for these injections is the deltoid in adults and older children and the outer thigh for younger children. The vaccine should never be given in the gluteal area.

30. What signs and symptoms should alert the clinician to the possibility of pericarditis, pericardial effusion, or pericardial tamponade?
- Tachycardia (to compensate for reduced stroke volume)
- Chest pain (worse when supine, better when leaning forward)
- Abdominal pain
- Tachypnea and increased work of breathing
- Peripheral vasoconstriction (cool extremities, pallor)
- Decreased systemic blood pressure
- Neck vein distention
- Hepatomegaly
- Rales
- Cardiac friction rub
- Distant or muffled heart sounds
- Weak apical impulse
- Pulsus parodoxus (a strong indicator of significant pericardial fluid accumulation requiring immediate intervention)

31. Describe the EKG findings in pericarditis.

Diminished precordial voltages, injury pattern changes (elevated ST segments, PR-segment depression, and diffuse T-wave inversions), and electrical alternans (variation of the QRS axis with each beat) may be seen.

32. What are diagnostic imaging findings in pericarditis?

Heart size may be symmetrically enlarged on chest x-ray. Echocardiography is the preferred diagnostic modality for identifying pericardial fluid.

33. What are the common infectious causes of pericarditis?

Bacterial causes include *S. aureus, Haemophilus influenza, Neisseria meningitidis, Streptoococcus pneumoniae*, and other streptococci. Atypical bacteria include *Mycoplasma tuberculosis* and other mycoplasmal species. Viral causes include coxsackie B, ECHO virus, rubella, Epstein-Barr virus, adenovirus, influenza. and mumps.

34. What are the typical manifestations of viral myocarditis in neonates and older children?

Because the symptoms of viral myocarditis are often nonspecific and variable, such as anorexia, lethargy, emesis, lightheadedness, shortness of breath, and cool extremities, the clinician needs to maintain a high index of suspicion. The triad of arrhythmia, fever, and cardiomegally is suggestive of viral myocarditis.

35. Describe the treatment for myocarditis.

The treatment of viral myocarditis is mainly supportive. Steroids may be considered in patients with viral myocarditis.

36. What is the generally accepted approach to febrile infants (temperature > 38.0°C rectally) under 1 month of age?

Unless an obvious bacterial or viral (herpes simplex virus) source of infection is present, a work-up to rule out bacteremia, urinary tract infection, and meningitis is appropriate for all such infants. The work-up includes blood, urine, and cerebrospinal fluid (CSF) cultures as well as a screening CBC, urinalysis, urine Gram stain, and CSF glucose, protein, cell count, and Gram stain. If diarrhea is present, investigation for bacterial enteritis is appropriate with a stool culture and screening Gram stain. If pneumonia is suspected, a chest x-ray is also appropriate.

37. What antibiotics should you choose for such an infant?

Antibiotic combinations to consider include ampicillin and gentamicin or ampicillin and cefotaxime.

38. Describe the approach to febrile children 30–90 days of age.

Attempts have been made to identify infants at low risk for serious bacterial illness (SBI). A variety of screening criteria have been published.

The **Rochester criteria** categorize infants under 60 days of age as being at low risk for SBI if they meet the following criteria:

- Previously healthy
- Appear well
- No focal infection
- Peripheral WBC count > 5,000 cells/ml and < 15,000 cells/ml
- Peripheral band count < 1,500 cells/ml
- ≤ 10 WBC/high-power field (HPF) on microscopic exam of spun urine
- ≤ 5 WBC/HPF on microscopic exam of stool smear if diarrhea

The recommended evaluation includes cultures of the blood, CSF, and urine.

The **Boston criteria** categorize infants 28–89 days of age as candidates for outpatient management, following a dose of IV antibiotics, if they meet the following criteria:

- No ear, soft tissue, bone, or joint infection on exam
- Peripheral WBC count < 20,000 cells/ml
- CSF WBC count < 10 cells/ml
- No urinary leukocyte esterase.
- No infiltrate on chest x-ray, if obtained.
- Not ill-appearing or dehydrated; taking fluids; normal vital signs for age and fever

• Reliable, cooperative parents who are available by phone.
• No antibiotics within the previous 48 hours
• No diphtheria-tetanus-pertussis (DTP) immunization within the last 48 hours
• No allergy to beta-lactam antibiotics

The **Philadelphia criteria** categorize infants between 29 and 56 days of age as being at low risk and as candidates for outpatient management without any antibiotics if they meet the following criteria:

• No bacterial infection on physical exam
• Normal Infant Observation Score (IOS)
• Peripheral WBC count < 15,000 cells/ml and a band-to-neutrophil ratio < 0.2
• Urine with < 10 WBC/HPF or negative bright-field microscopy
• CSF WBC count < 8 and negative CSF Gram stain
• Stool smear negative for blood with few or no WBCs
• No infiltrate on chest x-ray
• Reliable parents, living within 30 minutes of the hospital, with a working phone, willing to return for revisit check-ups on each of the following 2 days.

39. How does the height of the fever affect the likelihood of occult bacteremia in febrile children 3–24 months old?

The risk of occult bacteremia in children 3–24 months old is < 0.5% if the temperature is < 38.9°C. However, increasing temperature over 39.0 C is an independent predictor of bacteremia. The risk of occult bacteremia in children with temperatures > 41.0°C may be as high as 9.3%.

40. What organisms are responsible for occult bacteremia in this age group?

S. pneumoniae accounts for about 90% of occult bacteremia in this age group.

41. How often does occult bacteremia result in complications?

Most occult pneumococcal bacteremia does not result in serious disease. The risk of meningitis in children with occult pneumococcal bacteremia not treated with antibiotics has been estimated at about 4%. Other complications include cellulitis and pneumonia. Empirical treatment of occult pneumococcal bacteremia with antibiotics appears to reduce the risk of these complications.

The risk of complications associated with meningococcal bacteremia is much higher—about 50%. About 40% of children develop meningitis, and 3% develop extremity necrosis ; the mortality rate is 4%. Empirical treatment of occult meningococcal bacteremia appears to significantly lower the rate of these complications.

42. How helpful are screening tests in determining the likelihood of occult pneumococcal bacteremia in febrile children in this age group?

• WBC count, absolute neutrophil count (ANC), and band counts are usually higher in children with occult pneumococcal bacteremia than in those without occult pneumococcal bacteremia.
• A WBC count of 15,000 cell/ml has a prediction profile with a sensitivity of about 80–86%, a specificity of 70–77%, a positive predictive value of 5–6% and a negative predictive value of 99%. Applying these criteria would result in treating about 19 children for each child with pneumococcal bacteremia.
• An ANC of 9,000–10,000 cells/ml has a prediction profile with a sensitivity of 76%, a specificity of 78%, a positive predictive value of 8 %, and a negative predictive value of 99.2%. Applying these criteria probably would result in treating about 12 children for each child with pneumococcal bacteremia.

43. What about screening tests for occult meningococcal bacteremia?

WBC count is not a good screening tool for detecting occult meningococcal bacteremia. Seventy percent of patients may have WBC counts < 15,000 cells/ml. An elevated ANC and especially an elevated band count may be helpful in detecting occult meningococcal bacteremia. However, because the prevalence of occult menigococcal bacteremia is low, the positive predictive value of even the band count is low, and screening for occult meningococcal bacteremia may be inefficient.

44. Just so no one forgets—what is the gold standard test for detecting occult bacteremia?
The blood culture remains the gold standard for detection of occult bacteremia. Rapid detection culturing systems are available and may allow earlier treatment of such children.

45. What is the likely impact of vaccinating increasing numbers of children with conjugate pneumococcal vaccine?
Conjugate pneumococcal vaccine has demonstrated a 97.4% efficacy and significantly reduces the rate of invasive pneumococcal disease in vaccine recipients compared with non-recipients. As pneumococcal vaccination rates increase, the approach to fever in vaccinated children may change, possibly obviating much of the screening for occult bacteremia that currently takes place.

46. What factors can help guide the practitioner in assessing the likelihood of urinary tract infection (UTI) in children ?
Reported risk factors include age < 12 months (adjusted odds ratio [AOR] = 3.0), Caucasian race (AOR = 7.5), temperature ≥ 39.0°C (AOR = 2.6), fever for ≥ 2 days (AOR = 2.0), and absence of another source for fever (AOR = 2.4). The authors reporting these data found that using two or more risk factors as a cut-off for screening for UTI yielded a sensitivity of 95%, although the specificity was only 31%. The risk of UTI in the highest-risk children may be as high as 30%.

47. What tools can help to distinguish between toxic synovitis and septic arthritis?
• Guarding of the hip may be more pronounced in septic arthritis than in toxic synovitis.
• Temperature may be expected to be higher in children with septic arthritis than in those with toxic synovitis.
• WBC count and ESR are expected to be higher in children with septic arthritis.

48. What is the best test for the rapid diagnosis of septic arthritis?
Arthrocentesis remains the best test for rapid diagnosis of septic arthritis.

49. What are the usual signs and symptoms of meningitis in children?
The manifestations of meningitis are variable and depend on the age of the patient.
Young infants (0–3 months) may have irritability, altered sleep pattern, vomiting, lethargy, or fever. The neonate may have hypothermia. Shock, seizures, focal neurologic signs, and a bulging fontanelle are other signs of meningitis in this age group. Unfortunately, many of these signs and symptoms are nonspecific.
Older infants and young children (4–24 months) may have similar manifestations of meningitis. In addition, they may have nuchal rigidity and coma.
Children over 24 months, in addition to the signs and symptoms seen in younger children and infants, may manifest headache and neck pain.

50. What typical CSF findings help to differentiate between bacterial and viral meningitis?
• CSF WBC counts are typically higher in bacterial meningitis than in viral meningitis (200–20,000 cells/ml vs. 10–1,000 cells/ml, respectively).
• CSF protein is usually > 100mg/dl in bacterial meningitis and 40-100 mg/dl in viral meningitis.
• CSF glucose is usually < 30 mg/dl in bacterial meningitis and > 30 mg/dl in viral meningitis.
Note: Normal CSF in neonates may have a WBC count up to 30 cells/ml, protein up to 170 mg/dl, and glucose as low as 30 mg/dl.

51. What are the contraindications to performing a lumbar puncture (LP) in a child in whom meningitis is suspected?

Commonly cited contraindications include focal neurologic findings, evidence of increased intracranial pressure (e.g,. papilledema), and suspicion of a mass lesion by history or examination. If meningitis is suspected and LP is contraindicated, empirical antibiotics should be given immediately— not delayed for appropriate neuroimaging results. Although the CSF may be sterilized by appropriate antibiotics, screening cell counts and chemistries usually remain abnormal for some time.

52. What antibiotics should be given in the emergency department for the treatment of bacterial meningitis?

For children older than 1 month, therapy with vancomycin and ceftriaxone or cefotaxime should be initiated.

53. If corticosteroids are administered for bacterial meningitis, should they be given (a) 1 hour before antibiotics, (b) concurrently with antibiotics, (c) 24 hours after antibiotics are started, or (d) none of the above?

The decision to administer steroids in bacterial meningitis is controversial, but if administered, they should given concurrently with antimicrobials.

54. How often do CSF shunt infections occur?

Different series report that infections occur in 3–4% of ventricular shunts.

55. When are CSF shunt infections most likely to occur?

Most shunt infections result from endogenous spread of organisms present on the skin of the patient or operating room staff at the time of surgery. Seventy percent occur within 6 weeks of placement or revision and 90% within 6 months of placement.

56. What are the signs and symptoms of CSF shunt infection?

Children with CSF shunt infections may have signs of increased intracranial pressure due to shunt malfunction. Fever, inflammation along the shunt path or surgical incision, irritability, meningismus, alterations in mental status, seizures, vomiting, and abdominal tenderness are other indicators . Anemia, hematuria and splenomegaly may be seen in ventriculoatrial shunt infections.

57. What are the typical CSF findings in patients with CSF shunt infections?

Modest pleocytosis (< 150 WBC), slightly decreased glucose, and modest protein elevation. Eosinophilia has been noted in some patients with shunt infection.

58. What other conditions may mimic periorbital (preseptal) cellulitis?

Insect bites, allergic reactions, sinusitis, and conjunctivitis may mimic periorbital cellulitis. Allergic reactions may be bilateral, whereas periorbital cellulitis is usually unilateral. Moreover, an allergic reaction should be itchy, with the child often rubbing the eye, whereas cellulitis should be painful and tender. An allergic reaction or an insect bite should not be associated with the fever or ill appearance seen in periorbital cellulitis. An insect bite mark may be seen in some cases. Care must be taken to avoid excluding periorbital cellulitis as a possibility, however, because bites and allergic reactions may become superinfected and sinusitis and conjunctivitis may spread to the periorbital tissues. In the presence of fever, pain, tenderness, eyelid swelling, and eye redness, appropriate therapy should be instituted with either oral or intravenous antibiotics.

59. How can the clinician differentiate between periorbital cellulitis and orbital cellulitis?

Both periorbital and orbital cellulitis manifest with fever, pain, eyelid swelling, and eye redness. Orbital cellulitis, however, may have additional findings, including decreased eye movements, proptosis, visual impairment, and papilledema. Suspicion of orbital cellulitis requires an orbital CT scan and intravenous antibiotics.

BIBLIOGRAPHY

1. Alpern ER, Alessandrini EA, Bell LM, et al: Occult bacteremia from a pediatric emergency department: current prevalence, time to detection, and outcome. Pediatrics 106:505–551, 2000.
2. American Academy of Pediatrics: Kawasaki disease. In Pickering LK (ed): 2000 Red Book: Report of the Committee on Infectious Diseases, 25th ed. Elk Grove Villiage, IL, American Academy of Pediatric; 2000.
3. Baraff LJ: Management of fever without source in infants and children. Ann Emerg Med 36:602–614, 2000.
4. Baraff LJ, Oslund S, Prather M: Effect of antibiotic therapy and etiologic micro-organism on the risk of bacterial meningitis in children with occult bacteremia. Pediatrics 92:140–143, 1993.
5. Bernstein D: Myocarditis. In Behrman (ed): Nelson Textbook of Pediatrics, 16th ed. Philadelphia, W.B. Saunders, 2000, pp 1434–1435.
6. DelBeccaro MA, Champoux AN, Bockers T, et al: Septic arthritis versus transient sinovitis of the hip; the value of screening laboratory tests. Ann Emerg Med 21:1418–1422, 1992.
7. Fleisher GR, Ludwig S (eds): Textbook of Pediatric Emergency Medicine, 4th ed. Philadelphia, Lippincottt Williams & Wilkins, 2000.
8. Fow F: Neurosurgical emergencies. In:Selbst SM, Cronan K (eds): Pediatric Emergency Medicine Secrets. Philadelphia, Hanley & Belfus, 2001, pp 271–275.
9. Gorelick MH, Shaw KN: Clinical decision rule to identify febrile young girls at low risk for urinary tract infection. Arch Pediatr Adolesc Med 154:386–390, 2000.
10. Harper MB, Bachur R, Fleisher GR: Effect of antibiotic therapy on the outcome of outpatients with unsuspected bacteremia. Pediatr Infect Dis J 14:760-767, 1995.
11. Human rabies prevention—United States 1999. Recommendations of the Advisory Committee on Immunization Practices (ACIP). MMWR 48 (RR-1):1–21, 1999.
12. Jaskiewicz JA, McCarthy CA, Richardson AC, et al: Febrile infants at low risk for serious bacterial infection—an appraisal of the Rochester Criteria and implications for management. Febrile Infant Collaborative Study Group. Pediatrics 94:390–396, 1994.
13. Kuppermann N: Occult bacteremia in young febrile children. Pediatr Clin North Am 46:1073–1079, 1999.
14. Lee GM, Harper MD: Risk of bacteremia for febrile young children in the post-*Haemophilus influenzae* type B era. Arch Pedriatr Adolesc Med 152:624–628, 1998.
15. Mawn LA, Jordan DR, Donahue SP: Preseptal and orbital cellulitis: In Occuloplastic Surgical Update. Ophthalmol Clin North Am 13(4), 2000.
16. Negrini B, Kelleher KJ, Wald ER: Cerebrospinal fluid changes in aseptic versus bacterial meningitis. Pediatrics 105:316–319, 2000.
17. Ronan A, Hogg GG, Klug GL: Cerebrospinal fluid shunt infections in children. Pediatr Infect Dis J 14:782–786, 1995.
18. Rothrock SG, Harper ML, Green SM, et al: Do oral antibiotics prevent meningitis and serious bacterial infections in children with streptococcus pneumonae occult bacteremia? A meta-analysis. Pediatrics 99:438–444, 1997.
19. Saez-Llorens X, McCracken GH Jr: Antimicrobial and anti-inflammatory treatment of bacterial meningitis. Infect Dis Clin North Am 13:619–636, 1999.
20. Shaw KN, Gorelick M, McGowan KL, et al: Prevalence of urinary tract infection in febrile young children in the emergency department. Pediatrics 102(2):16, 1998.

49. SO YOU WANT TO BE A PEDIATRIC I.D. WIZ

Hal Charles Byck, M.D.

Test your knowledge. Total your points at the end of the chapter and see how you do. Each question is worth between 1 and 5 points. Answers are found at the end of the quiz.

1. Match the side effect with the antibiotic (1 point each).

1. Stevens-Johnson syndrome	a. Ceftriaxone
2. Tegretol toxicity	b. Chloramphenicol
3. Sodium overload	c. Bactrim
4. Neuromuscular blockade	d. Methicillin
5. Interstitial nephritis	e. Vancomycin
6. Aplastic anemia	f. Gentamicin
7. Gallbladder sludging	g. Erythromycin
8. Red man syndrome	h. Tetracycline
9. Worsening sunburn	i. Ticarcillin

2. Put these diseases in order of average incubation period from shortest to longest (1 point for knowing the shortest, 1 point for knowing the longest, 5 extra points if all are in correct order).

Primary syphilis
Subacute sclerosing panencephalitis
Rocky Mountain spotted fever
Varicella zoster
Rotavirus
Hepatitis B
Epstein Barr virus

3. Name the causative agent (genus/species) in each clinical scenario (2 points each).

1. Four-day-old infant presents with thick, purulent eye discharge over 24 hours associated with tense eyelid edema.

2. Seven-year-old presents with severe diarrhea for 10 hours with fever, seizures, and 16,000 white blood cell count with 40% neutrophils and 35% bands.

3. Three-month-old breastfed infant presents with lethargy, difficulty feeding and constipation. On exam, the patient is afebrile.

4. Eight-year-old vacationing in North Carolina presents with fever, severe headache, myalgia, and rash on wrists and ankles.

5. Ten-month-old with fever to 104° for 2 days, followed by defervescence and a rash on trunk lasting only 12 hours.

6. Fifteen-year-old works in pet store, comes in with a painful lump in the axilla and small papule on the ipsilateral forearm.

7. Two-month-old presents with anemia, copious drainage from nose, glomerulonephritis, large spleen and liver, and pneumonia alba.

8. Three-year-old comes in contact with another child with chicken pox and 15 days later develops chicken pox with bullae all over body.

9. Newborn is found to have osteomyelitis of right shoulder.

10. Nineteen-year-old rabbit hunter develops severe conjunctivitis with a preauricular lymph node.

4. Put the following vaccines in chronological order of initiation in U.S. (1 point for earliest, 1 point for latest, 5 points for getting all in order).

Measles   Influenza
Varicella   Rabies
Inactivated polio vaccine

5. Take the first letter of each answer and unscramble an infectious disease term (2 points for each correct answer, 5 points if you get the word).

1. Prevalence of toxoplasmosis is highest in what world city?
2. Causative agent of tinea versicolor.
3. Type of hepatitis with highest mortality rate.
4. Organism most commonly associated with bacteremia in patients with untreated galactosemia.
5. Reye syndrome has most commonly been associated with varicella and this other virus.
6. Primary drug used for prophylaxis of malaria.
7. This clinical disease is similar to Rocky Mountain spotted fever, although typically it does not present with a rash and is associated with anemia and leukopenia.
8. This class of organisms is responsible for up to 40% of summer and fall febrile illness in children.

6. Match the virus with the gastroenteritis syndrome (1 point each).

1. Astrovirus   a. Most commonly found on a cruise ship
2. Norwalk   b. Typically causes more prolonged gastroenteritis
3. Rotavirus   c. Common in Mexico in September–October and Nova Scotia in May
4. Enterovirus   d. Thought to be the fourth most common cause of viral gastroenteritis
5. Adenovirus   e. Clinically insignificant cause of gastroenteritis

7. Name the clinical agent that most commonly causes the following clinical findings (2 points each).

1. Acute myositis   6. Febrile seizures
2. Hemorrhagic   7. Acute anemia with low reticulocyte count in
   conjunctivitis   sickle cell anemia
3. Acute cerebellar ataxia   8. Perihepatitis
4. Endocarditis   9. Epidemic keratoconjunctivitis
5. Pseudoparalysis   10. Adrenal hemorrhage

8. Fungus from head to toe (2 points each).

1. Name the inflammatory ringworm plaque on scalp that can become pustular.
2. Most frequent sinus infected in paranasal aspergillosis.
3. Where is the infection of tinea barbae?
4. Tinea versicolor is most common on what part of the body?
5. Portal of entry of blastomycosis.
6. Fungus most commonly associated with homograft valve surgery.
7. Predominant invasion of what organ system occurs in disseminated histoplasmosis?
8. Most commonly involved joint in disseminated coccidiomycosis.
9. Athlete's foot is most common in which interdigital space?

9. Put these organisms in chronologic order of when they were first identified (1 point for earliest, 1 point for latest, 5 extra points for getting all correct).

Respiratory syncytial virus   Parvovirus B19
Mycobacterium tuberculosis   Human herpes virus 6
Influenza A

10. Which vaccines are absolutely contraindicated in the following cases? (1 point for each correct vaccine, 9 points possible total).
1. Known anaphylaxis to neomycin (name 3)
2. HIV (name 3)
3. Acute respiratory distress after ingestion of egg (name 3)

11. The ladder of difficulty

1 point each
1. Etiologic agent of endemic croup.
2. Infection most commonly associated with Bell's palsy.
3. Most common cause of common cold.
4. Drug of choice for streptococcal pharyngitis.

2 points each
1. Hepatitis other than A that does not have a chronic carrier state.
2. Common electroencephalographic abnormality seen with herpes encephalitis.
3. Two leading viral causes of exudate pharyngitis.
4. Leading cause of hemolysis throughout the world.

3 points each
1. Organism most commonly associated with migratory arthritis.
2. Beta-lactamase production is more common in *Moraxella catarrhalis*, *Streptococcus pneumoniae*, or *Haemophilus influenzae*.
3. Most common infectious cause of fetal demise secondary to nonimmune hydrops.
4. Common electrolyte abnormality seen with Rocky Mountain spotted fever.

4 points each
1. Antibiotic class which is contraindicated in infantile botulism.
2. Time frame needed to give varicella zoster immunoglobulin if person is exposed to varicella.
3. Most common bones affected in osteomyelitis (two answers).
4. Vitamin deficiency that needs to be treated in patients with measles.

5 points each
1. Most common clinical presentation of infection with *Cryptococcus neoformans*.
2. Why do laboratories generally *not* attempt to culture *Rickettsia rickettsii?*
3. Which, if any, of these bacterial gastroenteritis pathogens are not gram-negative bacilli?
   - *Salmonella* sp.   • *Shigella* sp.
   - *Yersina* sp.   • *Campylobacter* sp.
   - *Vibrio* sp.   • *Aeromonas* sp.
4. Agglutination of sheep red blood cells with serum is called what?.

ANSWERS

1. Side effect

Side effect	Antibiotic
1. Stevens-Johnson syndrome	Bactrim (c)
2. Tegretol toxicity	Erythromycin (g)
3. Sodium overload	Ticarcillin (i)
4. Neuromuscular blockade	Gentamicin (f)
5. Interstitial nephritis	Methicillin (d)
6. Aplastic anemia	Chloramphenicol (b)
7. Gallbladder sludging	Ceftriaxone (a)
8. Red man syndrome	Vancomycin (e)
9. Worsening sunburn	Tetracycline (h)

2. Disease

   1. Rotavirus
   2. Rocky Mountain spotted fever
   3. Varicella zoster
   4. Primary syphilis
   5. Epstein Barr virus
   6. Hepatitis B
   7. Subacute sclerosing panencephalitis

Incubation period

1–3 days
2–14 days, average 1 week
10–21 days, average 14–16 days
10–90 days, average 3 weeks
30–50 days
45–160 days, average 90 days
average 10.8 years

3.
   1. *Neisseria gonorrhoeae*
   2. *Shigella dysenteriae*
   3. *Clostridium botulinum*
   4. *Rickettsia rickettsii*
   5. Human herpes virus 6

   6. *Bartonella henselae*
   7. *Treponema pallidum*
   8. *Staphylococcus aureus*
   9. *Streptococcus agalactiae*
   10. *Francisella tularensis*

4. Vaccine

   1. Rabies

   2. Influenza
   3. Inactivated polio vaccine
   4. Measles
   5. Varicella

Order of initiation in U.S.

1885—Joseph Meister, first human to receive vaccine
Late 1940s
1953 by Jonas Salk
1963
1995, developed in Japan in 1973

5.
   1. **Paris**
   2. *Malassezia furfur*
   3. **D**
   4. *Escherichia coli*

   5. Influenza
   6. Chloroquine
   7. Ehrlichiosis
   8. Enterovirus

Unscrambled infectious disease term → **EPIDEMIC**

6. Viral gastroenteritis

   1. Astrovirus

   2. Norwalk
   3. Rotavirus

   4. Enterovirus
   5. Adenovirus

Description

Thought to be the fourth most common cause of viral gastroenteritis (d)
Most commonly found on a cruise ship (a)
Common in Mexico in September–October and Nova Scotia in May (c)
Clinically insignificant cause of gastroenteritis (e)
Typically causes more prolonged gastroenteritis (b)

7. Clinical finding

   1. Acute myositis
   2. Hemorrhagic conjunctivitis
   3. Acute cerebellar ataxia
   4. Endocarditis
   5. Pseudoparalysis
   6. Febrile seizures
   7. Acute anemia with low reticulocyte count in sickle cell anemia
   8. Perihepatitis
   9. Epidemic keratoconjunctivitis
   10. Adrenal hemorrhage

Clinical agent that causes

Influenza
Coxsackie
Varicella zoster
Staphylococcus aureus
Treponema pallidum
Human herpes 6
Parvovirus B19

Chlamydia trachomatis or *Neisseria gonorrhoeae*
Adenovirus
Neisseria meningitidis

8.
1. Kerion
2. Maxillary
3. Beard
4. Upper back
5. Lung
6. *Candida* sp.
7. Reticular endothelial system (liver, spleen, bone marrow)
8. Ankle and knee
9. Fourth

9.

Organism	First identified
1. *Mycobacterium tuberculosis*	1882 by Koch
2. Influenza A	1933 by Wilson Smith
3. Respiratory syncytial virus	1953 by Morris et al.
4. Parvovirus B19	1975 by Cossart
5. Human herpes virus 6	1986 by Salahuddin

10.
1. Varicella, measles-mumps-rubella, oral polio vaccine
2. Oral polio vaccine, bacille Calmette-Guérin, oral typhoid (yellow fever acceptable)
3. Influenza, yellow fever, oral polio vaccine

11. 1 point each
1. Parainfluenza 3
2. Lyme disease
3. Rhinovirus
4. Penicillin

2 points each
1. Hepatitis E
2. Temporal lobe spike
3. Adenovirus, Epstein Barr virus
4. Malaria

3 points each
1. Gonorrhea
2. Moraxella catarrhalis

3 points each *(cont.)*
3. Parvovirus B19
4. Hyponatremia

4 points each
1. Aminoglycoside
2. Seventy-two hours
3. Tibia and fibula
4. Vitamin A

5 points each
1. Meningitis
2. Danger of transmission to laboratory personnel
3. None
4. Heterophile antibody

SCORES

<30	30–60	60-90	90-110	>110
It's a good thing you bought this book!	Nothing to be ashamed of— keep reading.	You have great I.D. potential. Keep up the good work.	I.D. is for you. You must love it!	Do *not* do an I.D. fellowship, as you know all there is to know about infectious disease. Go into gastroenterology!

BIBLIOGRAPHY

1. Armstrong D, Cohen J: Infectious Diseases. London, Mosby, 1997.
2. Fergin R, Cherry JD: Textbook of Pediatric Infectious Diseases. Philadelphia, W.B. Saunders, 1998.
3. Katz SL, et al: Krugman's Infectious Diseases of Children, 10th ed. St. Louis, Mosby, 1998.
4. Long SS, et al: Principles and Practice of Pediatric Infectious Disease. New York, Churchill Livingstone, 1997.

50. EDITORS' FAST FACTS

Joel D. Klein, M.D., FAAP, and Theoklis E. Zaoutis, M.D.

1. What do the following acronyms mean?

HACEK: *Haemophilus, Actinobacillus, Cardiobacterium, Eikenella,* and *Kingella* species. These microorganisms are associated with culture-negative endocarditis.

SPACE: *Serratia, Pseudomonas, Acinetobacter, Citrobacter,* and *Enterobacter* species. These organisms produce beta lactamases when treated with beta-lactamase antibiotics. (This is bad.)

ESBL: extended-spectrum beta lactamase. Enzymes produced predominantly by *Escherichia coli* and *Klebsiella* species make these organisms resistant to broad-spectrum cephalosporins.

MIC: minimal inhibitory concentration. MIC values, which are commonly seen in susceptibility reports, represent the lowest concentration of antibiotic that will inhibit bacterial growth.

CRMO: chronic recurrent multifocal osteomyelitis. CRMO is a multifocal, culture-negative osteomyelitis of unclear etiology.

2. Which orthopedic infection shares a name with a famous NFL quarterback?

Brodie's abscess, named after the English surgeon Benjamin Collins Brodie (1783–1862). The quarterback (no relation to the abscess) is John Brodie.

3. From which chronic infection did Mickey Mantle suffer during his entire career?

Osteomyelitis.

4. Name six infectious diseases that can be diagnosed by examining a blood smear.

Babesiosis, ehrlichiosis, malaria, meningococcemia, mononucleosis, and hemolytic uremic syndrome.

5. Which infectious agents are most readily isolated from cultures of bone marrow?

Salmonella typhi and *Mycobacterium, Leishmania, Brucella,* and *Histoplasma* species.

6. What particular characteristic of infecting organisms is found in patients with chronic gramulomatous disease?

Infecting organisms are catalase-positive.

7. Explain the significance of a gram-negative rod described as oxidase-positive.

It probably belongs to *Pseudomonas* species.

8. Name three infectious causes of central nervous system calcifications in children.

Neurocysticercosis, cytomegalovirus infection, and toxoplasmosis.

Serology is an important aspect of diagnosing infectious mononucleosis. Answer the following questions about Epstein-Barr virus (EBV) serology.

9. Which of the following statements about antibodies to viral capsid antigen (VCA) is true: (a) IgM is undetectable after 3 months; (b) IgG is present during acute and convalescent phases; (c) antibodies to VCA are rarely found in children younger than 15 months; or (d) all of the above.

Answer: (a) and (b).

10. Which antibodies to which antigen are found in 70–90% of patients in the first 2 or 3 months of illness and in 20% of patients with past infections: (a) VCA, (b) Epstein-Barr virus–associated nuclear antigen (EBNA), (c) MBNA, or (d) early antigen (EA)?

Answer: (d).

11. Which antibody to which antigen develops after 2 months and persists for a lifetime: (a) VCA, (b) EBNA, (c) EA, or (d) EBV?

Answer: (b). The absence of EBNA after primary infection may suggest an immunodeficiency or a laboratory error.

12. What are heterophil antibodies?

They are a heterogeneous group of IgM antibodies that are not directed at EBV antigens. Heterophil antibodies are detectable at the end of the first week or beginning of the second week after onset of clinical symptoms and remain positive for up to 1 year. The test has a high specificity and a sensitivity approaching 90% in children over 4 years of age.

13. Name the stage of infectious mononucleosis based on the following serologic results.

1. Elevated VCA-IgG
   Elevated VCA-IgM
   Elevated EA antibody
2. High titers of VCA-IgG
   No or low titers of VCA-IgM
   No EBNA antibody
   EA antibody may be present
3. VCA-IgG antibody
   EBNA antibody
   EA- and VCA-IgM–antibody negative
4. Heterophil antibody present
   All other EBV serologies negative

Answers: 1, acute infection (0–3 months); 2, recent infection (3–12 months); 3, past infection (> 12 months); 4, repeat both tests.

14. Match the following hepatitis B serologic results with the stage of infection.

	HBsAg	ANTI-HBs	ANTI-HBcIgG
A	+	–	–
B	+		+
C	–	+	±

HBsAg = hepatitis B surface antigen, anti-HBs = antibody to hepatitis B surface antigen, anti-HBcIgG = antibody to hepatitis B core antigen.

Answers: A = acute hepatitis B infection, B = chronic hepatitis B infection, C = resolved old infection.

15. Which test should be performed for children born to mothers infected with hepatitis C?

Hepatitis C virus RNA polymerase chain reaction (PCR) at 1–2 months of age.

16. Which of the following interventions should be performed in a child baron to an HIV-positive mother: (a) an HIV DNA PCR at 1 and 4 months, (b) HIV antibody testing, (c) initiation of azidothymidine (AZT), (d) initiation of trimethoprim-sulfamethoxazole, or (e) initiation of amoxicillin directed against *Streptococcus pneumoniae*?

Answer: (a) and (c).

17. **Match the following organisms with the appropriate association.**
    a. *Candida parapsilosis*   1. Amphotericin-resistant
    b. *Candida lusitaniae*   2. Fluconazole-resistant
    c. *Candida krusei*   3. Thrush
    d. *Candida albicans*   4. Common in neonates
    e. *Candida dubliniensis*   5. HIV
    Answers: a, 4; b, 1; c, 2; d, 3; e, 5.

18. **Match the environmental hazard with the associated organism.**
    a. Rosebush   1. *Vibrio parahaemolyticus*
    b. Splinter   2. *Pseudomonas* spp.
    c. Aquarium   3. Sporothrix
    d. Hot tub   4. *Enterobacter* spp.
    e. Oyster shucking   5. *Mycobacterium marinum*
    Answers: a, 3; b, 4; c, 5; d, 2; e, 1.

19. **Match the following athletic teams with the fungus endemic to the region.**
    a. Arizona Diamondbacks   1. Blastomycosis
    b. Cincinnati Reds   2. Histoplasmosis
    c. Sacramento Kings   3. Coccidioidomycosis
    d. Green Bay Packers
    Answers: a and c, 3; b, 2; d, 1.

20. **In which of the following scenarios has antibiotic prophylaxis been proved effective: (a) subacute bacterial endocarditis, (b) otitis media, (c) sickle cell disease, (d) traveler's diarrhea, (e) nephrotic syndrome, and (f) open compound fracture of the femur?**
    Answers: b, c, d, and e.

INDEX

Page numbers in **boldface type** indicate complete chapters.